Neurocritical Care

What Do I Do Now?

SERIES CO-EDITORS-IN-CHIEF

Lawrence C. Newman, MD
Director, Brain Health
Atria Institute
Professor of Neurology
New York University Langone Health
New York, New York

Morris Levin, MD
Director, Headache Center
Professor of Neurology
University of California, San Francisco
San Francisco, California

OTHER VOLUMES IN THE SERIES
Epilepsy
Pain
Neuroinfections
Neurogenetics
Neurotology
Women's Neurology
Concussion
Pediatric Neurology, Second Edition
Stroke, Second Edition
Peripheral Nerve and Muscle Disease, Second Edition
Cerebrovascular Disease, Second Edition
Movement Disorders, Second Edition
Neuroimmunology, Second Edition
Neuro-Ophthalmology, Second Edition
Emergency Neurology, Second Edition
Headache and Facial Pain, Second Edition

Neurocritical Care

THIRD EDITION

EELCO F. M. WIJDICKS, MD, PhD, FACP, FNCS
Professor of Neurology, Mayo Clinic College of Medicine and Science
Consultant, Neurosciences Intensive Care Unit
Mayo Clinic Hospital, Saint Marys Campus
Rochester, Minnesota

ALEJANDRO A. RABINSTEIN, MD, FAHA, FNCS
Professor of Neurology, Mayo Clinic College of Medicine and Science
Consultant, Neurosciences Intensive Care Unit
Chair, Division of Neurocritical Care and Hospital Neurology
Mayo Clinic Hospital, Saint Marys Campus
Rochester, Minnesota

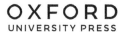

OXFORD
UNIVERSITY PRESS

Oxford University Press is a department of the University of Oxford.
It furthers the University's objective of excellence in research, scholarship,
and education by publishing worldwide. Oxford is a registered trade mark of
Oxford University Press in the UK and certain other countries.

Published in the United States of America by Oxford University Press
198 Madison Avenue, New York, NY 10016, United States of America.

© Mayo Foundation for Medical Education and Research 2025

All rights reserved. No part of this publication may be reproduced, stored in a retrieval system,
transmitted, used for text and data mining, or used for training artificial intelligence, in any form or
by any means, without the prior permission in writing of Oxford University Press, or as expressly
permitted by law, by license or under terms agreed with the appropriate reprographics rights
organization. Inquiries concerning reproduction outside the scope of the above should be sent
to the Rights Department, Oxford University Press, at the address above.

You must not circulate this work in any other form
and you must impose this same condition on any acquirer

Library of Congress Cataloging-in-Publication Data
Names: Wijdicks, Eelco F. M., 1954– author. | Rabinstein, Alejandro A., author.
Title: Neurocritical care / Eelco F. M. Wijdicks, Alejandro A. Rabinstein.
Other titles: What do i do now?
Description: 3rd edition. | New York, NY : Oxford University Press, 2025. |
Series: What do i do now? |
Includes bibliographical references and index.
Identifiers: LCCN 2024028581 | ISBN 9780197676875 (paperback) |
ISBN 9780197676899 (epub) | ISBN 9780197676882 | ISBN 9780197676905
Subjects: MESH: Nervous System Diseases—therapy | Trauma, Nervous System—therapy |
Critical Care—methods | Emergency Medicine | Intensive Care Units | Case Reports
Classification: LCC RC350.N49 | NLM WL 140 |
DDC 616.8/0428—dc23/eng/20241204
LC record available at https://lccn.loc.gov/2024028581

This material is not intended to be, and should not be considered, a substitute for medical or other
professional advice. Treatment for the conditions described in this material is highly dependent on
the individual circumstances. And, while this material is designed to offer accurate information with
respect to the subject matter covered and to be current as of the time it was written, research and
knowledge about medical and health issues is constantly evolving and dose schedules for medications
are being revised continually, with new side effects recognized and accounted for regularly. Readers
must therefore always check the product information and clinical procedures with the most up-to-date
published product information and data sheets provided by the manufacturers and the most recent
codes of conduct and safety regulation. The publisher and the authors make no representations or
warranties to readers, express or implied, as to the accuracy or completeness of this material. Without
limiting the foregoing, the publisher and the authors make no representations or warranties as to the
accuracy or efficacy of the drug dosages mentioned in the material. The authors and the publisher do
not accept, and expressly disclaim, any responsibility for any liability, loss, or risk that may be claimed
or incurred as a consequence of the use and/or application of any of the contents of this material.

DOI: 10.1093/med/9780197676875.001.0001

Printed by Integrated Books International, United States of America

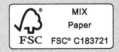

To our better halves and loved ones, Barbara-Jane and Carlota

To the admirable staff of the Neurosciences Intensive Care Unit in Mayo Clinic Hospital, Saint Marys Campus

Contents

Preface to the Third Edition xi

SECTION 1: ACUTE INTERVENTIONS

1   **Expanding Lobar Cerebral Hemorrhage** 3

2   **Reversing and Restarting Anticoagulation in Cerebral Hemorrhage** 13

3   **The Very First Priorities in Traumatic Brain Injury** 23

4   **Acute Subdural Hematoma With a Taxing Postoperative Course** 35

5   **Craniectomy's Triad of Complications** 45

6   **Grappling With Acute Bacterial Meningitis** 53

7   **Sorting Out and Treating Acute Encephalitis** 61

8   **The Presenting Features of Autoimmune Encephalitis** 73

9   **Escalating Dyspnea in Acute Neuromuscular Disease** 83

10   **Life-Threatening Complications of Intravenous Thrombolysis** 91

11   **When to Retrieve a Clot in Acute Stroke** 99

12   **A "Wake-Up" Major Stroke** 109

13   **Recognizing an Acute Embolus to the Basilar Artery** 119

14   **Timing of Hemicraniectomy in Swollen Ischemic Stroke** 129

15   **Worsening Cerebral Venous Thrombosis Despite Anticoagulation** 139

16   **Aneurysmal Subarachnoid Hemorrhage: From Good to Bad Grade** 147

17   **Delayed Cerebral Ischemia in Aneurysmal Subarachnoid Hemorrhage** 155

18   **Nonaneurysmal Subarachnoid Hemorrhage Turning Aneurysmal** 165

19 **Options in Acute Spinal Cord Compression Due to Cancer** 173

20 **Unanticipated Paraplegia After Aortic Repair** 181

21 **When Status Epilepticus Cannot Be Controlled** 189

22 **When Brain Metastasis Becomes a Neurocritical Emergency** 199

23 **The Surgical Urgency With Pituitary Apoplexy** 207

24 **Eclampsia and Its Neurologic Consequences** 215

25 **Targeted Temperature Management After Cardiopulmonary Resuscitation** 221

26 **Surviving Cardiac Arrest but Disabling Twitches** 227

27 **Hypertensive Emergency and Brain Edema** 233

28 **The Elusive Rapidly Progressive Brain Disease** 241

29 **Immune Checkpoint Inhibitors and Neuromuscular Disease** 249

30 **Neurotoxicity of CAR T-Cell Therapy** 257

31 **Failure to Awaken After Surgery** 265

32 **Stupor After Brain Surgery** 273

33 **When Antiseizure Medication Causes Harm** 279

34 **LVAD and Intracranial Hemorrhage** 287

SECTION 2: THE BASICS OF BRAIN MONITORING

35 **The Choice Between Spot and Continuous Electroencephalography** 297

36 **When to Place an Intracranial Pressure Monitor** 305

SECTION 3: CALLS, PAGES, TEXTS, AND OTHER ALARMS

37 **Alert With a Fixed and Dilated Pupil** 315

38 **Sorting Through Delirium** 323

39 **Antibiotic-Associated Toxic Encephalopathy** 333

40 **Alcohol Withdrawal With Extreme Agitation** 339

41 **Acute Alcohol-Related Neurologic Complications** 345

42 **Sudden Hypotension and Fever Spike** 353

43 **When Blood Pressure Is Too High** 361

44 **Acute White-Out on Chest X-Ray** 371

45 **Storming With Sweating, Fever, and Rigid Posturing** 379

46 **Common Cardiac Arrhythmias** 389

47 **Dysautonomia in Guillain-Barré Syndrome** 395

48 **Difficult Ventilator Weaning in Myasthenia Gravis** 403

49 **Decreasing Serum Sodium** 411

50 **Increasing Serum Sodium** 419

51 **Rising Serum Ammonia in Liver Cirrhosis** 427

SECTION 4: PRINCIPLES OF PROGNOSTICATION

52 **Prognostication After Severe Traumatic Brain Injury** 435

53 **Prognostication After Acute Ischemic Stroke and Cerebral Hemorrhage** 443

54 **Prognostication After Cardiopulmonary Resuscitation** 451

SECTION 5: LONG-TERM SUPPORT, END-OF-LIFE CARE, AND PALLIATION

55 **Decisions in Persistent Comatose States** 463

56 **When Withdrawal of Life-Sustaining Treatment Is Considered** 471

57 **Brain Death Determination: Slip-ups and Other Misreadings** 481

58 **When to Mention Organ Donation** 489

SECTION 6: THE OTHER SIDE OF NEUROCRITICAL CARE: COMMUNICATION CONUNDRUMS

59 **Patients Coming In and Going Out**   501

60 **When Families Do Not Agree With Our Approach and Care**   509

Index   517

Preface to the Third Edition

Learning from well-documented and reasoned cases can be effective. The task of the writer is to make it so, and our signature is to bring you as close to practice as we can and cut out all extraneous theoretical knowledge. Once we decide on a patient, we are often faced with decision after decision and so we took the publisher-suggested subtitle "what do I do now?" seriously—it sounded all too familiar to us.

A new edition of any book offers an opportunity to scrutinize the prior material and to make substantial changes. Though care of the neurocritically ill patient does not become rapidly archaic, several clinical trials and new clinical observations have prompted us to adjust our practices. We also greatly extended the number of patient examples and replaced older ones with (most) cases not published before. This third edition has nearly twice as many case histories as the first edition.

Several new topics deserve special mention. For example, this edition includes more complex cases of traumatic brain injury. We have included two additional complications in patients with traumatic brain injury. We recognize the urgent central and peripheral nervous system complications of new immunotherapy. We expanded the collection with a discussion on so-called "wake-up stroke," which often leads to several tests and difficult decision-making. We added the challenge of early prognostication in acute stroke and aneurysmal subarachnoid hemorrhage often based on the early clinical trajectory. Two chapters on communication conundrums in neurocritical care are new to this edition. An important part of our daily work is communication with each other, and the challenges are discussed. Family conferences are also part of our fabric, and we added a discussion on the principles of communication and how to manage major patient and physician disagreements when de-escalation of care is considered. All our other original cases remain, although we have, in many places, extensively rewritten the discussion to incorporate relevant new literature.

To present a work of synthesis we both closely edited our assigned chapters and went back and forth until we felt it was right. We acknowledge our colleagues Sara Hocker and Jen Fugate, who contributed to the prior edition, and we retained some of their contributions. We appreciate the great care and editing expertise of Lea Dacy. Gnanambigai Jayakumar from Newgen KnowledgeWorks was extraordinarily helpful.

In this new edition, we place more emphasis on how diagnostic and management decisions can go awry. When pertinent, we discuss new care paradigms, the latest support modalities, and new therapies, interventions, and technologies, but the main purpose is to convey a sense of what our specialty, in the trenches, is all about in 60 case studies.

We initially authored this book for rotating fellows and residents, and they have remained our target readership. But after receiving positive feedback from other practitioners, we suspect it might be suitable for all health care professionals acutely involved in the care of a critically ill neurologic patient, including advanced practice providers. This book is not a comprehensive text, nor is it a primer. This book should make the reader want to know more and that information can be found in recently published, new editions of neurocritical textbooks. (And at the risk of being brazen you may consider *Neurologic Complications of Critical Illness*, fourth edition, and *The Practice of Emergency and Critical Care Neurology*, third edition.) We may not have all the answers to the barrage of agonizing questions coming our way, but we surely hope this book will help to answer some. Our aim is to recount our patient-related experiences, what caught our attention, how we come to our decisions and when we need to move very quickly. Ideally, the reader will recognize these problems more easily in the future.

Our goal has always been to focus on relevant patient examples and to concentrate on the welter of decisions that matter to us. We come across many situations where we are unable to understand the cause of deterioration, unable to diagnose properly, and even surprised by autopsy findings. That "real world" is never fully reflected in books, which may give the false impression that our diagnostic travails always lead to a resolution. Moreover, this book is not an airbrushed collection of success stories or proudly discovered esoteric rarities, and there are patients with a bad outcome and near misses. In this book we seriously attempt to get to the core of what we (and so many others) do.

This is a new edition of the work we both started over a decade ago. We are not only colleagues but also good friends, know each other well, repeatedly discuss care of patients and our judgments, and challenge each other to do better. But we also surround ourselves with an absolutely, positively caring multidisciplinary team and have come to believe that neurocritical care is one of the most interesting specialties because it covers the broadest canvas. We appreciate the immediacy, intensity, and need for appropriate triage. The excitement of discovery never goes away, nor do we want it to. The upshot of all this is that, to cite the Doctors Mayo, "Once you start studying Medicine (read: Neurocritical Care), you never get through with it." There is plenty more that we can learn.

EFMW and AAR

SECTION 1

ACUTE INTERVENTIONS

1 Expanding Lobar Cerebral Hemorrhage

A 78-year-old woman with hypertension and acute severe headache and confusion was transferred to our emergency department. In the outside emergency department, her level of alertness was normal, and her major neurological deficit was left-sided weakness and neglect. Her blood pressure was 183/92 mmHg. An emergency computed tomography (CT) scan showed a large right temporal lobe hematoma (estimated volume 70 cm^3) with mass effect (Figure 1.1A). CT angiography showed a spot sign (Figure 1.1B). Coagulation studies were normal. During transport, she became sleepier. On our examination, she opened her eyes to pain, still demonstrated several hand positions to command, had intact pupil and corneal reflexes, and had a Cheyne-Stokes breathing pattern (FOUR Score E1, M4, B4, R3). There were concerns about an obstructed airway as well as episodic oxygen desaturations.

What do you do now?

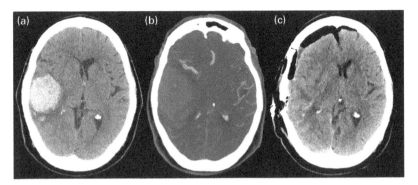

FIGURE 1.1 (A) CT scan shows a right temporal lobe hematoma with shift of midline structures. (B) CT angiogram soon thereafter shows a hyperdensity in the hematoma ("spot sign"). We see that the hemorrhage shadow is now larger, suggestive of active bleeding. (C) Postoperative CT shows hematoma evacuation.

This situation clearly warrants a call to a neurosurgeon. But there is a bigger story to tell when it comes to neurosurgical evacuation of a cerebral hematoma. Generally, a clot above the tentorium is situated in the deep gray matter of the brain, which is difficult for the neurosurgical suction device to reach without causing collateral damage. However, in our patient, the clot was superficial and thus more easily approachable. Lobar hematomas in the white matter occur in one in four patients with hemorrhages and, because they are closer to the bone, are more easily (and more safely) evacuated by neurosurgeons. This is a crucial point in any discussion on the benefits of neurosurgical management in cerebral hemorrhage—how far into normal brain tissue must an instrument traverse to reach its target lesion? And do the so-called "minimally invasive" instruments cause less harm?

Neurosurgical options in cerebral hemorrhage include evacuation of the hematoma, placement of a ventriculostomy, and, in some cases, decompressive craniectomy. Without surgical removal of a large expanding lobar hematoma, mortality is high, and survivors have a poor outcome. To do nothing may be justified in patients with a prior poor functional state, coma, and simultaneous loss of upper brainstem reflexes, but anyone else with an expanding lobar hematoma (at least 50 cm^3) should undergo hematoma evacuation, which carries a reasonable chance of recovery. However, this surgery is a complicated procedure—not just a matter of "let's get the hematoma out"—and more than a few neurosurgeons are reluctant to commit. Several factors will influence neurosurgical decisions (Box 1.1). The young and active have an advantage.

Decisions to proceed with surgery are ultimately determined by neurosurgeons (with their biases), and we cannot really force their hands. Moreover, there is robust evidence that neurosurgical evacuation through an open craniotomy does not improve outcome in stable deep hemorrhages and is questionably effective even in very superficially located hemorrhages. Indeed, this has been unequivocally proven in the two Surgical Trial in Intracerebral Hemorrhage (STICH) studies, but again, it might be worth trying in a rapidly worsening patient. We think a nuanced understanding of these and other clinical trials and recent cohorts is necessary.

It is an ugly truth that intracerebral hemorrhage (ICH) has major consequences. Four in 10 patients with ICH die, and many survivors remain disabled. The medical treatment of ICH is limited, but we can provide general supportive care, hyperosmolar therapy for treatment of cerebral edema, control of severe hypertension, and correction of coagulation abnormalities when needed. Some hematoma enlargements do not translate into measurable clinical differences. There are several theories of why cerebral hematomas expand: (1) perihematomal hypoperfusion might be associated with reduced tissue integrity and reduced resistance to hematoma expansion; (2) the hematoma mass effect triggers the rupture of adjacent pathological small vessels, resulting in further bleeding ("an avalanche"); (3) high systolic blood pressure and variability of blood pressure with large swings upward, increasing blood flow, and, obviously, prior use of anticoagulants nearly always will lead to some expansion of the hematoma, and sometimes substantially—doubling or tripling in size.

BOX 1.1 **Factors Favoring Surgery for ICH**

Worsening clinical signs
Absence of severe comorbidities
Absent or corrected coagulopathy
Lobar hematoma (<1 cm from brain surface)
Absent brainstem injury
Absent intraventricular hemorrhage
Good rehabilitation potential

Hemostatic therapy reduces hematoma expansion, but it may not result in better functional outcomes. We do not know how quickly we need to act, and often we may be too late. Speed of hematoma growth as noted on serial CT scans (more than 10 mL/h), the presence of a spot sign (as in our patient), and anticoagulation (Chapter 2) all predict enlargement and worse outcome. Other CT characteristics predicting an unstable hematoma are irregular shape, mixed clot density and fluid levels typically seen with anticoagulation or low platelets, and small satellite hemorrhages surrounding or connected to the main clot. Again, there is no proof that these patients will benefit from early surgery. The challenge for clinical researchers is to identify patients who might benefit. Multiple studies comparing medical and surgical management of spontaneous ICH have shown disappointing results. Although many patients still have a poor outcome, occasionally patients with signs of clinical and radiological brainstem compression or displacement recover well after emergency evacuation. If patients have potential for a good recovery, surgery should at least be considered.

The largest trials evaluating surgical evacuation for spontaneous ICH were the STICH studies. Over 500 patients—with similar numbers of hematomas in the putamen/thalamus and lobar locations—were randomized to surgical or medical treatment within 3 days of ICH onset (median time to surgery was 30 hours). Six months later, only one-quarter of patients in both groups had achieved good recovery or, at least, had only moderate disability. Surgery did not improve the overall outcome of patients with spontaneous ICH, thus confirming the results of previous, smaller trials. Subgroup analyses in the STICH I population, however, disclosed that patients who were not comatose and had superficial lobar hematomas (<1 cm from the brain surface) did better when they underwent surgery. The STICH II trial thus evaluated craniotomy in patients with lobar hematoma (10–100 mL) and no associated intraventricular hematoma but found no significant differences in outcome except in a post hoc analysis that identified benefit in lobar clots located within 1 cm of the cortical surface. Again, we must remember that these trials evaluating surgery in ICH have typically not enrolled rapidly deteriorating patients.

We know a few other things about surgery for ICH. Deep-seated hematomas do not benefit from evacuation via a traditional open craniotomy, but some case series and one randomized study suggested that stereotactic surgery with needle aspiration is useful in deep-seated hematoma. Ultra-early hematoma evacuation as a concept made a lot of sense but a clinical trial testing this strategy had to be terminated because of increased deaths among patients operated on within hours. This was explained by difficulties in maintaining hemostasis and frequent postoperative rebleeding. Ongoing clinical trials are investigating whether minimally invasive surgery may improve outcome. If it works, we suspect this type of surgery will be elective and restricted to nondeteriorating patients. For now, most U.S. centers remove ICH traditionally through a craniotomy and corticectomy, but there is growing interest in newer devices that could remove hematomas with "minimal" violation of brain tissue. The Early Minimally Invasive Removal of Intracerebral Hemorrhage (ENRICH) trial was designed to evaluate the "minimally invasive trans-sulcal parafascicular surgery" approach using the BrainPath* and Myriad* devices (NICO Corporation, Indianapolis, IN). In other words, moving a blunt instrument thought the natural folds and slipping through white matter tracks while using a navigation system.

In the positive ENRICH trial, surgery was performed within 24 hours of ictus and can be considered for 30–80 mL lobar ICH with a goal of reducing hematoma volume to <15 mL in patients aged 18–80 years without significant premorbid disability and so it is clear that the population which benefited is narrowly defined. There was no benefit in deep seated (ganglionic) supratentorial cerebral hemorrhages. ENRICH was the first of its kind. A number of other minimally invasive surgical trials are underway and will provide more relevant clinical information. It is yet unclear how many neurosurgical practices will acquire this or other devices. These newer technologically advanced instruments may make the difference in outcomes (if the timing is right).

Neurosurgical evacuation is standard practice in certain circumstances. We do know that sizable cerebellar hematomas must be evacuated to avoid obstructive hydrocephalus and brainstem compression, which can be fatal or result in irreversible damage. Delaying evacuation of the clot in these patients is bad management. Another indication for surgical evacuation is an ICH secondary to a vascular anomaly (such as an arteriovenous malformation; a dural AV fistula; cavernous malformation; or an aneurysm) and because of the substantial risk of recurrent bleeding. Suspicion of amyloid angiopathy does not contraindicate surgery. (In the past, neurosurgeons worried about the fragility of the arteries.) Some patients with pathologically confirmed amyloid angiopathy recover well after surgery, especially those younger than 75 years, without intraventricular hemorrhage, and without dementia. We must always consider hemorrhage into a new metastasis and look for it, if time allows, with MR imaging.

Another neurosurgical issue is the placement of a ventriculostomy in a patient with cerebral hematoma and obstructive hydrocephalus. This intervention may result in clinical improvement when obstructive hydrocephalus worsens and there is no other explanation for the decline in consciousness (e.g., enlarging thalamic hematoma). A clot clogging the drainage catheter may create complications. The Clot Lysis Evaluation of Accelerated Resolution of Intraventricular Hemorrhage (CLEAR) III trial investigated the value of thrombolytics infused through the ventriculostomy catheter to accelerate the resolution of the intraventricular hemorrhage and improve functional outcomes in patients with ICH volumes less than 30 ml. The intervention (12 doses of 1 mg of rtPA and 8 hours apart) was safe but had no major impact on the chances of functional recovery despite increased survival. We may consider this treatment when the intraventricular clot burden is large and the patient does not make any headway.

Finally, and perhaps most importantly, there is the issue of timing of surgical intervention. In reality, waiting for the patient to decline before offering surgery often results in not offering surgery at all. Once the patient is "too poor for surgery," the opportunity is gone.

So, what did we decide to do with our patient? We intubated the patient, gave 10 mg of intravenous labetalol to reduce systolic blood pressure to below 140 mmHg, and urgently consulted a neurosurgeon. We discussed the situation with the family, since the patient was not able to sustain attention sufficiently to participate in the conversation, and we told them that we had a favorable experience with early intervention but without hard proof of benefit. We mentioned that delaying surgery would not be a good option. After the family provided informed consent, our neurosurgical team performed a craniotomy and clot evacuation (Figure 1.1C). Improvement was slow, but she eventually became independent in daily functioning.

When considering surgery for ICH, we need to consider a range of factors related to the location and volume of the ICH itself, the patient's chances of recovery, and the patient's preferences, which often must be discussed with the family or proxy. When the decision is to proceed with surgery, the patient must first be fully stabilized (i.e., adequate ventilation and oxygenation, control of hypertension below a systolic blood pressure of 140–160 mmHg, and reversal of anticoagulation, as discussed in Chapter 2). Realistic expectations should be discussed with the family. In cases of deep ganglionic hematomas, neurosurgical evacuation in stuporous or comatose patients may only shift patients from certain death to severe disability, without improving function ("life-saving procedure"). Even patients who make it to a neurorehabilitation center may not have a substantial functional improvement. While patients with a lobar hematoma can improve after clot removal, as illustrated by our example, surgery is hardly a standard approach for these patients. Of course, careful patient selection is the key to optimizing functional results, but we cannot always tell which patients are the best candidates for surgical treatment. The first 24- to 48-hour prognostication (in the absence of secondary brainstem injury), almost by definition, is a "guesstimate," and prognosticating just after admission is seldom possible (leaving aside the multiple occasions when we disagree with the assessment of the transferring physician, who may have underestimated or overestimated the severity). Yet, if clot evacuation or ventriculostomy is considered, one should not wait until the patient worsens further. By then, it may be too late although there might still be benefit if one pupil is "blown". For some catastrophic cases, and certainly when hemorrhages are deep and sizable, we can agree upon a neurosurgical red line. But not for others. Newer less invasive instrumentation may even more so blur this line.

KEY POINTS TO REMEMBER

- Surgery cannot be recommended as a routine intervention for stable patients with spontaneous ICH and no mass effect.
- Surgery is a strong consideration in worsening patients with a lobar ICH, especially patients with good rehabilitation potential and superficial location with no intraventricular hemorrhage.
- Surgery is indicated in patients with large cerebellar hematomas and considerable mass effect or obstructive hydrocephalus.
- Surgery is indicated when ICH is due to underlying vascular anomalies or tumor.

Further Reading

Balami, J. S., and A. M. Buchan. "Complications of Intracerebral Hemorrhage." [In eng]. *Lancet Neurol* 11, no. 1 (Jan 2012): 101–18. https://doi.org/10.1016/s1474-4422(11)70264-2.

Brouwers, H. B., Y. Chang, G. J. Falcone, et al. "Predicting Hematoma Expansion After Primary Intracerebral Hemorrhage." [In eng]. *JAMA Neurol* 71, no. 2 (Feb 2014): 158–64. https://doi.org/10.1001/jamaneurol.2013.5433.

Fisher, C. M. "Pathological Observations in Hypertensive Cerebral Hemorrhage." [In eng]. *J Neuropathol Exp Neurol* 30, no. 3 (Jul 1971): 536–50. https://doi.org/10.1097/00005072-197107000-00015.

Huang, X., Z. Yan, L. Jiang, et al. "The Efficacy of Stereotactic Minimally Invasive Thrombolysis at Different Catheter Positions in the Treatment of Small- and Medium-Volume Basal Ganglia Hemorrhage (SMITDCP I): A Randomized, Controlled, and Blinded Endpoint Phase 1 Trial." [In eng]. *Front Neurol* 14 (2023): 1131283. https://doi.org/10.3389/fneur.2023.1131283.

Kuramatsu, J. B., S. T. Gerner, W. Ziai, et al. "Association of Intraventricular Fibrinolysis With Clinical Outcomes in Intracerebral Hemorrhage: An Individual Participant Data Meta-Analysis." [In eng]. *Stroke* 53, no. 9 (Sep 2022): 2876–86. https://doi.org/10.1161/strokeaha.121.038455.

Last, J., M. Perrech, C. Denizci, et al. "Long-Term Functional Recovery and Quality of Life After Surgical Treatment of Putaminal Hemorrhages." [In eng]. *J Stroke Cerebrovasc Dis* 24, no. 5 (May 2015): 925–29. https://doi.org/10.1016/j.jstrokecerebrovasdis.2014.12.001.

Mendelow, A. D., B. A. Gregson, H. M. Fernandes, et al. "Early Surgery Versus Initial Conservative Treatment in Patients with Spontaneous Supratentorial Intracerebral Haematomas in the International Surgical Trial in Intracerebral hemorrhage (STICH): A Randomized Trial." [In eng]. *Lancet* 365, no. 9457 (Jan 29–Feb 4 2005): 387–97. https://doi.org/10.1016/s0140-6736(05)17826-x.

Morris, N. A., J. M. Simard, and S. Chaturvedi. "Surgical Management for Primary Intracerebral Hemorrhage." [In eng]. *Neurology* 103 (2024): e209714. doi:10.1212/WNL.0000000000209714.

Morotti, A., G. Boulouis, D. Dowlatshahi, et al. "Intracerebral Haemorrhage Expansion: Definitions, Predictors, and Prevention." [In eng]. *Lancet Neurol* (Oct 26, 2022). 22, no. 2 (Feb 2023): 159–71. https://doi.org/10.1016/s1474-4422(22)00338-6.

Pagani-Estévez, G. L., P. Couillard, G. Lanzino, et al. "Acutely Trapped Ventricle: Clinical Significance and Benefit From Surgical Decompression." [In eng]. *Neurocrit Care* 24, no. 1 (Feb 2016): 110–17. https://doi.org/10.1007/s12028-015-0145-6.

Pradilla, G., J. J. Ratcliff, A. J. Hall, et al. "Trial of early minimally invasive removal of intracerebral hemorrhage." [In eng]. *N Engl J Med* 390, no. 14 (2024): 1277–89. doi:10.1056/ NEJMoa2308440.

Rabinstein, A. A., J. L. Atkinson, and E. F. Wijdicks. "Emergency Craniotomy in Patients Worsening Due to Expanded Cerebral Hematoma: To What Purpose?" [In eng]. *Neurology* 58, no. 9 (May 14 2002): 1367–72. https://doi.org/10.1212/wnl.58.9.1367.

Ratcliff, J. J., A. J. Hall, E. Porto, et al. "Early Minimally Invasive Removal of Intracerebral Hemorrhage (Enrich): Study Protocol for a Multi-Centered Two-Arm Randomized Adaptive Trial." [In eng]. *Front Neurol* 14 (2023): 1126958. https://doi.org/10.3389/fneur.2023.1126958.

Teo, K. C., S. M. Fong, W. C. Y. Leung, et al. "Location-Specific Hematoma Volume Cutoff and Clinical Outcomes in Intracerebral Hemorrhage." [In eng]. *Stroke* 54, no. 6 (Jun 2023): 1548–57. https://doi.org/10.1161/strokeaha.122.041246.

Zhang, Y., X. Wang, C. Schultz, et al. "Postoperative Outcome of Cerebral Amyloid Angiopathy-Related Lobar Intracerebral Hemorrhage: Case Series and Systematic Review." [In eng]. *Neurosurgery* 70, no. 1 (Jan 2012): 125–30; discussion 30. https://doi.org/10.1227/NEU.0b013e31822ea02a.

2 Reversing and Restarting Anticoagulation in Cerebral Hemorrhage

A 70-year-old man with a mechanical aortic valve on warfarin and aspirin developed sudden speech difficulty, right arm weakness, and numbness. On arrival to an outside emergency department, he was alert but had mild dysarthria and right-sided hemiparesis and hypesthesia. Computed tomography (CT) scan showed a localized thalamic hematoma without ventricular extension but with some mass effect (Figure 2.1). The international normalized ratio (INR) was 4.3. He received fresh frozen plasma (FFP) 2 units) and intravenous (IV) vitamin K (10 mg).

After transfer to our neurosciences intensive care unit, the patient had further neurological deterioration, mainly decline in responsiveness (only eye opening to voice now), impaired vertical eye movements, severe dysarthria, and flaccid hemiplegia. He was still able to protect his airway, but he developed a Cheyne-Stokes breathing pattern. Repeat CT scan of the brain showed enlargement of the thalamic hematoma and rupture into the third ventricle. His systolic blood pressure had climbed to 200 mmHg. The INR remained at 4.0.

What do you do now?

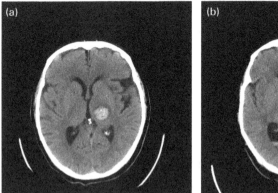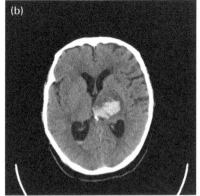

FIGURE 2.1 Serial CT scans show a left thalamic hematoma with local mass effect (A) and subsequent hematoma expansion with intraventricular extension and more left to right shift of brain tissue (B).

Anticoagulation-associated cerebral hemorrhages do expand, particularly if anticoagulation is excessive and outside the set range. The mere presence of blood thinners (and, to a lesser extent, dual antiplatelet agents) increases the chance of a poor outcome simply because blood does not clot or clots insufficiently. Avoiding this expansion—or even reducing its size by small amounts—can be an effective way to diminish the chance of a poor outcome by reducing the morbidity from additional brain tissue destruction or preventing displacement-associated brainstem injury. Larger clots also increase the chance of more surrounding cerebral edema. Everyone agrees that a first step in patients anticoagulated with warfarin should be rapidly restoring the INR to a normal value (INR <1.3) and, in the case of direct oral anticoagulants (DOACs), to counter its effect with specific reversal agents. Some have found that a door-to-treatment time of 60 minutes or less was associated with decreased mortality and discharge to hospice. However, it is not conclusively established that rapid reversal of anticoagulant effects effectively reduces expansion of the hematoma and "stops" the bleeding. So, there is the proverbial "horse out of the barn" explanation—treatment is futile in some patients because these anticoagulation-associated hemorrhages are often rapidly unstable at onset.

There are many other unknowns. This is a good opportunity to review the state of the art of anticoagulation reversal. As a starting point, the reversal options are summarized in Box 2.1.

One approach is to reverse the antagonistic effect of warfarin on vitamin K, and IV vitamin K will reactivate factors II, VII, IX, and X. Using both vitamin K and FFP accomplishes the reversal, but only after several hours. Moreover, vitamin K, 10 mg IV, is not sufficient by itself and may even take up to 24 hours to achieve full effect. FFP replaces the depleted coagulation factors, but multiple studies have shown that the target INR is not reached within 2 to 4 hours in most patients. Additionally, compatibility testing and thawing of plasma realistically take 30 to 60 minutes, delaying treatment too much. Second and equally problematic, if the INR is not rapidly corrected with FFP, physicians may infuse more units of FFP, leading to transfusion-associated circulatory overload, pulmonary edema, and, in the worst-case scenario, unnecessary endotracheal intubation and mechanical ventilation. There is no consensus on the number of FFP units

---

BOX 2.1 **Anticoagulation Reversal in ICH**

Warfarin
Prothrombin complex concentrate: 30–50 IU/kg (preferred)
Fresh frozen plasma (2–4 units) (much less preferred)
Vitamin K (10 mg IV) (in all patients)

Heparin
Protamine 1 mg per 100 U of heparin (maximal dose 50 mg preferred)

Low-molecular-weight heparin (LMWH)
If within 8 hours, 1 mg protamine for each 1 mg of enoxaparin
Between 8 and 12 hours, 0.5 mg protamine for each 1 mg of enoxaparin
Protamine not useful when administered after 12 hours of last dose of LMWH
Protamine does not reverse fondaparinux

IV thrombolysis
Tranexamic acid, 10–15 mg/kg over 20 minutes
Cryoprecipitate, 0.15 U/kg if fibrinogen is <150 mg/dL

Thrombocytopenia
Platelet transfusion if platelets <100 × 10^9/L

needed, although weight-based calculation may reduce complications. As a rule, a dose of 10 to 20 mL of FFP per kilogram of body weight produces a sufficient 10% increase in coagulation factors. A typical unit is 250 ml; thus 3 to 4 units are often needed. This remains the least preferable approach and should be avoided if possible.

The best option to correct warfarin-induced coagulopathy—and this is now first-line standard practice—is use of four-factor prothrombin complex concentrates (PCCs) that contain human-derived clotting factors. The three-factor PCC contains little factor VII, but the four-factor PCC provides full replacement of factor VII. The dose of PCC is determined by the INR and the weight of the patient—higher (50 IU/kg) with higher INR (>4), lower (30 IU/kg) with lower INR (2–3). Some US practices prefer a fixed-dose regimen such as 1500 units. PCC is easy to use and quickly prepared; it requires minimal infused volume, and it replaces clotting factors nearly completely. Risk of thrombotic events directly caused by PCC is not very well established and likely small.

Intracerebral hemorrhages may occur in hospitalized patients on IV heparin or on low-molecular-weight heparin (LMWH), for example, subcutaneous enoxaparin every 12 hours. Protamine reverses unfractionated heparin fully but only 60% of LMWH and none of the effect of fondaparinux. Serum anti-factor Xa—the main factor inhibited by LMWH—can be measured but may take a while. It is more important to establish the exact time of LMWH administration and consider protamine if its administration was close to the hemorrhage onset.

Patients with thrombocytopenia (when <100 × 10^9/L) need platelet transfusions. One apheresis platelet collection is equivalent to six pooled random-donor platelet concentrates, also known as a "six-pack." One unit should increase the platelet count in adults by 30 to 60 × 10^9/L. Platelet transfusion to sustain platelets at least above 50 × 10^9/L remains a major hurdle in patients on chemotherapy for solid tumors and in patients with serious hematologic malignancies.

Reversal of IV thrombolysis can be accomplished with tranexamic acid and cryoprecipitate if fibrinogen is less than 150 mg/dL. Because IV thrombolysis has such a short half-life (terminal half-lives of tenecteplase and alteplase are shorter than 2 hours), the cerebral hemorrhage must have occurred close to administration of thrombolysis to even consider these reversal methods.

Direct oral anticoagulants (DOACs) are more commonly used. Dabigatran, which targets factor IIa, is currently approved in the United States, and the factor Xa inhibitor rivaroxaban is approved for venous thromboembolism after orthopedic surgery, stroke prevention, and atrial fibrillation. Apixaban is the most commonly used DOAC in the United States. It is an Xa inhibitor approved for venous thromboembolism in Europe and approved for atrial fibrillation in the United States. (all factor Xa inhibitors such as apixaban, rivaroxaban and edoxaban end with -xaban and is clever naming) The anticoagulation effects of DOACs persist over many hours (half-life, 12–15 hours); thus, reversal therapy is needed unless the last dose of the DOAC was given more than 1 to 2 days before the ictus.

Two DOAC reversal agents are available. Andexanet alfa, acting as an Xa decoy, reverses the anticoagulant effects of direct factor Xa inhibitors, and idarucizumab is a specific antidote for dabigatran (Table 2.1).

A few practical tips are in order. First, we can measure thrombin time with dabigatran (thrombin inhibitor). If thrombin time is normal, no hemostatically meaningful dabigatran is present. We can also measure anti–factor Xa levels with apixaban, rivaroxaban, and edoxaban. If normal, then we can assume no hemostatically meaningful factor Xa inhibition is present. But time does not allow us to do these measurements when treating a life-threatening hemorrhage. Second, four-factor PCC may still be highly effective and much less expensive. (The total estimated cost for reversal treatment is $12,000–24,000 for treatment with andexanet alfa

TABLE 2.1 **Reversal of DOACs**

DOAC	Reversal Agent
Dabigatran (Pradaxa®)	Idarucizumab IV, 5 g IV (two divided doses) or Four-factor PCC, 25–50 U/kg
Apixaban (Eliquis®) Rivaroxaban (Xarelto®)	Andexanet alfa IV, 400 mg IV, and 480 mg IV in 2 hours or Four-factor PCC, 25–50 U/kg

and $7000 for treatment with four-factor PCC.) The need for more doses can be determined by anti-Xa values. After administering the bolus, anti–factor Xa activity decreases rapidly. When drugs are taken in the morning, we advise 50 U/kg, and 25 U/kg of PCC if taken the prior day. (Some prefer 1500 U flat also for DOAC reversal.) For surgical patients, four-factor PCC remains the preferred reversal method. If surgery to evacuate the hematoma or place a ventriculostomy is delayed by more than 4 hours after infusion, redosing of four-factor PCC can be considered. Third, andexanet alfa has other major disadvantages such as preparation time, which can take up to an hour. A clinical trial in patients with cerebral hemorrhage on DOACs (ANNEXa I) compared andexanet alfa versus standard care—which included administration of four-factor PCC in around 80% of cases. Andexanet alfa met the primary endpoint of achieving better hemostasis but was associated with more thrombotic events and there were no differences in functional outcomes. Also be warned, never use both due to the thrombosis risk!

And finally, let us look at reversal of antiplatelet agents. Next to aspirin, the most used is clopidogrel, followed by ticagrelor. Aspirin, 75 to 325 mg orally daily, has a short half-life and is dose dependent: 3 hours with doses of 300 to 600 mg and 10 hours with larger doses. Clopidogrel has a duration of action between 5 and 10 days (remainder of platelet lifespan after inhibition). Ticagrelor is administered as a 180-mg load, followed by 90 mg twice daily. There are no specific reversal agents for aspirin, but the FDA has accepted for priority review the Biologics License Application for Bentracimab as the first drug to reverse ticagrelor (intravenous bolus of 6 g over 10 minutes, followed immediately by a 6-g intravenous loading infusion over 4 hours and then a 6-g intravenous maintenance infusion over 12 hours). Approval is expected by early 2025. Platelet infusions are an option, but their effects remain to be seen. As alluded to, one apheresis unit (six-pack) substantially increases platelets (30,000–60,000), but the crucial issue is whether they work appropriately and do not get inactivated after infusion. In the Platelet Transfusion Versus Standard Care After Acute Stroke due to Spontaneous Cerebral Hemorrhage Associated with Antiplatelet Therapy (PATCH) trial, platelet transfusion in cerebral hemorrhage not only offered no benefit but also was associated with doubling of the mortality and higher rates of disability. Another option is desmopressin, 0.3 to 0.4 mcg/kg in a single IV dose, which increases the von Willebrand factor, factor VIII, and procoagulant platelets, but the clinical effect remains unproven. Most neurosurgeons administer one or two "six-packs" or even desmopressin before surgery or ventriculostomy placement, but in this situation, the benefits and risks are also unknown, and once such practices start, they are hard to change.

So, what lesson did we learn, and what would be better the next time? Initial management must focus on rapid correction of the coagulopathy. Equally important is aggressive control of blood pressure using labetalol, hydralazine, or an IV infusion of nicardipine or clevidipine, with the assumption that controlling blood pressure additionally reduces further expansion. In one recent study, reversal of INR to less than 1.3 within 4 hours and achieving systolic blood pressure less than 160 mmHg at 4 hours correlated with lower rates of hematoma enlargement. There is little time to waste.

Finally—and this is by no means a trivial question—should anticoagulation be resumed after the patient recovers and still needs protection against future emboli? The Restart or Stop Antithrombotics Randomized Trial (RESTART) found that resumption of antiplatelet therapy had no major impact on the rate of recurrent intracerebral hemorrhage or the occurrence of thromboembolic events over a median follow-up of 3 years. In another study, the Apixaban after Anticoagulation-associated Intracerebral Hemorrhage in Patients with Atrial Fibrillation (APACHE-AF) trial, a higher percentage of patients on apixaban had nonfatal stroke or vascular death than patients without resumption over a median follow-up of 1.9 years, but the difference was small (26% vs. 24%). The Start or Stop Anticoagulants Randomised Trial (SoSTART) showed that 8% of the patients assigned to start anticoagulation therapy had recurrence of intracerebral hemorrhage, as compared with 4% of the patients who did not start anticoagulation. All these data are somewhat askew, and there is no clear consensus on what to do. The tradeoff depends on the individual risk of thromboembolism (higher with prosthetic valves) and recurrent hemorrhage (higher with suspected cerebral amyloid angiopathy). One retrospective analysis, mostly in patients with atrial fibrillation alone, found that a 1- or 2-month pause was justified. However, we generally wait just 7 days before restarting warfarin in patients with a mechanical valve irrespective of its location (aorta or mitral valve).We strongly warn against bridging with IV heparin because in our own patient cohort the risk of rebleeding was higher. Another cohort study of patients with a mechanical valve and cerebral hemorrhage found that the risk of stroke only increased after 30 days of discontinuation suggesting a possible time window beyond which embolization is much more likely. But we do not think there is a compelling reason to wait that long. While restarting warfarin may be unnecessary in other cases, early resumption (DOAC or warfarin) is certainly needed in patients with echocardiographic finding of an atrial thrombus and perhaps in patients with marked atrial or ventricular dilatation.

What did we do in our case? We immediately and effectively reversed the persistent anticoagulation with four-factor PCC. Hours later the patient required a ventriculostomy and the placement was completed without hemorrhagic complications. With supportive care and time, the patient recovered with moderate disability. Warfarin was reinitiated without problems 12 days after hematoma onset and following removal of the ventricular drain.

One thing is obvious: if we ever want to make an impact, anticoagulation must be reversed fast. It is even a question whether we need to know the INR value before treating if we know the patient is taking warfarin. DOAC reversal should be based on available history (time of last dose) using the best available agents. We fully support the American Heart Association (belated) call to action and development of a "bundle of care" in cerebral hemorrhage (CODE-ICH). We have too often seen worsened patients when arriving in our neurosciences intensive care where we, with the benefit of hindsight, found suboptimal care and missed opportunities.

KEY POINTS TO REMEMBER

- Four-factor PCC is the most effective way to reverse warfarin.
- FFP may also be an option, but it works more slowly to correct INR, and excess fluids may cause complications.
- IV vitamin K should always be administered along with the hemostatic agent.
- IV heparin can be quickly reversed with protamine.
- LMWH is partially reversed with protamine if administered within 8 hours.

- Platelet transfusion does not improve outcome in patients with cerebral hemorrhage on antiplatelet therapy.
- Whenever possible, use idarucizumab for reversal of dabigatran.
- For reversal of Xa inhibitors, andexanet alfa provides better hemostasis but with increased risk of subsequent thromboembolism. Four-factor PCC is a reasonable alternative.
- Neurosurgical evacuation of hematoma should remain an option, but only after anticoagulation is reversed.

Further Reading

Baharoglu, M. I., C. Cordonnier, R. Al-Shahi Salman, et al. "Platelet Transfusion Versus Standard Care After Acute Stroke Due to Spontaneous Cerebral Haemorrhage Associated with Antiplatelet Therapy (Patch): A Randomised, Open-Label, Phase 3 Trial." [In eng]. *Lancet* 387, no. 10038 (Jun 25, 2016): 2605–13. https://doi.org/10.1016/s0140-6736(16)30392-0.

Barra, M. E., R. Forman, B. Long-Fazio, et al. "Optimal Timing for Resumption of Anticoagulation After Intracranial Hemorrhage in Patients With Mechanical Heart Valves." *J Am Heart Assoc* 13, no. 10 (May 21 2024): e032094. doi:10.1161/JAHA.123.032094. Epub 2024 May 18. PMID: 38761076; PMCID: PMC11179836.

Bershad, E. M., and J. I. Suarez. "Prothrombin Complex Concentrates for Oral Anticoagulant Therapy-Related Intracranial Hemorrhage: A Review of the Literature." [In eng]. *Neurocrit Care* 12, no. 3 (Jun 2010): 403–13. https://doi.org/10.1007/s12028-009-9310-0.

Chaudhary, R., A. Singh, R. Chaudhary, et al. "Evaluation of Direct Oral Anticoagulant Reversal Agents in Intracranial Hemorrhage: A Systematic Review and Meta-Analysis." [In eng]. *JAMA Netw Open* 5, no. 11 (Nov 1 2022): e2240145. https://doi.org/10.1001/jamanetworkopen.2022.40145.

Claassen, D. O., N. Kazemi, A. Y. Zubkov, et al. "Restarting Anticoagulation Therapy After Warfarin-Associated Intracerebral Hemorrhage." [In eng]. *Arch Neurol* 65, no. 10 (Oct 2008): 1313–8. https://doi.org/10.1001/archneur.65.10.1313.

Connolly, S. J., Sharma, M., Cohen, A.T.; "ANNEXA-I Investigators. Andexanet for Factor Xa Inhibitor-Associated Acute Intracerebral Hemorrhage." [in eng] *N Engl J Med.* 2024 May 16;390(19):1745–1755. doi: 10.1056/NEJMoa2313040. PMID: 38749032.

Frontera, J. A., J. J. Lewin, 3rd, A. A. Rabinstein, et al. "Guideline for Reversal of Antithrombotics in Intracranial Hemorrhage: A Statement for Healthcare Professionals From the Neurocritical Care Society and Society of Critical Care Medicine." [In eng]. *Neurocrit Care* 24, no. 1 (Feb 2016): 6–46. https://doi.org/10.1007/s12028-015-0222-x.

Hickey, M., M. Gatien, M. Taljaard, et al. "Outcomes of Urgent Warfarin Reversal With Frozen Plasma Versus Prothrombin Complex Concentrate in the Emergency Department." [In eng]. *Circulation* 128, no. 4 (Jul 23 2013): 360–64. https://doi.org/10.1161/circulationaha.113.001875.

Imberti, D., G. Barillari, C. Biasioli, et al. "Emergency Reversal of Anticoagulation with a Three-Factor Prothrombin Complex Concentrate in Patients With Intracranial Hemorrhage." [In eng]. *Blood Transfus* 9, no. 2 (Apr 2011): 148–55. https://doi.org/10.2450/2011.0065-10.

Kuramatsu, J. B., S. T. Gerner, P. D. Schellinger, et al. "Anticoagulant Reversal, Blood Pressure Levels, and Anticoagulant Resumption in Patients With Anticoagulation-Related Intracerebral Hemorrhage." [In eng]. *Jama* 313, no. 8 (Feb 24 2015): 824–36. https://doi.org/10.1001/jama.2015.0846.

Lee, S. B., E. M. Manno, K. F. Layton, and E. F. Wijdicks. "Progression of Warfarin-Associated Intracerebral Hemorrhage After INR Normalization With FFP." [In eng]. *Neurology* 67, no. 7 (Oct 10 2006): 1272–74. https://doi.org/10.1212/01.wnl.0000238104.75563.2f.

Li, Q., A. Yakhkind, A. W. Alexandrov, et al. "Code ICH: A Call to Action." [In eng]. *Stroke* 55, no. 2 (Feb 2024): 494–505. doi:10.1161/STROKEAHA.123.043033. Epub 2023 Dec 15.

Sakusic, A., A. A. Rabinstein, B. Anisetti, et al. "Timing of Anticoagulation Resumption and Risk of Ischemic and Hemorrhagic Complications in Patients With ICH and Mechanical Heart Valves." [In eng]. *Neurology* 103, no. 4 (Aug 27 2024): e209664. doi:10.1212/WNL.0000000000209664. Epub 2024 Aug 5.

Sheth, K. N., N. Solomon, B. Alhanti, et al. "Time to Anticoagulation Reversal and Outcomes After Intracerebral Hemorrhage." [In eng]. *JAMA Neurol* 81, no. 4 (Feb 9 2024): 363–72. doi:10.1001/jamaneurol.2024.0221. Epub ahead of print. PMID: 38335064; PMCID: PMC11002694.

SoSTART Collaboration. "Effects of Oral Anticoagulation for Atrial Fibrillation After Spontaneous Intracranial Haemorrhage in the UK: A Randomised, Open-Label, Assessor-Masked, Pilot-Phase, Non-Inferiority Trial." [In eng]. *Lancet Neurol* 20, no. 10 (Oct 2021): 842–53. https://doi.org/10.1016/s1474-4422(21)00264-7.

Troyer, C., W. Nguyen, A. Xie, and D. Wimer. "Retrospective Review of Andexanet Alfa Versus 4-Factor Prothrombin Complex Concentrate for Reversal of DOAC-Associated Intracranial Hemorrhage." [In eng]. *J Thromb Thrombolysis* 55, no. 1 (Jan 2023): 149–55. https://doi.org/10.1007/s11239-022-02715-4.

3 The Very First Priorities in Traumatic Brain Injury

Thrown from his motorcycle in a motocross race, a 27-year-old helmeted patient was run over across the torso by another motorcycle. There is a puncture wound to the forehead. A paramedic intubated him. On arrival to the emergency department, the patient is comatose. His eyes do not open to pain. Pupils are small and react minimally to light. Due to concern of associated spine injury, staff cannot assess oculocephalic reflexes. The other brainstem reflexes are intact. There is extensor posturing. Computed tomography (CT) scan shows evidence of multiple contusions in the frontal and temporal lobes (Figure 3.1) and a frontal bone fracture. There is no evidence of a subdural or epidural hematoma. CT of the cervical spine is normal. Initial examination and additional CT scans do not reveal other systemic injuries or fractures, and his vital signs are stable. Arterial blood gas is normal.

What do you do now?

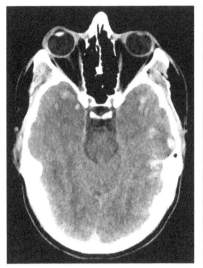 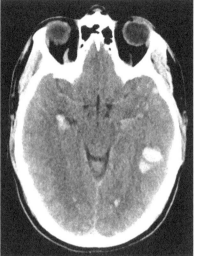

FIGURE 3.1 Multiple hemorrhagic lesions (contusions) on admission CT scan of the brain.

After patients with traumatic brain injury (TBI) arrive in the emergency bay, staff quickly assess and further stabilize them; they then undergo a series of tests. It is difficult to imagine a place more harried than the emergency department in the throes of a trauma team alert. Physicians managing or comanaging care must fully understand the consequences of a comatose patient presenting with a traumatic brain injury. Therapeutic interventions follow in rapid succession. Nonetheless, limited options are available in neurocritical care and neurosurgery, and these have not changed in half a century. Specific neuroprotection in TBI is, unfortunately, a string of disappointments and major setbacks, and thus, the care remains guided by simple (but no less important) core fundamentals.

Still, in the early hours after TBI, anything that can go wrong often does. At least five crucial developments can occur in the very first hours after presentation, typically in the emergency room bay.

First issue: Determine the urgency of neurosurgical intervention and categorize CT scans of TBI patients into penetrating vs. closed injury. Focus attention on the presence of hemorrhagic contusions and epidural or subdural hematomas, which may produce significant mass effect.

Isolated shear lesions on CT may indicate a large prevalence of shear lesions on magnetic resonance imaging (MRI). MRI can quantify the degree of white matter injury with diffusion tensor imaging and connecting networks with functional MRI, but data are insufficient to predict functional outcome (and even awakening).

Urgent neurosurgical indications are often obvious at the time of arrival and usually involve the presence of a large cerebral contusion creating brain tissue displacement. A neurosurgeon must explore a depressed skull fracture; indeed, the presence of an acute subdural or epidural hematoma on admission CT scan is always neurosurgical terrain. These hematomas can emerge quickly, and a normal CT scan after any significant trauma may not mean much. We repeat the CT scan if the clinical examination has changed and, in particular, does not fit the neuroimaging findings. The threshold for repeating a CT scan should be lower in intoxicated or sedated (e.g., as a result of transport) patients, to avoid falsely attributing a poor neurological examination to these confounders.

The expectation of universally poor outcomes has driven management of penetrating, traumatic gunshot injury to the brain. This incorrect premise has resulted in exclusion of these patients from clinical trials in TBI. Most experience of gunshot injury is in the military and approaches are not necessarily applicable to civilian injury. Management includes early decompressive craniectomy, prevention of cerebrospinal fluid leak with skull base repair, attention to cerebrovascular injuries and vasospasm, and a multispecialty approach to cranial reconstruction. Outcome in these young individuals can be acceptable with overall mortality in the 10% to 20% range. Moreover, neurorehabilitation programs have made substantial progress, but patients need to get there.

The management of civilian gunshot wounds is similar to that of nonpenetrating trauma. Removal of any large intracerebral hematoma with mass effect and reconstructive repair of the bone and dura should begin immediately. Regard the wound as contaminated and administer broad-spectrum antibiotics (vancomycin with third-generation cephalosporin) early. Perform CT angiography when anticipating injury to the cerebral vasculature, but short of endovascular or surgical occlusion, there are few therapeutic options. If a full bullet track runs through both hemispheres of the brain on CT or if the patient has lost one or more brainstem reflexes, aggressive ICP management is of little benefit. A bolus of mannitol, 1 g/kg, can determine whether improvement is possible, but if there is no observed response, it is unlikely. Patients with gunshots to the head consistently have higher mortality rates and unfavorable outcomes compared with blunt TBI, even if matched for baseline characteristics.

Second issue: Is the patient actively bleeding? Patients may be on oral anticoagulation, which requires immediate reversal because of the possibility of urgent surgery. Use four-factor prothrombin complex concentrate [PCC] plus vitamin K if the patient is on warfarin; Andexanet alfa or four-factor PCC if on anti-Xa inhibitors, such as apixaban and rivaroxaban; and idarucizumab if on direct thrombin inhibitors, such as dabigatran. In patients previously anticoagulated with warfarin, neurosurgeons usually prefer seeing an international normalized ratio of less than 1.4 before surgery.

Third issue: As mentioned earlier, major confounders are often present. A toxicology screen is helpful, but a careful history remains most valuable. Alcohol abuse accounts for many major TBIs. Alcohol intoxication is present in up to 70% of trauma patients of which 30% meet criteria for alcohol use disorder, but only 1% develop alcohol withdrawal syndrome. In trauma, phenobarbital-treated patients are less likely to develop complicated alcohol withdrawal delirium or experience medication side effects compared to patients treated mostly with benzodiazepines. There is some push for early preemptive use of phenobarbital in high risk TBI patients but this heavily sedating drug must be very carefully titrated and checked with levels if deemed too high, (see also Chapter 40). Another common confounder is anoxic-ischemic brain injury—patients may have been lying face down, in debris, apneic. Even performing endotracheal intubation in the field might have been a struggle, and often intubations are faulty, requiring immediate correction of the tube position or replacement. In our experience, coexisting anoxic-ischemic brain injury, viewable on MRI, may occasionally account for failure to improve after surgical evacuation of a subdural hematoma or failure to improve despite control of intracranial pressure (ICP).

Fourth issue: Any comatose patient after TBI is at substantial risk of increased ICP. Options for monitoring are an intraparenchymal probe or a ventriculostomy. Most major trauma centers use intraparenchymal probes. A ventriculostomy allows cerebrospinal fluid removal with increased ICP, but in patients with a small ventricle size and risk of further compression, this is a second target of approach. Ventricular ICP monitors may have to be recalibrated often and they may be unreliable. Placement of a parenchymal ICP monitor provides not only an ICP value but also the cerebral perfusion pressure (CPP), calculated using the mean arterial blood pressure (MAP). The abbreviated formula is CCP = MAP − ICP. The Brain Trauma Foundation currently defines optimal ICP and CPP as ICP less than 22 mmHg and CPP between 60 and 70 mmHg.

Indications for intracranial monitoring include patients with a severe TBI defined as coma or decerebrate or decorticate posturing and with an abnormal CT scan (contusions, shear lesions, early brain edema). Any patient who will require deep sedation—usually when pulmonary injury is present—is best managed by monitoring ICP. But, in all honesty, it turns out that if physicians follow a strict guideline-based management protocol, the ICP value does not add much to decisions based on clinical and radiological assessment, and knowing ICP values did not improve outcome when assessed in a prospective randomized trial. (The critique has been that conducting the TBI and ICP management trial in lower-resource countries limited the generalizability of its results.) In addition, the merit of multimodal monitoring in the management of TBI remains unconfirmed. We often try to persuade neurosurgeons to place an ICP monitor and also a brain oximetry monitor in comatose patients with TBI—with variable luck. Such a diversity of opinions among neurosurgeons remains a prevailing tendency in management of TBI. This also applies to multimodal monitoring, and proponents of such comprehensive monitoring may need more convincing reasons to justify its universal use.

Fifth issue: Treatment of increased ICP first requires mundane interventions such as head elevation, adequate oxygenation, avoidance of hypercarbia, and treatment of posttraumatic seizures, which may require prolonged electroencephalographic (EEG) monitoring, but also reducing intrathoracic (positive end-expiratory pressure values <15 mmHg) and intra-abdominal pressure. Fentanyl, 1 mcg/kg/h; atracurium, 0.5 mg/kg/h; and propofol titrated up to 80 mcg/kg/min might be necessary to sedate patients adequately and have them synchronize with the mechanical ventilator. Although commonly used in TBI, the effect of opiates on ICP is variable, and we have seen patients with reduced intracranial compliance

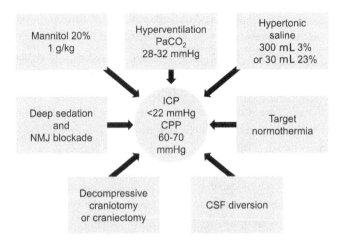

FIGURE 3.2 Optimizing conditions and treatment for increased intracranial pressure. CPP, central perfusion pressure; CSF, cerebrospinal fluid; NMJ, neuromuscular junction.

in which the ICP increased after the administration of these drugs. Seizures require treatment, and baseline EEG might be necessary if focal seizures have occurred. It is frequent practice to treat a more severely injured stuporous or comatose patient with intravenous levetiracetam (a 7-day course of antiseizure therapy can reduce early seizures but does not change the risk of subsequent posttraumatic epilepsy).

Initially, we treat raised ICP (Figure 3.2) with hyperventilation (arterial PCO_2 in the low 30s) and mannitol (1–2 g/kg) or 3% saline solution. The use of highly concentrated hypertonic saline requires the placement of a central venous catheter, but waiting for placement can markedly delay initial treatment of ICP; alternatively, it can be administered urgently through a femoral vein. Hypertonic saline administered in higher concentrations (23%) can be effective even after mannitol or lower concentrations of hypertonic saline have failed to reduce ICP. One should expect that in equivalent osmolar doses, mannitol and hypertonic saline have comparable effects on ICP and CPP.

Any unsuccessful control of ICP requires further management by decompressive craniectomy—either bifrontal craniectomy or hemicraniectomy. In extreme situations, patients with refractory ICP have benefited from abdominal decompression. A randomized trial using bifrontotemporoparietal decompressive surgery (DECRA) found no improvement in outcome, but patient selection in this trial has received criticism because patients could be candidates for surgery after only 15 minutes of high ICP. Moreover, very few neurosurgeons would opt for a bilateral approach initially. Another trial (RESCUEicp) using higher ICP targets for decompression by means of large hemicraniectomy or bifrontal craniectomy showed mixed results: at 6 months the surgery group had lower mortality but at the expense of more survivors with persistent disorders of consciousness and severe disability; the rates of good functional recovery did not differ from the control arm. So surgery is hardly a panacea in patients with TBI and refractory intracranial hypertension. But it is a valid option, particularly for young patients when other interventions to control the ICP have failed. Timing is an unresolved issue, with aggressive neurosurgeons rapidly moving in while others practice avoidance.

A long-standing discussion has been whether treatment of TBI should be "ICP or CPP driven." Studies have found no difference between these two approaches. However, treatment of CPP alone with less attention to increased ICP may be a wrong approach. It is not just cerebral perfusion that matters, and increasing ICP will eventually lead to brainstem displacement and permanent brainstem injury.

Avoidance of fever is an accepted treatment principle. Hypothermia may reduce ICP, but randomized controlled trials have clearly shown that it does not improve clinical outcomes in patients with severe TBI and increased ICP. Therefore, we rarely resort to hypothermia for ICP management in trauma patients.

Treatment of TBI also involves other immediate aspects of care (Box 3.1). Sequential pneumatic compression applied to the legs reduces the risk of deep venous thrombosis. When deemed safe, we add chemoprophylaxis with heparin or low-molecular weight heparin. In the most severe cases, prophylactic placement of a vena cava filter might be a better option than waiting for pulmonary emboli to occur. Treatment with subcutaneous heparin may not always suffice. There is little consensus on how to identify those patients at high risk of fatal pulmonary emboli. Inferior vena cava filter placement, however, is frequent practice in anticipation of long-term care in polytraumatized patients.

> **BOX 3.1 Initial Priorities After Traumatic Brain Injury**
>
> **Need for ICP control?**
> Osmotic diuretics (mannitol 20%, 1 g/kg; or hypertonic saline 300 mL of 3%, or 30 mL of 23.4%)
> Hyperventilation (short-term targeting PaCO2 around 30 mmHg)
> Evacuation of new contusion or subdural hematoma
> Ventriculostomy for cerebrospinal fluid drainage
> Pharmacological neuromuscular paralysis and deep sedation (induced coma)
> Decompressive unilateral or bilateral hemicraniectomy
>
> **Need for seizure control?**
> Levetiracetam, loading dose of 60 mg/kg mg IV, if seizures, cerebral contusion, increased ICP, or skull fractures. Continue levetiracetam 750 -1000 mg bid.
>
> **Need for better oxygenation?**
> Maintain hemoglobin level at least at 7 g/dL. Avoid multiple transfusions.
> Placement of brain tissue oxygen monitor (if feasible)
> Endotracheal intubation and mechanical ventilation
> Careful use of positive end-expiratory pressure
> Propofol (or midazolam) infusion for sedation

Gastrointestinal prophylaxis is essential for mechanically ventilated patients at substantial risk of gastrointestinal bleeding. We place these patients on a proton pump inhibitor or H2 blocker (a component of the "ventilator bundle").

Treatment in TBI involves recognition and prompt treatment of infections, including ventilator-associated pneumonia (VAP), urinary tract infections, and catheter (line)-associated sepsis—all complications requiring appropriate treatment. A single dose of 2 gram of ceftriaxone is included in some ventilator bundles for the prevention of VAP in patients with acute brain injury who require mechanical ventilation. Early tracheostomy (and reducing time on the ventilator), close monitoring of intravascular catheters and prompt removal when infected or no longer necessary, surveillance for the development of deep venous thrombosis in upper and lower extremities, and early placement of a gastrostomy may all reduce complications and improve the chances of survival and functional outcome in general.

Oxygen to the brain is dependent on the arterial oxygen content (and cerebral blood flow) and is highly dependent on the degree of oxygen binding to hemoglobin. Whether to correct a low hemoglobin and when has been a topic of contention. The HEMOTION and TRAIN trials had different results, but for now a liberal red-cell transfusion strategy is not more effective as restrictive transfusion strategy in patients with TBI. ("restrictive" is hemoglobin transfusion threshold of 7 g/dl, or a "liberal" is transfusion with a threshold 9 or 10 g/dl). We have not changed our practice to go beyond a target of 7–8 g/dl. In fact prevention is key (reducing blood draws).

Our patient was treated with a combination of osmotic agents and other standard measures to reduce ICP, and he started to become more awake a week later. Eventually the patient was successfully extubated and enrolled in a neurorehabilitation program. We will return to this topic in Chapter 52 on prognosis.

KEY POINTS TO REMEMBER

- Place an ICP monitor in any comatose patient with early CT scan abnormalities.
- Maintain ICP less than 22 mmHg and CPP between 60 and 70 mmHg (CPP = MAP − ICP).
- Mannitol remains the most commonly used first line osmotic agent.
- Hypertonic saline requires central access and effectively lowers ICP.
- Decompressive craniectomy is an effective last-resort measure for refractory ICP, but with dubious impact on outcome.
- Treat infections without delay.
- Think early about other prophylactic measures (preintubation ceftriaxone, gastrointestinal protection and surveillance for deep venous thrombosis).

Further Reading

Bodanapally, U. K., C. Sours, J. Zhuo, and K. Shanmuganathan. "Imaging of Traumatic Brain Injury." [In eng]. *Radiol Clin North Am* 53, no. 4 (Jul 2015): 695–715, viii. https://doi.org/10.1016/j.rcl.2015.02.011.

Carney, N., A. M. Totten, C. O'Reilly, et al. "Guidelines for the Management of Severe Traumatic Brain Injury, Fourth Edition." [In eng]. *Neurosurgery* 80, no. 1 (Jan 1 2017): 6–15. https://doi.org/10.1227/neu.0000000000001432.

Chesnut, R., S. Aguilera, A. Buki, et al. "A Management Algorithm for Adult Patients With Both Brain Oxygen and Intracranial Pressure Monitoring: The Seattle International Severe Traumatic Brain Injury Consensus Conference (SIBICC)." [In eng]. *Intensive Care Med* 46, no. 5 (May 2020): 919–29. https://doi.org/10.1007/s00134-019-05900-x.

Chesnut, R. M., N. Temkin, N. Carney, et al. "A Trial of Intracranial-Pressure Monitoring in Traumatic Brain Injury." [In eng]. *N Engl J Med* 367, no. 26 (Dec 27 2012): 2471–81. https://doi.org/10.1056/NEJMoa1207363.

Cooper, D. J., J. V. Rosenfeld, L. Murray, et al. "Decompressive Craniectomy in Diffuse Traumatic Brain Injury." [In eng]. *N Engl J Med* 364, no. 16 (Apr 21 2011): 1493–502. https://doi.org/10.1056/NEJMoa1102077.

Hutchinson, P. J., A. G. Kolias, I. S. Timofeev, et al. "Trial of Decompressive Craniectomy for Traumatic Intracranial Hypertension." [In eng]. *N Engl J Med* 375, no. 12 (Sep 22 2016): 1119–30. https://doi.org/10.1056/NEJMoa1605215.

Kamel, H., B. B. Navi, K. Nakagawa, et al. "Hypertonic Saline Versus Mannitol for the Treatment of Elevated Intracranial Pressure: A Meta-Analysis of Randomized Clinical Trials." [In eng]. *Crit Care Med* 39, no. 3 (Mar 2011): 554–59. https://doi.org/10.1097/CCM.0b013e318206b9be.

Lazaridis, C., and P. Das. "Penetrating Firearm-Inflicted Injury—The Neglected Traumatic Brain Injury." [In eng]. JAMA Neurol. 2023 Oct 1;80(10):1013–1014. https://doi.org/10.1001/jamaneurol.2023.3030.

Le Roux, P., D. K. Menon, G. Citerio, et al. "Consensus Summary Statement of the International Multidisciplinary Consensus Conference on Multimodality Monitoring in Neurocritical Care: A Statement for Healthcare Professionals From the Neurocritical Care Society and the European Society of Intensive Care Medicine." [In eng]. *Intensive Care Med* 40, no. 9 (Sep 2014): 1189–209. https://doi.org/10.1007/s00134-014-3369-6.

Mangat, H. S., Y. L. Chiu, L. M. Gerber, et al. "Hypertonic Saline Reduces Cumulative and Daily Intracranial Pressure Burdens After Severe Traumatic Brain Injury." [In eng]. *J Neurosurg* 122, no. 1 (Jan 2015): 202–10. https://doi.org/10.3171/2014.10.Jns132545.

Mansour A, Powla PP, Alvarado-Dyer R, Fakhri F, Das P, Horowitz P, Goldenberg FD, Lazaridis C. Comparative Analysis of Clinical Severity and Outcomes in Penetrating Versus Blunt Traumatic Brain Injury Propensity Matched Cohorts. *Neurotrauma Rep.* 2024 Apr 3;5(1):348-358. doi: 10.1089/neur.2024.0009.

Ng, C., M. Fleury, H. Hakmi, et al. "The Impact of Alcohol Use and Withdrawal on Trauma Outcomes: A Case Control Study." [In eng]. Am J Surg 222, no. 2 (2021): 438–45.

Stocchetti, N., M. Carbonara, G. Citerio, et al. "Severe Traumatic Brain Injury: Targeted Management in the Intensive Care Unit." [In eng]. *Lancet Neurol* 16, no. 6 (Jun 2017): 452–64. https://doi.org/10.1016/s1474-4422(17)30118-7.

Turgeon AF, Fergusson DA, Clayton L, et al. HEMOTION Trial Investigators on behalf of the Canadian Critical Care Trials Group, the Canadian Perioperative Anesthesia Clinical Trials Group, and the Canadian Traumatic Brain Injury Research Consortium. Liberal or Restrictive Transfusion Strategy in Patients with Traumatic Brain Injury. *N Engl J Med.* 2024 Aug 22;391(8):722-735. doi: 10.1056/NEJMoa2404360. Epub 2024 Jun 13.

Taccone FS, Rynkowski Bittencourt C et al TRAIN Study Group. Restrictive vs Liberal Transfusion Strategy in Patients with Acute Brain Injury: The TRAIN Randomized Clinical Trial. *JAMA.* 2024 Oct 9. doi: 10.1001/jama.2024.20424. Epub ahead of print.

Wang, M., C. Falank, V. Simboli, et al. "Should We Phenobarb-it-All?" A Phenobarbital-Based Protocol for Non-Intensive Care Unit Trauma Patients at High Risk of or Experiencing Alcohol Withdrawal." *Am Surg* 90, no. 6 (Jun 2024): 1531–9. doi: 10.1177/00031348241244639.

Wijdicks, E. F. M. "10 or 15 or 20 or 40 mmHg? What Is Increased Intracranial Pressure and Who Said So?" [In eng]. *Neurocrit Care* 36, no. 3 (Jun 2022): 1022–26. https://doi.org/10.1007/s12028-021-01438-3.

4　Acute Subdural Hematoma With a Taxing Postoperative Course

A 21-year-old male was in motorcycle-car collision and immediately comatose. First responders found a major bleeding scalp laceration and a right dilated pupil. A large periorbital hematoma was developing. He had obstructive respiration, for which he was intubated. A bradycardia of 40 beats per minute was noted. Computed tomography (CT) scan (Figure 4.1) showed right large cerebral convexity and smaller left frontal convexity extra-axial hematomas. There was extension along the falx and tentorial leaflets with significant midline shift. A left parietal fracture was noted. He was immediately taken to the operating room for evacuation of the right subdural hematoma. Following the procedure, he was transported to the CT scanner while remaining under general anesthesia. Head CT now demonstrated a large left hemispheric epidural hematoma (Figure 4.2).

What do you do now?

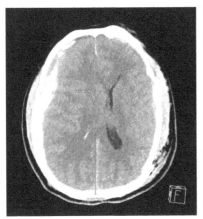 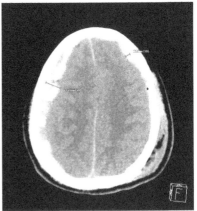

FIGURE 4.1 Initial right subdural hematoma with midline shift (and some on the left).

Clearly, the patient had to be emergently transported back to the operating room, where the left-sided epidural clot was evacuated (Figure 4.2). On admission to our neurosciences intensive care unit (neuro-ICU), his examination demonstrated persistent anisocoria with asymmetric pupillary reactivity (large minimally reactive pupil on the right but smaller reactive pupil on the left). Other cranial nerve reflexes were present. Motor responses to pain were trace extension on both arms. A follow-up magnetic resonance imaging (MRI) scan did not show diffuse axonal injury except for injury in the corpus callosum. Over a number of weeks, he remained comatose. He started to flex or withdraw to pain, but

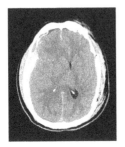 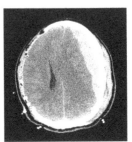 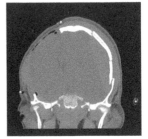

FIGURE 4.2 Postoperative CT after evacuation of right subdural hematoma leaving an open skull and now showing a new left epidural hematoma under a fractured skull.

his outcome remained uncertain. The family wanted to remain in a holding pattern. We were very uncertain how this would end.

This patient highlights two major situations that we must face. First, traumatic brain injury is dynamic, and the traumatic process is rarely established within the first 24 hours. His left-sided skull fracture already predicted development of an epidural hematoma. For that reason, neurosurgeons repeat CT scans after a certain period (4–6 hours) has passed and certainly after evacuation of a subdural hematoma with shift, which could relieve pressure on the other side. Moreover, delayed epidural hematoma has been noted in patients whose condition deteriorates after correction of hypotension, which increases cerebral perfusion pressure and, thus, facilitates recurrent bleeding.

Delayed development of subdural hematomas occurs more commonly than delayed epidural hematomas. Hematomas can indeed occur after removal of a contralateral subdural hematoma from release of its tamponade effect. Patients with associated skull fractures that traverse the middle meningeal artery or major dural vessels, such as the transverse sinus, have a one in two chance of delayed expansion requiring surgical intervention. Of the total population of head injury patients admitted to emergency departments, an estimated 3% to 5% have epidural hematoma. The clinical presentation is dramatic, with rapid onset of coma. The pupil ipsilateral to the epidural hematoma dilates and becomes fixed to light, and the opposite pupil soon demonstrates lack of reactivity because acute, substantial mass effect results in direct compression, traction, or compression of the opposite oculomotor nerve against the clivus.

Generally, neurologic examination guides management, although surgical decisions are largely based on CT scan findings. Multiple CT scans are necessary to judge an evolving contusion, epidural hematoma, or subdural hematoma accurately. Careful review of the CT scan should include review of bone windows of specific areas that can be affected. Fracture sites are associated with vascular injury, and this includes basal skull fracture and fractures in the sphenoid sinus. The presence of an epidural hematoma on CT scan almost always requires neurosurgical intervention. A satisfactory outcome depends on whether there is presurgical obliteration of the basal cisterns and whether there is a brain tissue shift of greater than 5 mm, measured at the location of the septum pellucidum.

Surgery for acute subdural hematoma is typically decided based on size and degree of mass effect. The choice to operate remains arbitrary, but any patient with neurologic deterioration requires neurosurgical intervention. Evacuation of large subdural hematomas causing loss of multiple brainstem reflexes, particularly absent pupil, and corneal reflexes, is unlikely to result in improved outcome. However, fixed pupils should not necessarily dissuade a neurosurgeon from proceeding with evacuation.

Extra-axial hematomas can be watched closely but are typically evacuated in most patients even before admission to the neuro-ICU. The Collaborative European Neurotrauma Effectiveness Research in Traumatic Brain Injury (CENTER-TBI) cohort with details on 1407 patients found that acute surgical evacuation was done in 24% (craniotomy in 73% and decompressive craniectomy in 27%). One in 10 patients underwent craniectomy or craniotomy after initial conservative treatment. Unsurprisingly, practice varies markedly across centers (with rates of early surgery ranging from 5% to 50%). The arbitrary choice of surgery vs. watchful waiting may reflect the low level of evidence for certain presentations. Initial management of acute subdural hematoma may remain conservative if the thickness of the hematoma is similar to the thickness of the skull bone and no midline shift is noted. However, if enlargement correlates with clinical deterioration, timely craniotomy is essential to achieve a potentially successful outcome. Subdural hematoma may grow due to repeated, intermittent rupture of weak neovessels.

How do neurosurgeons approach a subdural hematoma? According to the guidelines, surgical evacuation is indicated if the thickness of the hematoma exceeds 10 mm or the midline shift exceeds 5 mm, regardless of level of consciousness. Surgical evacuation of acute subdural hematoma can be categorized into two distinct types based on the removal of a bone flap: craniotomy and decompressive craniectomy. Brain swelling is the main reason to leave the bone flap off. Because decompressive craniectomy is associated with complications and requires subsequent cranioplasty (which poses additional risks), others argue that replacing the bone flap on the skull is a better option. We now know that leaving the bone flap off correlates more often with local infections, but overall, the outcome between craniotomy and craniectomy does not seem to be different.

When do neurosurgeons decide not to intervene? It is uncertain when the benefit of early surgery diminishes or disappears except in the case of a patient with loss of two or more brainstem reflexes after aggressive resuscitation (blood pressure support, osmotic agents). Some neurosurgeons hesitate when antithrombotic agents have been used before the traumatic brain injury or when platelet transfusions have proven ineffective in correcting thrombocytopenia. Age matters, and patients older than 70 years are more likely to have poor outcomes; approximatively one-third of patients die during admission, and another third are discharged with severe disability. The Richmond Acute Subdural Hematoma (RASH) score is a validated prognostic model that uses readily available factors in an emergent setting to predict postoperative outcomes in patients who present with traumatic subdural hematoma. The RASH score (Table 4.1)

TABLE 4.1 **RASH Grading Scale — Range From 0 (good) to 8 (poor)**

Age (years)	
≤59	0
60–79	1
≥80	2
GCS Severity	
Mild (≥14)	0
Moderate (9–13)	1
Severe (≤8)	2
Pupillary response	
Unresponsive, unilateral	1
Unresponsive, bilateral	2
Midline shift >5 mm	1
Loss of consciousness	2
TOTAL	0–8

GCS, Glasgow Coma Scale; RASH, Richmond Acute Subdural Hematoma.
From Dincer, A., A. N. Stanton, K. J. Parham, et al. "The Richmond Acute Subdural Hematoma Score: A Validated Grading Scale to Predict Postoperative Mortality." *Neurosurgery* 90, no. 3 (2022): 278–86FN.

ranges from 0 to 8, with the predicted postoperative mortality percentage calculated by multiplying the RASH score by 10. However, it is ill-advised to use the score to inform decisions on surgery, and most neurosurgeons will proceed after a candid discussion with family members.

Any patient who undergoes emergency evacuation for a subdural hematoma should have a postoperative CT scan. We occasionally encounter rebleeding of the surgical site, demanding reoperation. The challenge is to recognize this potential early complication, which might be difficult to judge in a patient who has returned to the unit intubated and mechanically ventilated with no obvious new signs of tissue shift (e.g., extensor posturing and a new fixed wide pupil or new anisocoria at the site of the subdural hematoma). Some refilling and residual hemorrhage are expected, and the drains are often filled with blood. Often, we repeat a CT scan in 1 to 2 hours to note progression of reaccumulation, if any. One such example is shown in Figure 4.3.

Back to our patient: an immediately present extradural hematoma is an uncommon (1%) complication following decompressive craniectomy for subdural hematoma evacuation. Pathophysiological mechanisms include coagulopathies, hyperosmolar therapy, vascular damage caused by the sudden restoration of normal perfusion pressures and delayed arterial bleeding. Few signs indicate development of delayed epidural hematoma following craniotomy. Risk is greater with skull fracture, intraoperative brain edema, profound intraoperative dehydration, and aggressive cerebrospinal fluid aspiration.

The next expected issue was that our patient later developed persistent focal seizures. In patients surgically treated for acute subdural hematoma, the presence of postoperative seizures or epileptiform abnormalities on electroencephalography (EEG) studies is common, and these patients often fail to regain full alertness after surgery. Some have found that the impact of early postoperative seizures on functional recovery becomes less significant over time. Other studies reporting on patients who had undergone emergent evacuation showed postoperative focal deficits without accompanying electrographic epileptiform activity, but treatment with antiepileptic drugs eventually resulted in clinical improvement. Long-term monitoring with EEG may also reveal electrographic seizures in a delayed fashion.

Bottom line: Do what you can in young individuals and try not to be too discouraged by poor postoperative findings. We do not yet know if our patient will thrive, hold a job, and enjoy the simple pleasures of life,

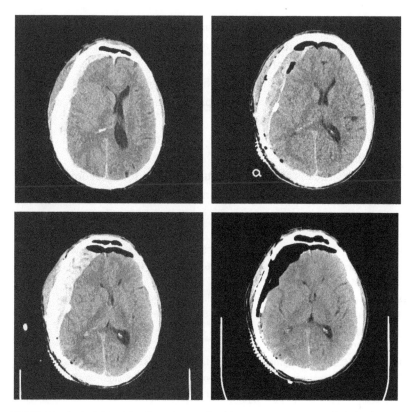

FIGURE 4.3 Acute right subdural hematoma and rapid reoccurrence postoperatively leading to a re-operation.

but youthful resilience often surprises us. In the elderly (arbitrarily defined as age above 70), we often surmise that things are unlikely to go well, but we should still look for mitigating circumstances (e.g., excellent premorbid highly functioning state) to justify an aggressive approach. If patients in this age group do not visibly improve, the predicted high mortality by the RASH score may tell us if our first impression was right.

> **KEY POINTS TO REMEMBER**
>
> - Surgical evacuation is indicated if the thickness of the hematoma exceeds 10 mm or the midline shift exceeds 5 mm, regardless of level of consciousness.

- Surgical evacuation will not change outcome with fixed pupils and one or two other absent brainstem reflexes and after a large dose of osmotic agents.
- CT scan findings in the first 24 hours are not static, and many abnormalities can enlarge or appear; therefore, a second CT is needed 6 to 8 hours later.
- Failure to awaken fully may have many causes, including seizures.
- Carefully look at the postoperative CT scan for reaccumulation that could warrant a reoperation.

Further Reading

Bullock, M. R., R. Chesnut, J. Ghajar, et al. "Surgical Management of Acute Subdural Hematomas." [In eng]. *Neurosurgery* 58, no. 3 Suppl (Mar 2006): S16–24; discussion Si–iv.

Dincer, A., A. N. Stanton, K. J. Parham, et al. "The Richmond Acute Subdural Hematoma Score: A Validated Grading Scale to Predict Postoperative Mortality." [In eng]. *Neurosurgery* 90, no. 3 (Mar 1 2022): 278–86. https://doi.org/10.1227/neu.0000000000001786.

Driver, J., A. C. DiRisio, H. Mitchell, et al. "Non-Electrographic Seizures Due to Subdural Hematoma: A Case Series and Review of the Literature." [In eng]. *Neurocrit Care* 30, no. 1 (Feb 2019): 16–21. https://doi.org/10.1007/s12028-018-0503-2.

Fukamachi, A., H. Koizumi, Y. Nagaseki, and H. Nukui. "Postoperative Extradural Hematomas: Computed Tomographic Survey of 1105 Intracranial Operations." [In eng]. *Neurosurgery* 19, no. 4 (Oct 1986): 589–93. https://doi.org/10.1227/00006123-198610000-00013.

Hutchinson, P. J., H. Adams, M. Mohan, et al. "Decompressive Craniectomy Versus Craniotomy for Acute Subdural Hematoma." [In eng]. *N Engl J Med* 388, no. 24 (Jun 15 2023): 2219–29. https://doi.org/10.1056/NEJMoa2214172.

Rabinstein, A. A., S. Y. Chung, L. A. Rudzinski, and G. Lanzino. "Seizures After Evacuation of Subdural Hematomas: Incidence, Risk Factors, and Functional Impact." [In eng]. *J Neurosurg* 112, no. 2 (Feb 2010): 455–60. https://doi.org/10.3171/2009.7.Jns09392.

Solomou, G., J. Sunny, M. Mohan, et al. "Decompressive Craniectomy in Trauma: What You Need to Know." [In eng]. *J Trauma Acute Care Surg* (Aug 14 2024). doi:10.1097/TA.0000000000004357. Epub ahead of print.

Su, T. M., T. H. Lee, W. F. Chen, et al. "Contralateral Acute Epidural Hematoma After Decompressive Surgery of Acute Subdural Hematoma: Clinical Features and

Outcome." [In eng]. *J Trauma* 65, no. 6 (Dec 2008): 1298–302. https://doi.org/
10.1097/TA.0b013e31815885d9.

Trevisi, G., C. L. Sturiale, A. Scerrati, et al. "Acute Subdural Hematoma in the
Elderly: Outcome Analysis in a Retrospective Multicentric Series of 213 Patients."
[In eng]. *Neurosurg Focus* 49, no. 4 (Oct 2020): E21. https://doi.org/10.3171/
2020.7.Focus20437.

van Essen, T. A., H. F. Lingsma, D. Pisică, et al. "Surgery Versus Conservative
Treatment for Traumatic Acute Subdural Haematoma: A Prospective, Multicentre,
Observational, Comparative Effectiveness Study." [In eng]. *Lancet Neurol* 21, no.
7 (Jul 2022): 620–31. https://doi.org/10.1016/s1474-4422(22)00166-1.

5 Craniectomy's Triad of Complications

A 40-year-old roofer slipped and fell from a 20-foot height onto concrete and immediately became unconscious. He was intubated in the field, and on arrival, he had a wide pupil with extensor posturing due to large subdural hematoma with a 2-cm midline shift and multiple smaller contusions. An emergency craniectomy followed with evacuation of a subdural hematoma under considerable pressure. He gradually awakened and improved in his motor responses. Follow-up computed tomography (CT) scans showed an evolving fluid collection or subdural hygroma (Figure 5.1) that expanded over several days. He also developed a fever. The wound looked dry, and there was no evidence of cerebrospinal fluid (CSF) leak.

What do you do now?

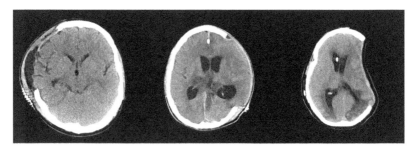

FIGURE 5.1 Three major complications after craniectomy: left: subdural hygroma; middle: craniectomy associated hydrocephalus; right: the syndrome of the trephined.

Craniectomy—for whatever indication—will leave a large part of the brain, usually shielded by the skull, unprotected. Such denudation substantially changes the anatomy and, together with opening of the dura (even if then closed), can lead to several (partly unavoidable) complications. The decision to proceed with decompressive craniectomy in an acute subdural hematoma (without closing the dura) simply depends on whether there is significant brain swelling, and that is a neurosurgical decision made in the operating room. If there is no swelling, the outcome of patients with craniectomy or craniotomy is similar.

Three complications from craniectomy stand out: (1) growing fluid collections and subdural hygroma with a tendency to expand over days, on the same side of the craniectomy and occasionally on the opposite side; (2) hydrocephalus; and (3) the "syndrome of the trephined." These complications are most often (but not exclusively) observed after craniectomy following traumatic brain injury and may first appear on serial CT within 7 to 10 days after the procedure. The clinical presentation of these complications is nonspecific, and therefore, the findings first become apparent on a "routine" follow-up CT.

A neurosurgeon reading this vignette may quickly argue that this triad is in fact a quartet or quintet. CSF skin leaks do occur regularly, and most are "fixed" with a single stitch. Others continue to seep and need more aggressive management. A new-onset fever spike with the appearance of purulent CSF leak is a worrisome, potentially major complication but fortunately uncommon. Moreover, in up to 10% of patients, wound complications or infections occur following craniectomy, and occasionally, plastic surgeons need to assist with wound revision and closure.

But first, contrary to what we are led to believe, we must emphasize that we have no good understanding of the pathophysiology of CSF dynamics in each of these altered conditions. Interventions may even be counter-productive. Once a substantial portion of skull is removed from a bruised and compressed brain, all the CSF equations and formulas become meaningless.

Extradural or subdural hygromas are extra-axial CSF accretions. The traditional explanation is that decompressive craniotomy perturbs pulsative CSF dynamics and allows egress into the extra-axial compartments, but this has been questioned. Arachnoid rents function as ball-valve mechanisms and gradually enlarge the buildup until it becomes symptomatic. Contralateral subdural fluid collections are more often symptomatic than ipsilateral fluid collections and pose a different type of challenge. Several mechanisms have been proposed. For example, a rapid release of intracranial pressure (ICP) with outward-bulging brain tissue could create a pressure gradient and cause the contralateral subdural space to accumulate effusions. Subdural hygromas may combine with large extradural collections if the dura is left partly open by the neurosurgeon to mitigate swelling, and this may become a mix of CSF and seroma and thus essentially an external hydrocephalus.

Another important sequela of craniectomy is the development of posttraumatic hydrocephalus (PTH)—with new neurologic symptoms consistent with hydrocephalus and imaging of ventriculomegaly (Figure 5.1, middle). CT studies have found that half of the patients show posttraumatic ventriculomegaly at discharge, but less than 5% develop PTH requiring ventriculoperitoneal (VP) shunt treatment. Another study found PTH in 40% of patients after craniectomy for traumatic brain injury, with one in four patients requiring a shunt. This diversity in numbers is a strong indicator of neurosurgical preference. Most PTH patients have measurable improvement following VP shunt surgery. Those with poor clinical status before treatment, halted neurological recovery, or low-pressure hydrocephalus do poorly, whereas patients with high-pressure hydrocephalus have greater chance of improvement following shunt placement.

PTH often develops insidiously and is challenging to diagnose. But early diagnosis and treatment of PTH could significantly improve patient outcomes. It is commonly seen in comatose patients, making it more difficult to recognize clinically. Early cranioplasty within 90 days may reduce this complication, suggesting that (1) decreased resistance to CSF outflow follows craniectomy, and (2) the expanded ventricles, via the cerebral mantle, obstruct the lumen of the cortical subarachnoid space and increase the resistance to CSF outflow.

Accumulation of extra-axial fluid may continue after ventriculostomy placement. One large study suggested the following term: craniectomy-associated progressive extra-axial collections with treated hydrocephalus (CAPECTH), essentially a form of external hydrocephalus. It is defined as progressively enlarging extra-axial CSF accretion despite high-output ventricular drainage (>300 cm^3/d) and no ventricular enlargement on imaging. This accretion accounts for clinical deterioration in nearly a third of patients. In the remaining patients, accretion sustained the poor clinical status of the patients and impeded recovery. The ventriculostomy should be removed, but the only solution, again, is early bone-flap replacement (cranioplasty) to reestablish normal ICP dynamics and resolve the underlying perturbation in CSF hydrodynamics. As noted earlier, this condition may not occur exclusively in patients with a ventriculostomy, and extra-axial and extradural collections may contain CSF if the dura was left open. Drainage may reduce compression, but early cranioplasty rather than prolonged drainage should be the next step.

Other complications are the syndrome of the trephined and the so-called sinking skin flap syndrome. How do they differ? The syndrome of the trephined is merely associated with skin depression where skull is missing and often asymptomatic. The sinking skin flap syndrome is indeed the more serious of the two. Clinically, it presents with new profound focal neurologic deficits and rapid decline in consciousness to deep coma, particularly when sitting up. CT scan will reveal downward displacement of brain tissue and filling of the usually open basal cisterns. Under normal physiological conditions, due to the protective effect of the calvarium, atmospheric barometric changes are usually insufficient to affect intracranial physiology significantly. With an intact skull, the ICP is negative in the upright position, but when part of the skull is missing, ICP equalizes with atmospheric pressure. In a retrospective series of decompressive craniectomies, the incidence of this problem was 1%. These symptoms are rapidly reversible in a Trendelenburg position. Again, cranioplasty is needed to resolve the complication.

And finally, there is the major risk of a wound infection or, worse, epidural empyema. CSF leakage, venous sinus entry, duration of operation (>4 hours), and number of operations (more than one) are associated with neurosurgical site infections after craniotomy. CSF leakage can cause the retrograde entry of pathogenic bacteria and intracranial infection, which can increase ICP and further worsen CSF leakage in turn. The longer the CSF leakage, the greater the chance of surgical site infection. Preventive treatment for CSF leakage during surgery is particularly important, and lumbar drains are often successfully employed. The drain height is adjusted to drain 10 to 20 mL/h, and the lumbar drain is generally left in place for 5 days. Limited reports have shown success in dealing with CSF leaks using tissue adhesives and dural substitutes without spinal drainage. Cutaneous organisms such as coagulase-negative staphylococci, *Staphylococcus aureus*, and *Propionibacterium acnes* are the main culprits in postneurosurgical meningitis. However, aerobic gram-negative bacilli (GNB) can cause some of these infections. Most infectious disease experts recommend 21 days of directed antibiotic treatment in GNB meningitis and 10 to 14 days for *S. aureus* meningitis.

Our patient gradually improved, and cultures remained negative. CT scan gradually improved with no further measures, reemphasizing that observation could be enough in most instances.

Neurointensivists often must manage these patients on neurosurgical services and take on a primary role. Therefore, it should be part of our repertoire to recognize these complications.

KEY POINTS TO REMEMBER

- Postcraniectomy fluid collections tend to expand over days. No further action may be needed, although in more severe cases early cranioplasty is warranted.
- Postcraniectomy hydrocephalus is best managed with shunting.

- Once the syndrome of the trephined and sinking skin flap syndrome appear, cranioplasty is indicated more urgently and may facilitate rehabilitation and even shorten time to recovery.
- Many CSF leaks resolve spontaneously or with a single stitch, but we should monitor for wound infection or meningitis, often only seen on magnetic resonance imaging or proven by culture.

Further Reading

Beucler, N., and A. Dagain. "Historical Vignette Portraying the Difference Between the 'Sinking Skin Flap Syndrome' and the 'Syndrome of the Trephined' in Decompressive Craniectomy." [In eng]. *World Neurosurg* 162 (Jun 2022): 11–14. https://doi.org/10.1016/j.wneu.2022.03.027.

Chen, C. H., C. Y. Chang, L. J. Lin, et al. "Risk Factors Associated With Postcraniotomy Meningitis: A Retrospective Study." [In eng]. *Medicine (Baltimore)* 95, no. 31 (Aug 2016): e4329. https://doi.org/10.1097/md.0000000000004329.

Di Rienzo, A., R. Colasanti, M. Gladi, et al. "Sinking Flap Syndrome Revisited: The Who, When and Why." [In eng]. *Neurosurg Rev* 43, no. 1 (Feb 2020): 323–35. https://doi.org/10.1007/s10143-019-01148-7.

Diaz-Segarra, N., and N. Jasey. "Improved Rehabilitation Efficiency After Cranioplasty in Patients With Sunken Skin Flap Syndrome: A Case Series." [In eng]. *Brain Inj* 38, no. 2 (Jan 2024): 61–67.

Heinonen, A., M. Rauhala, H. Isokuortti, et al. "Incidence of Surgically Treated Post-Traumatic Hydrocephalus 6 Months Following Head Injury in Patients Undergoing Acute Head Computed Tomography." [In eng]. *Acta Neurochir (Wien)* 164, no. 9 (Sep 2022): 2357–65. https://doi.org/10.1007/s00701-022-05299-3.

Honeybul, S., and K. M. Ho. "Incidence and Risk Factors for Post-Traumatic Hydrocephalus Following Decompressive Craniectomy for Intractable Intracranial Hypertension and Evacuation of Mass Lesions." [In eng]. *J Neurotrauma* 29, no. 10 (Jul 1 2012): 1872–78. https://doi.org/10.1089/neu.2012.2356.

Hussein, K., R. Bitterman, B. Shofty, et al. "Management of Post-Neurosurgical Meningitis: Narrative Review." [In eng]. *Clin Microbiol Infect* 23, no. 9 (Sep 2017): 621–28. https://doi.org/10.1016/j.cmi.2017.05.013.

Hutchinson, P. J., H. Adams, M. Mohan, et al. "Decompressive Craniectomy Versus Craniotomy for Acute Subdural Hematoma." [In eng]. *N Engl J Med* 388, no. 24 (Jun 15 2023): 2219–29. https://doi.org/10.1056/NEJMoa2214172.

Lu, V. M., L. P. Carlstrom, A. Perry, et al. "Prognostic Significance of Subdural Hygroma for Post-Traumatic Hydrocephalus After Decompressive Craniectomy in the Traumatic Brain Injury Setting: A Systematic Review and Meta-Analysis."

[In eng]. *Neurosurg Rev* 44, no. 1 (Feb 2021): 129–38. https://doi.org/10.1007/s10
143-019-01223-z.

Mustroph, C. M., C. M. Stewart, L. M. Mann, et al. "Systematic Review of Syndrome
of the Trephined and Reconstructive Implications." [In eng]. *J Craniofac Surg* 33,
no. 6 (Sep 1 2022): e647–e52. https://doi.org/10.1097/scs.0000000000008724.

Nalbach, S. V., A. E. Ropper, I. F. Dunn, and W. B. Gormley. "Craniectomy-
Associated Progressive Extra-Axial Collections With Treated Hydrocephalus
(CAPECTH): Redefining a Common Complication of Decompressive
Craniectomy." [In eng]. *J Clin Neurosci* 19, no. 9 (Sep 2012): 1222–27. https://doi.
org/10.1016/j.jocn.2012.01.016.

Salunke, P., R. Garg, A. Kapoor, et al. "Symptomatic Contralateral Subdural
Hygromas After Decompressive Craniectomy: Plausible Causes and Management
Protocols." [In eng]. *J Neurosurg* 122, no. 3 (Mar 2015): 602–9. https://doi.org/
10.3171/2014.10.Jns14780.

Svedung Wettervik, T., A. Lewén, and P. Enblad. "Post-Traumatic Hydrocephalus—
Incidence, Risk Factors, Treatment, and Clinical Outcome." [In eng]. *Br J
Neurosurg* 36, no. 3 (Jun 2022): 400–406. https://doi.org/10.1080/02688
697.2021.1967289.

Sveikata, L., L. Vasung, A. El Rahal, et al. "Syndrome of the Trephined: Clinical
Spectrum, Risk Factors, and Impact of Cranioplasty on Neurologic Recovery in
a Prospective Cohort." [In eng]. *Neurosurg Rev* 45, no. 2 (Apr 2022): 1431–43.
https://doi.org/10.1007/s10143-021-01655-6.

Vedantam, A., J. M. Yamal, H. Hwang, et al. "Factors Associated With Shunt-
Dependent Hydrocephalus After Decompressive Craniectomy for Traumatic Brain
Injury." [In eng]. *J Neurosurg* 128, no. 5 (May 2018): 1547–52. https://doi.org/
10.3171/2017.1.Jns162721.

6 Grappling With Acute Bacterial Meningitis

A 50-year-old woman presented initially to her family physician with progressive ear pain treated with eardrops. Over a matter of days, she developed increasing headache and a fever. A visiting family member found her unresponsive. On arrival, she was comatose and intubated. There was marked neck stiffness and intermittent downward gaze with notably small pupils (1–2 mm). Magnetic resonance imaging (MRI) showed communicating hydrocephalus, pus pockets, and significant enhancement of the meninges (Figure 6.1). She was initiated on ceftriaxone, vancomycin, ampicillin, and preceded by dexamethasone for concerns for meningitis. Blood cultures were positive for *Streptococcus pneumoniae*. Lumbar puncture opening pressure was 360 mm H_2O and after 20 mL of turbid and viscous cerebrospinal fluid (CSF) was removed the CSF closing pressure was 150 mmH_2O. Cell count showed 7000/mcL with 82% neutrophils.

What do you do now?

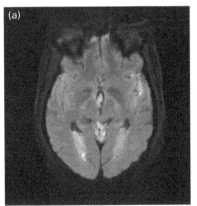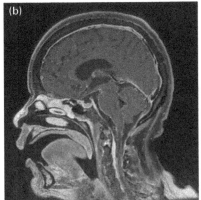

FIGURE 6.1 MRI shows layering material within the occipital horns consistent with ventriculitis and pus/exudate (A). Note marked meningeal enhancement (B).

One of the more dreaded clinical scenarios is a patient rapidly deteriorating from bacterial meningitis, despite adequate and immediate broad-spectrum antibiotic coverage. Anyone who has experienced this situation will wonder what accounts for the deterioration in our patient despite receiving antibiotics in adequate doses. To understand these questions better, we must review some basic facts on acute bacterial meningitis. *S. pneumoniae* (or *pneumococcus*) is the most common cause of bacterial meningitis in adults. Fatality has declined in pneumococcal meningitis, but not in low-income countries where vaccinations are lagging.

Generally, CSF gram stain and cultures, and sometimes blood cultures, readily and rapidly identify the bacteria in most cases. An infection with *Listeria monocytogenes* should be considered in elderly (>60 years) patients and patients with alcoholic cirrhosis. Adding ampicillin (or ciprofloxacin) to an initial, already broad empiric regimen with vancomycin and a third-generation cephalosporin potentially eradicates *L. monocytogenes*. Film arrays (i.e., BioFire® FilmArray® Meningitis/Encephalitis Panel) are capable of simultaneous detection and identification of multiple bacterial, viral, and yeast nucleic acids extracted from CSF.

An overwhelming infection can result in rapid, permanent brain injury. The brain may be an "innocent bystander" from the invading bacteria, as leukocytes, macrophages, and microglia release neurotoxic free radicals, proteases, cytokines, and other substances that result in neuronal cell death. Corticosteroids could mitigate this response. A randomized controlled trial of patients with predominantly *S. pneumoniae* meningitis offers compelling evidence that early treatment with intravenous (IV) dexamethasone (10 mg every 6 hours for 4 days) improves outcome with a 10% reduction in mortality, but only if dexamethasone was started shortly before or combined with the first dose of antibiotics. The data in meningococcal meningitis in adults remain uncertain; one European study shows no benefit from corticosteroids. Uncertainty also remains about the appropriate duration of administration, the dose, and potential other beneficial mechanisms of corticosteroids in a fulminant infection (e.g., reducing brain edema, reducing inflammation and vasculitis, reducing the effects of associated septic shock).

Corticosteroid use in patients with acute bacterial meningitis, however, remains widespread practice irrespective of the organism. The lingering concern remains that reduction of the blood-brain barrier permeability (because of reduced inflammation) also reduces penetration of antibiotics (particularly vancomycin). Additional use of rifampicin may overcome this effect, but this drug is used infrequently. In day-to-day practice, we encounter inconsistent use of pre-antibiotic corticosteroid administration, unfortunately due to simple carelessness rather than legitimate concerns.

The main priorities of early treatment of bacterial meningitis are summarized in Box 6.1. The antibiotic treatment is well defined, but the most important priority is to treat as soon as there is the slightest suspicion. We should administer antibiotics within the first 30 to 60 minutes

---

BOX 6.1 **First Treatment Priorities in Bacterial Meningitis**

Ceftriaxone, 2 g IV every 12 hours

Vancomycin, 20 mg/kg every 12 hours

Ampicillin, 2 g every 6 hours (for patients >60 years)

Dexamethasone, 10 mg IV every 6 hours for 4 days

Ventriculostomy or lumbar drain for acute hydrocephalus

Mannitol, 1 g/kg (or hypertonic saline 23% 30 ml), with acute brain edema

TABLE 6.1 **Why Is the Patient With Bacterial Meningitis Deteriorating?**

Issue	Remedy
Wrong antibiotic	Add ampicillin for *Listeria monocytogenes*
Wrong diagnosis	Consider epidural abscess
Complication	Consider nonconvulsive status epilepticus, hydrocephalus, or new cerebral infarcts
Aggressive treatment needed	Ventriculostomy, osmotic therapy for brain edema, removal of cerebellar abscess
Inadequate source control	Treat pneumonia, otitis media, mastoiditis, sinusitis

after arrival in the emergency department—that is, before neuroimaging, before lumbar puncture, and before an obligatory blood culture. Only corticosteroids come before antibiotics computed tomography (CT) scanning follows immediately, to exclude other diagnoses and to assess for acute hydrocephalus, which may need CSF diversion with a ventriculostomy. This simple directive should be automatic in any physician encountering these patients. So, memorize the following: *get a blood culture, give several drugs IV (10 mg of Dexamethasone, 2 gram of Cefriaxone, 20 mg/kg of Vancomycin and for the elderly 2 gram of Ampicillin) and do an urgent CT and CSF.*

We must always consider the multiple causes of deterioration in bacterial meningitis, which are summarized in Table 6.1. Several of these are treatable. A cerebral venous thrombosis of the cavernous sinus after a suppurative mastoiditis is a major medical emergency that requires immediate surgical intervention by an otolaryngologist. In other patients, the appearance of epidural empyema—commonly associated with frontal sinusitis and sinus surgery and mimicking bacterial meningitis—may be difficult to recognize and can be missed on a noncontrast CT scan of the brain, and MRI is definitive (Figure 6.2). Otitis media contributes to 10% to 20% of cases. Its course can be protracted, characterized only by a several-week history of localized headache and low-grade fever. Focal neurological signs can be absent initially but often become apparent when focal seizures appear. Epidural empyema a neurosurgical emergency and

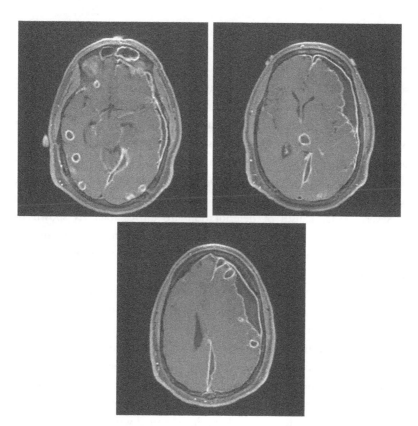

FIGURE 6.2 MRI shows multiple intracranial abscesses and an empyema in a patient with nonspecific malaise, fever, and headaches.

requires craniotomy. Microabscesses are more difficult to treat; when they rupture into the ventricles, exploratory surgery may be needed. Abscesses in the posterior fossa are particularly worrisome and require neurosurgical drainage.

Back to our patient. We know that the main site of CSF reabsorption is the arachnoid granulations and that these outpouchings into the sagittal sinus can fill with pus; thus, bacterial meningitis can cause acute hydrocephalus (Figure 6.1). Hydrocephalus is a manifestation of a more severe infection and correlates with higher fatality rates. Blocked CSF pathways may also occur at the foramina of Magendie and Luschka in ventriculitis. Use of a ventricular drain could result in neurological improvement. However, if there is ventricular pus, the hydrocephalus in meningitis often causes loculations and compartments that a single catheter cannot drain. Lumbar drainage is an option only if there is no cerebral edema or tonsillar descent that could worsen with placement of the lumbar drain. In most series of bacterial meningitis, acute hydrocephalus despite placement of a ventriculostomy denotes a greater likelihood of poor outcome.

Cerebral edema is mostly cytotoxic and has a particularly rapid onset with subsequent loss of some brainstem reflexes. Immediate, aggressive use of osmotic agents and high-dose intravenous corticosteroids may turn the tide, but many patients progress further to loss of all brainstem reflexes.

Several other causes of deterioration are untreatable. As shown in our case, ischemic lesions may develop due to vasospasm, vasculitis, or vasculopathy. Cortical infarctions are common and widespread and rarely lead to swelling or mass effect. These abnormalities on CT scan are often mislabeled as "cerebritis." Thrombotic vasculopathy may lead to ischemia. MRI is the best means to diagnose these complications and may be useful for prognostication. There is some debate whether cerebral infarcts result from vasculitis or thrombotic vasculopathy (or both) because autopsy studies have not found inflammatory cells in the vessel wall or thrombi. We also have encountered secondary deterioration due to multiterritorial cerebral infarctions, after clear early clinical improvement. Some have reported virtual total recovery only to deteriorate 2 weeks later. High-dose IV corticosteroids did not change the (overall poor) outcome. The mechanism remains unexplained. We and others are also considering cerebral vasospasm from inflammatory cells surrounding the arteries. CTA is needed when cerebral infarcts emerge. It is unknown if endovascular treatment of vasospam is beneficial.

In our patient, acute hydrocephalus was considered symptomatic, and a lumbar drain was placed draining 20 cc every 2 hours. She underwent a mastoidectomy for source control. She gradually awoke within a few days of antibiotics and could be extubated. She recovered fully in weeks. She was treated just in time and had a good outcome despite (albeit mild) hydrocephalus.

Outcome is different in fulminant forms of acute bacterial meningitis, which may be difficult to treat effectively, and major secondary manifestations (i.e., cerebral infarcts) may make recovery much less likely.

Sepsis and multiorgan failure may lead to mortality in acute-phase bacterial meningitis, and of course, this complication is the worst one. We are still close to a 20% mortality prevalence. *L. monocytogenes* meningitis has a worse prognosis. Yet, we suspect that early withdrawal of intensive care unit care is a common reason for death in patients remaining comatose after fulminant meningitis. Early withdrawal of support in not yet adequately treated central nervous system infections is inappropriate and self-defeating; even seemingly moribund patients may survive, and some may even recover to independent functionality.

KEY POINTS TO REMEMBER

- Detection of responsible bacteria may come from blood culture and CSF. Despite negative CSF gram tests, film arrays are often helpful with detection and identification of multiple bacterial nucleic acids extracted from CSF.
- Treat aggressively with corticosteroids and broad-spectrum antibiotics as early as possible.
- In patients who fail to improve despite adequate antibiotic therapy, MRI may be useful to explain the reason.
- Patients may not improve due to cerebral infarcts or severe meningeal inflammation causing hydrocephalus.
- Cerebral edema may require osmotic agents and additional high-dose corticosteroids.
- Patients may need time to recover after a severe bout, and early transition to palliative care is inappropriate, except for patients with refractory sepsis and multiorgan failure.

Further Reading

Assiri, A. M., F. A. Alasmari, V. A. Zimmerman, et al. "Corticosteroid Administration and Outcome of Adolescents and Adults With Acute Bacterial Meningitis: A Meta-Analysis." [In eng]. *Mayo Clin Proc* 84, no. 5 (May 2009): 403–9. https://doi.org/10.1016/s0025-6196(11)60558-2.

Brouwer, M. C., S. G. Heckenberg, J. de Gans, et al. "Nationwide Implementation of Adjunctive Dexamethasone Therapy for Pneumococcal Meningitis." [In eng].

Neurology 75, no. 17 (Oct 26 2010): 1533–39. https://doi.org/10.1212/WNL.0b013 e3181f96297.

Hasbun, R. "Progress and Challenges in Bacterial Meningitis: A Review." [In eng]. *Jama* 328, no. 21 (Dec 6 2022): 2147–54. https://doi.org/10.1001/jama.2022.20521.

Hutchinson VA, Braksick SA, Campeau NG, Wijdicks EFM. Biphasic Clinical Trajectory in Pneumococcal Meningitis from Cerebral Infarcts. [In eng]. *Neurocrit Care.* 2024 Apr 17. doi: 10.1007/s12028-024-01967-7. Epub ahead of print.

Kasanmoentalib, E. S., M. C. Brouwer, A. van der Ende, and D. van de Beek. "Hydrocephalus in Adults With Community-Acquired Bacterial Meningitis." [In eng]. *Neurology* 75, no. 10 (Sep 7 2010): 918–23. https://doi.org/10.1212/ WNL.0b013e3181f11e10.

Lucas, M. J., M. C. Brouwer, and D. van de Beek. "Delayed Cerebral Thrombosis in Bacterial Meningitis: A Prospective Cohort Study." [In eng]. *Intensive Care Med* 39, no. 5 (May 2013): 866–71. https://doi.org/10.1007/s00134-012-2792-9.

McGill, F., R. S. Heyderman, S. Panagiotou, et al. Acute bacterial meningitis in adults. *Lancet* 388, no. 10063 (Dec 17 2016): 3036–47.

Mourvillier, B., F. Tubach, D. van de Beek, et al. "Induced Hypothermia in Severe Bacterial Meningitis: A Randomized Clinical Trial." [In eng]. *Jama* 310, no. 20 (Nov 27 2013): 2174–83. https://doi.org/10.1001/jama.2013.280506.

Muralidharan, R., F. J. Mateen, and A. A. Rabinstein. "Outcome of Fulminant Bacterial Meningitis in Adult Patients." [In eng]. *Eur J Neurol* 21, no. 3 (Mar 2014): 447–53. https://doi.org/10.1111/ene.12328.

Muralidharan, R., A. A. Rabinstein, and E. F. Wijdicks. "Cervicomedullary Injury After Pneumococcal Meningitis With Brain Edema." [In eng]. *Arch Neurol* 68, no. 4 (Apr 2011): 513–16. https://doi.org/10.1001/archneurol.2011.61.

van de Beek, D., J. de Gans, A. R. Tunkel, and E. F. Wijdicks. "Community-Acquired Bacterial Meningitis in Adults." [In eng]. *N Engl J Med* 354, no. 1 (Jan 5 2006): 44–53. https://doi.org/10.1056/NEJMra052116.

van de Beek, D., C. Cabellos, O. Dzupova, et al. "ESCMID Guideline: Diagnosis and Treatment of Acute Bacterial Meningitis." [In eng]. *Clin Microbiol Infect* 22, no. Suppl 3 (May 2016): S37–62.

van Ettekoven, C. N., F. D. Liechti, M. C. Brouwer, M. W. Bijlsma, and D. van de Beek. "Global Case Fatality of Bacterial Meningitis During an 80-Year Period: A Systematic Review and Meta-Analysis." [In eng]. *JAMA Netw Open* 7, no. 8 (Aug 1 2024): e2424802. doi:10.1001/jamanetworkopen.2024.24802.

7 Sorting Out and Treating Acute Encephalitis

A 60-year-old woman came to the emergency department for evaluation of acute fever and confusion. She had psoriasis and rheumatoid arthritis, for which she was treated with weekly doses of methotrexate and efalizumab and had recently received corticosteroid injections in her knees. She first noticed spiking fevers a week earlier. Along with the fevers, she complained of malaise and headache. Her primary internist suspected a urinary infection and started her on levofloxacin 2 days previously. She became more confused over the preceding 24 hours and was found in the neighbor's garage at night. We have been called to examine her in the emergency department. She is tachycardic and has a temperature of 39.2°C. She is drowsy and confused, and her responses fluctuate. Her neck is rigid. Brainstem reflexes are preserved, and she has no lateralizing signs. Computed tomography (CT) scan shows low-attenuation changes in the right temporal and insular regions (Figure 7.1A and B).

What do you do now?

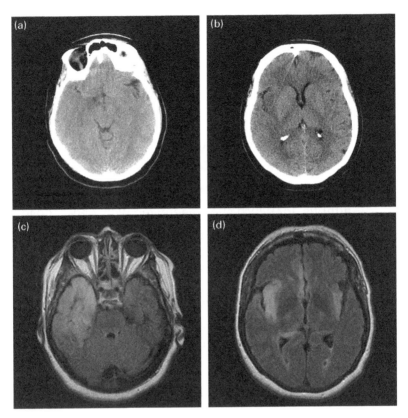

FIGURE 7.1 Brain imaging in our patient with acute HSV-1 encephalitis. CT scan (A and B) shows low-attenuation changes in the right temporal lobe and right insular region. Note also the slightly relative hyperdense appearance in the Sylvian fissure, which may be confused for a fresh thrombus in the middle cerebral artery (A). The areas of brain swelling are much better visualized on the FLAIR sequence of the MRI (C and D), which also reveals the characteristic asymmetric bilaterality of the inflammation in the insular regions.

We suspect encephalitis in a patient who presents with headache, fever, confusion, and, in more advanced cases, changes in the level of consciousness. Seizures (focal or generalized) are a common presentation. Examination may show neck stiffness or focal deficits, but their absence is not infrequent. In fact, when the patient is seen early in the course of the disease, the diagnosis may just be "confusion." While brain magnetic resonance imaging (MRI) is virtually always abnormal in herpes simplex virus type 1 (HSV-1) encephalitis (as illustrated by the classic temporal and insular areas of swelling in our patient) and some radiological findings are more common with specific forms of encephalitis (Table 7.1), changes on MRI can be nonspecific. Most importantly, a negative MRI certainly does not exclude the diagnosis of encephalitis. In fact, brain MRI is most commonly negative with nonherpetic viral etiologies. Cerebrospinal fluid (CSF) should show pleocytosis and increased protein concentration, and a normal CSF strongly points toward an alternative diagnosis. Nowadays, multiplex polymerase chain reaction (PCR) can screen for multiple infectious agents on CSF with results available within 1 to 2 hours. However, this rapid

TABLE 7.1 **Encephalitis and Neuroimaging**

Cause	Characteristic Radiological Features
Herpes simplex virus	Lesions in temporal lobes, insula, and operculum
Varicella zoster virus	Multifocal infarctions and irregularities (vasculitic pattern) of arterial lumen
	Cerebellitis (cerebellar enhancement) in children
Cytomegalovirus	Ventriculitis (subependymal enhancement) Brainstem lesions
West Nile virus	Myelitis[a], patchy foci in white matter, thalami, tegmentum, and substantia nigra
Tuberculosis	Basilar meningitis[b]
Fungal infections	Abscess formation[c]
Autoimmune limbic encephalitis	Lesions in mesial temporal lobes
Acute disseminated encephalomyelitis	Bilateral white matter T2 hyperintense lesions Corpus callosum involvement
Progressive multifocal leukoencephalopathy (JC virus)	Bilateral, confluent T2 hyperintense lesions in temporo-occipital white matter with involvement of U fibers and cortical sparing

[a] Presentation with acute flaccid paralysis may occur with or without radiological signs of myelitis.

[b] Also, with fungal meningoencephalitis.

[c] *Aspergillus* species is characterized by infarctions and hemorrhages.

screening may sometimes fail, and negative results should be interpreted with caution in patients with high suspicion for infection. Metagenomic next-generation sequencing is a powerful tool that permits detection of even very atypical microorganisms. Yet, it is susceptible to false-positive results from contamination. In some encephalitides, the viral load is too low (or may have peaked and cleared rapidly) and serology may diagnose the virus (we have seen this repeatedly in West Nile encephalitis). Generally, IgM and IgG capture enzyme linked immunosorbent assays (ELISAs) are the most useful and most widely used tests for the diagnosis of arboviral encephalitis.

Recognizing a clinical presentation consistent with the diagnosis of acute encephalitis is just the first step. Encephalitis can be infectious, postinfectious, or noninfectious (Table 7.2). Autoimmune (paraneoplastic or not) and radiation-induced encephalitis are examples of noninfectious causes. Defining the precise cause of the acute encephalitis is a much more arduous task that requires almost encyclopedic knowledge of neurological and infectious diseases, and working with a more knowledgeable infectious disease consultant is needed. Equally important is to narrow the differential diagnosis depending on the season, geographic area, specific exposures (including recent travel history), and risk factors. Despite extensive evaluations, all too often a specific cause is never identified.

Viral infection is the most common cause of acute encephalitis in adults. Epidemic outbreaks can be produced by the seasonal spread of arboviruses (i.e., viruses transmitted by arthropod vectors, such as mosquitoes). Most of these agents are constrained to specific geographical locations, but there are exceptions, such as the West Nile virus, or H1N1, that have been identified as a cause of outbreaks of encephalitis in all continents. Viral encephalitis can also be sporadic and can occur in both immunocompetent and immunosuppressed patients. We and other have seen HSV encephalitis after brain surgery from reactivation.

HSV-1 is the most frequent cause of sporadic viral encephalitis in immunocompetent patients. HSV-1 encephalitis has a predilection for the temporal lobes, insula, and operculum. Consequently, it should be suspected when a febrile patient develops confusion or drowsiness associated with seizures or focal deficits and brain lesions in those locations. Aphasia, amnesia, hallucinations, agitation, visual field deficits, and apraxia can be seen. When present, the typical distribution of signal abnormality on brain

TABLE 7.2 **Causes of Acute Encephalitis, Diagnostic Test, and Treatment**

Cause	Diagnostic Test	Management
Viral infections		
HSV-1	CSF PCR	Acyclovir
VZV	CSF PCR	Acyclovir ± steroids
CMV	CSF PCR	Ganciclovir + foscarnet. Exclude HIV
WNV	Serum IgM[a]	Supportive
Influenza	Viral culture, antigen, and PCR of respiratory tract specimen	Oseltamivir
Other arboviruses	CSF serology	Supportive
JC virus (PML)	CSF PCR	Immune reconstitution HAART if HIV
HIV	CSF PCR (viral load)	HAART
Measles	Serum and CSF Ab PCR of nasopharynx, urine, brain	Ribavirin if life-threatening
Mumps	Serum and CSF Ab	Supportive
Rabies	Serum and CSF Ab (if unvaccinated)	Supportive
	IMF of viral antigen in nuchal biopsy	
	Brain pathology	
Bacterial infections	Serum Ab CSF culture	Appropriate antibacterial drugs[b]
Mycobacterium tuberculosis	CSF AFB smear and culture CSF PCR (Gen-Probe Amplified)[c]	Isoniazid, rifampin, pyrazinamide, ethambutol + steroids

(continued)

TABLE 7.2 **Continued**

Cause	Diagnostic Test	Management
Rickettsioses and ehrlichiosis	Serum Ab	Doxycycline (add fluoroquinolone and rifampin if *Coxiella*)
	Morulae within PMN cells in blood smears (*Ehrlichia* only)	
Syphilis and spirochetes	Serum RPR, FTA-ABS	Penicillin G
	CSF VDRL (specific but not sensitive)	
	CSF FTA-ABS (sensitive but not specific)	
Lyme	Serum and CSF Ab (ELISA + Western blot)	Ceftriaxone
Fungal infections[d]		
Aspergillosis	Serum antigen Tissue culture	Voriconazole or amphotericin B or caspofungin
Blastomycosis	Urine antigen Tissue culture	Amphotericin B
Coccidioidomycosis	Serum and CSF Ab CSF culture	Fluconazole
Cryptococcosis	CSF India ink stain Serum and CSF antigen Serum and CSF cultures	Amphotericin B + flucytosine followed by fluconazole
Histoplasmosis	Urine and CSF antigen CSF Ab	Amphotericin B followed by fluconazole
Protozoal infections		
Amebiasis	Serum Ab Brain biopsy (pathology and culture)	Trimethoprim-sulfamethoxazole + rifampin + ketoconazole Check HIV serology

TABLE 7.2 **Continued**

Cause	Diagnostic Test	Management
Malaria	Thick and thin blood smears	Quinine Avoid corticosteroids
Toxoplasmosis	Serum Ab MRI findings Response to therapy	Pyrimethamine + sulfadiazine or clindamycin Check HIV status

Ab, antibodies; AFB, acid-fast bacillus; CMV, cytomegalovirus; CSF, cerebrospinal fluid; ELISA, enzyme-linked immunosorbent assay; FTA-ABS, fluorescent treponemal antibody absorption; HAART, highly active antiretroviral therapy; HIV, human immunodeficiency virus; HSV-1, herpes simplex virus type 1; IgM, immunoglobulin M; IMF, immunofluorescence; MRI, magnetic resonance imaging; PCR, polymerase chain reaction; PML, progressive multifocal leukoencephalopathy; PMN, polymorphonuclear; RPR, rapid plasma reagin; VDRL, Venereal Disease Research Laboratory; VZV, varicella-zoster virus; WNV, West Nile virus.
[a] Serum antibodies are more sensitive than CSF antibodies.
[b] Bacterial infections that may present with acute encephalitis include *Bartonella*, *Listeria* (which characteristically causes a rhombencephalitis), *Mycoplasma*, and *Tropheryma whippelii*.
[c] Sensitivity may not be optimal.
[d] Intrathecal amphotericin B may be necessary in severe cases.

MRI (Figure 7.1 C and D) strongly supports the diagnosis. The diagnosis should be confirmed by detection of the virus in CSF. PCR can be used to detect HSV-1 DNA in the CSF with great sensitivity and specificity. If PCR is negative but the clinical-radiological presentation strongly suggests HSV-1 infection, the test should be repeated on a new CSF sample after 3 to 5 days while continuing treatment with intravenous [IV] acyclovir.

Electroencephalography (EEG) should be performed in patients with HSV-1 encephalitis. Patients with encephalitis often exhibit fluctuating levels of alertness and awareness. In these cases, we often pursue continuous EEG monitoring. Also consider continuous EEG monitoring in comatose patients with encephalitis. Nonconvulsive seizures are not uncommon but should be differentiated from lateralized periodic discharges (LPDs). When LPDs are frequent or tend to become rhythmic, we favor the use of anti seizure medication to prevent seizures. However, in these cases, we do not escalate their doses to eliminate the discharges because the value of this approach is unproven and often provokes drug toxicity. LPDs tend to be quite refractory and should be interpreted as a manifestation of the structural injury caused by the encephalitis.

Testing for autoimmune encephalitis (paraneoplastic or not) is done in cases without a proven infectious cause. The existence of autoimmune profiles in diagnostic order sets facilitates testing because it includes the great majority of antibodies that must be checked. Because the antibodies are not specific for a certain neurological presentation and most can cause encephalitis, we prefer to be inclusive when choosing which tests to order. Also, test the antibodies in both the serum and CSF. Recognizing autoimmune encephalitis has important implications. The diagnosis indicates the need to search for an underlying tumor (though keeping in mind that a sizable proportion of cases will not be related to a tumor). Knowing the precise antibody (or antibodies, since more than one antibody can coexist) is also useful. For instance, anti-N-methyl D-aspartate receptor antibodies strongly correlate with ovarian teratomas in young women, and excision of the teratoma is necessary to achieve good response to immune therapy in these cases. More details on autoimmune encephalitis are found in Chapter 8.

The role of brain biopsy has been relegated to very few selected cases thanks to the high yield of PCR. Brain biopsy in unexplained encephalitis is only considered once all noninvasive diagnostic alternatives have been exhausted and the patient continues to decline despite treatment with adequate doses of acyclovir. It is also advisable to search for other biopsy targets before invading the brain. Detailed physical examination with special attention to the skin and lymph node chains; CT scans of the chest, abdomen, and pelvis; and a positron emission tomography scan can deliver a more accessible site for tissue sampling. Brain biopsy should be guided by MRI findings, and we favor inclusion of a meningeal sample. When neuroimaging is normal or unchanged, the yield of random brain biopsy is much lower, but pathology may still be diagnostic in these cases. The most salient problem regarding the evaluation of encephalitis is how much of it may be without results.

All patients with presumed acute encephalitis should be started immediately on IV acyclovir (10 mg/kg ideal body weight IV every 8 hours; longer intervals between doses in case of reduced glomerular filtration rate). This antiviral agent is the first choice for treating HSV-1, HSV-2, and varicella-zoster virus. Cytomegalovirus infection requires the combination of ganciclovir and foscarnet; these patients should also be tested for HIV infection. Ganciclovir and foscarnet are also the treatment for human herpesvirus type 6 infection in immunosuppressed patients. No antiviral has proven effective against West Nile virus infection. HIV-infected patients must receive highly active antiretroviral therapy (HAART). In cases of progressive multifocal leukoencephalopathy (JC virus), the treatment may consist of reversing immunosuppression to reconstitute an immune response. Directly isolated allogeneic virus-specific T-cell treatment for progressive multifocal leukoencephalopathy shows reduced mortality and improved functional outcome. The main treatment measures for infectious causes of encephalitis are summarized in Table 7.2.

Patients who develop severe brain swelling might require intracranial pressure monitoring. Intraparenchymal monitors are preferable when the ventricles are compressed by brain edema. Head-of-bed elevation and osmotic agents (mannitol, hypertonic saline) are the first step in cases of intracranial hypertension. The most severe cases may demand decompressive hemicraniectomy, but this is highly uncommon. Corticosteroids do not have a role in the treatment of viral encephalitis and should be avoided when untreated fungal infection is a possibility.

When acute encephalitis requires admission to an intensive care unit (ICU), the key issues are recognition and treatment of seizures requiring continuous EEG monitoring, mechanical ventilation in patients unable to protect the airway, and treatment of brain swelling and medical complications. Even when the cause of the encephalitis is not treatable, aggressive supportive care increases the chance of a favorable outcome.

Our patient was immediately started on IV acyclovir in the emergency department. An MRI of the brain (Figure 7.1C and D) was obtained to delineate the degree of temporal lobe swelling before proceeding with lumbar puncture. The CSF contained 14 white blood cells (predominantly lymphocytes), a protein concentration of 58 mg/dL, and normal glucose level. Shortly after arrival to the neurological ICU she was intubated because of progressive stupor and inability to maintain airway patency. Levofloxacin was stopped (it can reduce seizure threshold) and she was prophylactically started on IV levetiracetam. EEG demonstrated frequent LPDs arising from the right temporal region but no electrographic seizures. Within hours we received confirmation that the PCR for HSV-1 was positive in the CSF. She began to improve within the following 5 days. Two weeks later she was discharged home, where she continued recovering and completed a 21-day course of acyclovir. Her systemic immunosuppressive regimen was permanently stopped. Six months later she had regained full function.

KEY POINTS TO REMEMBER

- Always consider the diagnosis of encephalitis in a febrile and confused patient, regardless of the presence of meningeal signs or focal deficits.
- Start IV acyclovir in patients with suspected viral encephalitis.
- PCR for HSV-1 should be performed in all CSF samples of patients with presumed encephalitis. If PCR is negative but the diagnosis is still suspected (clinical or radiological localization to the temporal lobes or insular/opercular region), IV acyclovir should be continued, and PCR should be repeated after 3 to 5 days.
- MRI with gadolinium is the most informative neuroimaging modality for patients with suspected encephalitis.
- Patients with HSV-1 encephalitis should have an EEG. In patients with fluctuating consciousness the option of continuous EEG monitoring should be considered to exclude frequent nonconvulsive seizures.

Further Reading

Barnett, G. H., A. H. Ropper, and J. Romeo. "Intracranial Pressure and Outcome in Adult Encephalitis." [In eng]. *J Neurosurg* 68, no. 4 (Apr 1988): 585–88. doi.org/10.3171/jns.1988.68.4.0585.

Bhimani, A. D., D. D. Cummins, R. Kalagara, S. Chennareddy, and Z. L. Hickman. "A Rare Case of Herpes Simplex Virus Encephalitis from Viral Reactivation Following Surgically Treated Traumatic Brain Injury." [In eng]. *Brain Inj* (Jul 4 2024): 1–6. doi:10.1080/02699052.2024.2370834.

Bloch, K. C., C. Glaser, D. Gaston, and A. Venkatesan. "State of the Art: Acute Encephalitis." [In eng]. *Clin Infect Dis* 77, no. 5 (Sep 11 2023): e14–33. https://doi.org/10.1093/cid/ciad306.

Burki T. West Nile virus in the USA. *Lancet.* 2024, no.404. Jul 13:108-109. doi: 10.1016/S0140-6736(24)01435-1.

Graus, F., M. J. Titulaer, R. Balu, et al. "A Clinical Approach to Diagnosis of Autoimmune Encephalitis." [In eng]. *Lancet Neurol* 15, no. 4 (Apr 2016): 391–404. https://doi.org/10.1016/s1474-4422(15)00401-9.

Mahan, M., M. Karl, and S. Gordon. "Neuroimaging of Viral Infections of the Central Nervous System." [In eng]. *Handb Clin Neurol* 123 (2014): 149–73. https://doi.org/10.1016/b978-0-444-53488-0.00006-7.

McGrath, N., N. E. Anderson, M. C. Croxson, and K. F. Powell. "Herpes Simplex Encephalitis Treated With Acyclovir: Diagnosis and Long Term Outcome." [In eng]. *J Neurol Neurosurg Psychiatry* 63, no. 3 (Sep 1997): 321–26. https://doi.org/10.1136/jnnp.63.3.321.

Möhn, N., Grote-Levy, L., Wattjes, M.P., et al. "Directly isolated allogeneic virus-specific T cells in progressive multifocal leukoencephalopathy." [In eng]. *JAMA Neurol* 2024 doi.org/10.1001/jamaneurol.2024.3324

Singh, T. D., J. E. Fugate, S. Hocker, et al. "Predictors of Outcome in HSV Encephalitis." [In eng]. *J Neurol* 263, no. 2 (Feb 2016): 277–89. https://doi.org/10.1007/s00415-015-7960-8.

Singh, T. D., J. E. Fugate, and A. A. Rabinstein. "The Spectrum of Acute Encephalitis: Causes, Management, and Predictors of Outcome." [In eng]. *Neurology* 84, no. 4 (Jan 27 2015): 359–66. https://doi.org/10.1212/wnl.0000000000001190.

Tunkel, A. R., C. A. Glaser, K. C. Bloch, et al. "The Management of Encephalitis: Clinical Practice Guidelines by the Infectious Diseases Society of America." [In eng]. *Clin Infect Dis* 47, no. 3 (Aug 1 2008): 303–27. https://doi.org/10.1086/589747.

Venkatesan, A., B. D. Michael, J. C. Probasco, et al. "Acute Encephalitis in Immunocompetent Adults." [In eng]. *Lancet* 393, no. 10172 (Feb 16 2019): 702–16. https://doi.org/10.1016/s0140-6736(18)32526-1.

Wilson, M. R., and K. L. Tyler. "The Current Status of Next-Generation Sequencing for Diagnosis of Central Nervous System Infections." [In eng]. *JAMA Neurol* 79, no. 11 (Nov 1 2022): 1095–96. https://doi.org/10.1001/jamaneurol.2022.2287.

8 The Presenting Features of Autoimmune Encephalitis

A 27-year-old woman without any prior psychiatric history suddenly developed extreme anxiety, pressured and erratic speech, racing thoughts, flight of ideas, and visual hallucinations. She was initially admitted to a psychiatric service with a presumed acute psychotic break but then developed runs of tachycardia up to 140 beats per minute (bpm) and developed a fever. Cerebrospinal fluid (CSF) analysis revealed a pleocytosis of 43 nucleated cells and 93% lymphocytes. CSF glucose and protein were normal, and the gram stain and herpes simplex virus (HSV) polymerase chain reaction (PCR) were negative. Brain magnetic resonance imaging (MRI) was normal. Orofacial movements and fine motor movements of the hands were noted. She became increasingly agitated and combative, requiring restraints. One week into her illness, she became unresponsive to loud voices, and a painful stimulus prompted only minimal withdrawal. An electroencephalogram (EEG) demonstrated frequent bitemporal seizures lasting 1 minute each. Several hours after achieving seizure control, she became agitated and spoke fluently, although her speech was all over the place and without any context. EEG showed a pattern known as extreme delta brush (Figure 8.1).

What do you do now?

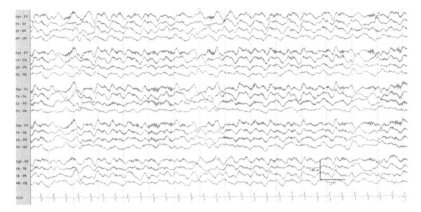

FIGURE 8.1 Electroencephalogram showing frontally maximal high-voltage beta activity superimposed on frontally maximal delta waves called "extreme delta brush."

Patients rarely transfer from a psychiatry ward to the neurosciences intensive care unit (neuro-ICU), but when it occurs, we often diagnose autoimmune encephalitis. Studies have shown that about half of these patients were initially misdiagnosed with primary psychiatric disorders and first admitted to psychiatric wards. A new field of "autoimmune psychiatry" seems be emerging with autoimmune encephalitis being diagnosed in patients with schizophrenia, bipolar disorder, and depression. For sure, acute psychotic breaks in young individuals now will be evaluated more thoroughly, particularly in those with diagnoses of de novo acute catatonia. We do not know the proportion of patients whose acute psychiatric presentations actually have an autoimmune mechanism, and the current clinical impression is that it is quite small.

Autoimmune encephalitis has now been characterized as a group of potentially treatable disorders that frequently look and behave like any (sub)acute viral encephalitis. Whatever that meant in the past. In fact, a recent prospective population-based study of 203 patients with encephalitis found an immune-mediated cause in one in five, and over a third of these patients had measurable neuronal antibodies. As senior neurologists, we can now confidently say that we have been very wrong in the diagnosis of "viral" encephalitis in some cases in the past; it is probably still a new disease and one that has become much better characterized.

Keeping in mind the highly variable clinical spectrum of autoimmune encephalitis, we now suspect it in patients presenting with a rapidly progressive encephalopathy, especially one preceded by a viral prodrome. However, while some syndromes such as anti-N-methyl D-aspartate receptor (NMDAR) encephalitis are well described, the clinical spectrum of other antibody-mediated encephalopathies is being frequently refined and adjusted. Certain infections, particularly viral infections, may trigger an immune-mediated encephalitis, and thus, the presence of one does not necessarily exclude the other. A more recent, surprising find is that autoimmune encephalitis occurs in 27% of patients with prior herpes simplex encephalitis (HSE), usually within 2 months after HSE treatment. The neurological outcome is worse in young children. No patients tested positive for antibodies at onset of HSE, which suggests that herpes simplex likely triggered the immune response. This spectrum of disorders now also includes cryptogenic epilepsy and new-onset refractory status epilepticus. This entity of disorders fascinates many of us, and after our first clinical experience, we are wary of any unexplained encephalitis (Box 8.1).

BOX 8.1 **When to Consider Autoimmune Encephalitis**

Clinical:

Viral prodrome

Unexpected new psychiatric symptoms

History of systemic autoimmunity or serological markers of auto-immunity, such as antinuclear antibody or thyroid peroxidase antibody positivity

History of cancer

Antiepileptic drug resistance

Cryptogenic status epilepticus (including nonconvulsive status epilepticus)

Subacute onset of cryptogenic epilepsy

CSF: Elevated protein, pleocytosis, oligoclonal bands, elevated IgG index or synthesis rate

MRI: Often unrevealing initially and on repeat studies; may show thalami and brainstem lesions

EEG: Beta activity superimposed on frontally maximal delta

Often these disorders display additional supportive clinical features such as severe dysautonomia, automatism, dyskinesias, stereotypy or extreme non verbal catatonia with catalepsy type posturing. There may be personal or family history of autoimmunity, smoking history, or other risk factors for cancer. There is often evidence of inflammation on CSF analysis with a lymphocytic pleocytosis, elevated protein, oligoclonal bands, or elevated IgG index. Brain MRI can be normal but may sometimes show hyperintensities in a number of locations (Box 8.1). Functional imaging (fluorodeoxyglucose positron emission tomography [FDG PET]) may show hypermetabolism. Serologic markers of systemic autoimmunity, such as antinuclear antibody or thyroid peroxidase antibodies, may be present. Interesting is the presence of an extreme delta brush on EEG, a recently described EEG finding in 30% of patients with anti-NMDAR encephalitis—and was present in our patient. This EEG pattern has now definitively been linked to this encephalitis.

When we encounter these patients, particularly among the elderly or those with cancer risk factors, we also consider a paraneoplastic disorder. Antibodies directed against intracellular onconeural proteins (ANNA-1, ANNA-2, Anti-Ma1/Ma2) classically correlate with paraneoplastic disorders of the central nervous system, while antibodies directed against plasma membrane proteins (NMDAR, AMPAR, LGl1, CASPR2, GABA-B, mGluR5) may or may not be paraneoplastic. If no antibody is identified, a trial of immunosuppression may still be worthwhile if there is no other explanation for the syndrome. Once an antibody is found, it should prompt a directed search for an associated malignancy (Table 8.1).

Furthermore, if a cancer not known to be associated with the antibody is found, we should look for another occult malignancy more typically associated with the antibody. Computed tomography (CT) scans of the chest, abdomen, and pelvis are recommended for initial screening and, when negative, may be followed by FDG PET-CT. If a germ cell tumor is suspected, CT and FDG PET-CT are inadequate, and testicular or pelvic ultrasounds or MRI of the pelvis is needed. Ovarian teratomas strongly correlate with anti-NMDAR encephalitis and may be difficult to identify with pelvic MRI or transvaginal ultrasound. Exploratory laparoscopy may be the only means of correct identification; this is important because the neurological syndrome is often refractory to treatment until the teratoma is

TABLE 8.1 **Antibodies Linked to Encephalitis With or Without Malignancies**

Antibody	Common Cancer Association
ANNA-1 (Anti-Hu)	SCLC
ANNA-2 (Anti-Ri)	Breast, gynecological, SCLC
Anti-CV2/CRMP-5	SCLC, thymoma
Anti-amphiphysin	SCLC, breast adenocarcinoma
Anti-Ma proteins	Testicular (Ma2); breast, colon, testicular (Ma1)
Anti-VGKC complex (mainly Lgl1)	SCLC, thymoma or adenocarcinoma of breast or prostate
Anti-NMDAR	Ovarian teratomas, testicular germinoma, neuroblastoma
Anti-AMPAR	Thymic tumors, lung carcinoma, breast adenocarcinoma
Anti-GABA$_A$R	No clear association, although some patients may have thymoma
Anti-GABA$_B$R	SCLC or another neuroendocrine tumor of lung
Anti-DPPX	No clear association
Anti-glycine	Rare associations with cancer
Anti-mGluR5	Hodgkin lymphoma
Anti-dopamine 2	No clear association
Anti-GAD65	Thymoma; renal cell, breast, or colon adenocarcinoma

SCLC, small cell lung cancer.

resected. Blind ovariectomy is another story and there insufficient support for such radical action. It not known, when microscopic teratoma is found, that its removal will improve outcome.

The specific treatment objectives are to disable antibodies through immunosuppression and to knock out production with treatment of the underlying malignancy. First-line immunosuppression in these critically ill adults is usually high-dose IV methylprednisolone and either IV immunoglobulin (IVIG) or plasma exchange. Rituximab and cyclophosphamide are considered second-line agents when there is an insufficient response to first-line treatments. Early treatment speeds recovery, reduces neurological disability, and decreases relapses.

Once in the neuro-ICU, patients often become wildly agitated with severe movement abnormalities. In some cases, intubation and IV midazolam or propofol infusion are necessary to control agitation. Dysautonomia (consistent with paroxysmal sympathetic hyperactivity) can be pronounced and may respond well to IV dexmedetomidine. In other cases, we have had to control refractory status epilepticus for months punctuated by multiple, unsuccessful anesthetic weaning attempts until seizures finally burned out.

What did we do for our patient? We rapidly controlled her agitation and associated dysautonomia with a dexmedetomidine infusion. Because treatment of the immunological response can be the only successful means of controlling agitation or seizures, we promptly initiated therapy with 5 days of IV methylprednisolone, 5 days of IVIG, and rituximab at a dose of 375 mg/m^2. She received further treatment with scheduled lorazepam, and we ultimately controlled her dysautonomia with high-dose gabapentin, eventually liberating her from the dexmedetomidine infusion. One week after sending the studies—an expected delay for the return of test results—her serum and spinal fluid were positive for NMDAR antibodies. MRI of the pelvis identified an ovarian teratoma, which was resected the following day. Maintenance immunosuppression consisted of (1) daily prednisone administration at 1 mg/kg and tapered off over 12 months; (2) weekly IVIG infusions tapered off over 3 months; and (3) rituximab, 375 mg/m^2 every week for 4 weeks.

She had a good outcome. Because anti-NMDAR antibody encephalitis can be a monophasic disease, particularly in the setting of resected teratoma, she is currently being observed off immunosuppressants. She has not had recurrent seizures and ultimately transitioned to levetiracetam monotherapy. Fifteen months after diagnosis, she has had marked improvement, although she continues to have some mood lability. Her case is not exceptional; outcomes can be very good with early diagnosis and treatment. However, we must not forget that autoimmune encephalitis requiring ICU admission is a profoundly serious disease. In our experience, at least a quarter of survivors are left with substantial cognitive sequelae.

Other experiences with outcome are also mixed. For sure a long recovery time is anticipated. Early plasma exchange alone has 5.6-fold increased odds of good outcome, but combinations have lesser beneficial impact (2.7-fold increased odds of good outcome with corticosteroids and IVIG; 2.8-fold with corticosteroids, IVIG, and therapeutic apheresis), though that may be because of selection bias (i.e., more severe cases being treated with combination therapy). Rituximab with a monophasic course also correlates with 5.9-fold reduced odds of relapse after follow-up of 24 months or more. Furthermore, there has been emerging use of escalation to second-line therapies such as IV/intrathecal methotrexate, subcutaneous/IV bortezomib, and IV tocilizumab. We still lack head-to-head comparative clinical trials, and treatment remains trial and error.

Finally, incorrect diagnosis of autoimmune disorders is also common, leading to exposure to potentially harmful immunosuppressive drugs. The disorders that may mimic autoimmune encephalitis are often neoplasms, including glioblastoma, located in the mesial temporal lobes, and lymphoma, particularly if the response to corticosteroids is robust. A broad spectrum of rare genetic disorders are also potential mimickers. An additional problem is that some autoantibody titers can be nonspecifically positive. The leading experts Dalmau and Graus suggest the following remedies:

(1) Become familiar with the syndromes and favor clinical reasoning over antibody results. (2) Use CSF and serum testing; if forced to pick one, use CSF. (3) Be aware that a positive test result does not always mean presence of antibodies; thus, request antibody confirmation by at least 2 techniques (brain tissue immuno-histochemistry and cell immunofluorescence method). (4) Doubt any positive serum result that is accompanied by negative CSF antibodies. An exception is the antibodies against myelin oligodendrocyte glycoprotein (MOG) that are more frequently detected in serum and can associate with symptoms of autoimmune encephalitis.

These pioneers in the diagnosis of autoimmune encephalitides also warn against the rapid emergence of autoimmune psychosis, autoimmune epilepsy, autoimmune movement disorders, or autoimmune depression; these disorders may not exist or may be far more uncommon than claimed in the literature.

KEY POINTS TO REMEMBER

- Symptoms of autoimmune encephalopathy are diverse, but some distinguishing features are a psychotic break, catatonia, seizures, depressed level of consciousness, or a new movement disorder such as choreoathetosis.
- Seizures due to autoimmune encephalitis are often resistant to antiepileptic drugs, and patients may need anesthetics.
- Patients should be screened and treated for associated cancer.
- In young women with anti-NMDAR antibodies, consult a gynecologist and comprehensively search for an ovarian teratoma.
- First-line immune therapies include high-dose corticosteroids, IV immunoglobulin, and plasma exchange. In refractory cases, second-line immunosuppression with rituximab should be added.
- Response to immunotherapy and treatment of malignancy determine prognosis.

Further Reading

Armangue, T., F. Leypoldt, and J. Dalmau. "Autoimmune Encephalitis as Differential Diagnosis of Infectious Encephalitis." [In eng]. *Curr Opin Neurol* 27, no. 3 (Jun 2014): 361–68. https://doi.org/10.1097/wco.0000000000000087.

Armangue, T., M. Spatola, A. Vlagea, et al. "Frequency, Symptoms, Risk Factors, and Outcomes of Autoimmune Encephalitis After Herpes Simplex Encephalitis: A Prospective Observational Study and Retrospective Analysis." [In eng]. *Lancet Neurol* 17, no. 9 (Sep 2018): 760–72. https://doi.org/10.1016/s1474-4422(18)30244-8.

Berk, M., M. Leboyer, and I. E. Sommer, eds. *Immuno-Psychiatry: Facts and Prospects.* New York: Springer; 2021.

Dalmau, J., and F. Graus. "Antibody-Mediated Encephalitis." [In eng]. *N Engl J Med* 378, no. 9 (Mar 1 2018): 840–51. https://doi.org/10.1056/NEJMra1708712.

Dalmau, J., and F. Graus. "Antibody-Mediated Neuropsychiatric Disorders." [In eng]. *J Allergy Clin Immunol* 149, no. 1 (Jan 2022): 37–40. https://doi.org/10.1016/j.jaci.2021.11.008.

Dalmau, J., and F. Graus. "Diagnostic Criteria for Autoimmune Encephalitis: Utility and Pitfalls for Antibody-Negative Disease." [In eng]. *Lancet Neurol* 22, no. 6 (Jun 2023): 529–40. https://doi.org/10.1016/s1474-4422(23)00083-2.

Dinoto, A., P. Zara, S. Mariotto, et al. "Autoimmune Encephalitis Misdiagnosis and Mimics." [In eng]. *J Neuroimmunol* 378 (May 15 2023): 578071. https://doi.org/10.1016/j.jneuroim.2023.578071.

Graus, F., M. J. Titulaer, R. Balu, et al. "A Clinical Approach to Diagnosis of Autoimmune Encephalitis." [In eng]. *Lancet Neurol* 15, no. 4 (Apr 2016): 391–404. https://doi.org/10.1016/s1474-4422(15)00401-9.

Irani, S. R. "Autoimmune Encephalitis." [In eng]. *Continuum (Minneap Minn)* 30, no. 4 (Aug 1 2024): 995–1020.

Mittal, M. K., A. A. Rabinstein, S. E. Hocker, et al. "Autoimmune Encephalitis in the ICU: Analysis of Phenotypes, Serologic Findings, and Outcomes." [In eng]. *Neurocrit Care* 24, no. 2 (Apr 2016): 240–50. https://doi.org/10.1007/s12028-015-0196-8.

Nosadini, M., M. Eyre, E. Molteni, et al. "Use and Safety of Immunotherapeutic Management of N-Methyl-D-Aspartate Receptor Antibody Encephalitis: A Meta-Analysis." [In eng]. *JAMA Neurol* 78, no. 11 (Nov 1 2021): 1333–44. https://doi.org/10.1001/jamaneurol.2021.3188.

Titulaer, M. J., L. McCracken, I. Gabilondo, et al. "Treatment and Prognostic Factors for Long-Term Outcome in Patients With Anti-NMDA Receptor Encephalitis: An Observational Cohort Study." [In eng]. *Lancet Neurol* 12, no. 2 (Feb 2013): 157–65. https://doi.org/10.1016/s1474-4422(12)70310-1.

9 Escalating Dyspnea in Acute Neuromuscular Disease

A 21-year-old woman presented to our emergency department complaining of low back pain over the preceding 2 days and tingling in her legs since the previous afternoon. Subsequently, she noticed progressive weakness in her legs. On initial evaluation, she had mild proximal weakness in both legs. Deep tendon reflexes were absent in both legs and decreased in both arms. Sensory examination was normal. She had no signs of oropharyngeal weakness or ventilatory problems. Arterial blood gases revealed neither hypoxia nor hypercapnia. Chest film was normal. She was admitted to our intensive care unit for close monitoring.

Early the following morning, we noticed she was much weaker. She could hardly activate her iliopsoas muscles, and her arms could barely stay up against gravity. She was now completely areflexic. Restless and tachypneic, she reported difficulty breathing and could only speak a few words at a time before catching a breath.

What do you do now?

For this patient, endotracheal intubation and mechanical ventilation support were imminent. Procrastination may lead to emergency intubation (or come at full tilt with cardiopulmonary resuscitation). Once the vital signs are stabilized, we can work on the cause of dyspnea and the underlying neuromuscular cause of the patient's shortness of breath. Some core fundamentals are needed to understand this clinical situation.

An acute neuromuscular disorder should be suspected in any patient with acute respiratory failure who presents with marginal oxygenation, mixed hypoxia and hypercapnia, or predominant hypercapnia in combination with signs of oropharyngeal and appendicular muscle weakness. The most likely causes are Guillain-Barré syndrome (GBS) or myasthenia gravis; myopathy or a previously undiagnosed motor neuron disease is a less frequent but possible consideration. Patients with neuromuscular respiratory failure have a characteristic presentation that includes dyspnea, tachypnea, and tachycardia. Restlessness is a common feature; inability to speak in full sentences (staccato speech) and diaphoresis (typically seen as sweat on the forehead) denote their struggle to breathe. We can test this further by having the patient exhale and count after a deep inspiration. (It is best to use numbers such as 1000, 2000, 3000, etc., that take longer to pronounce, thus preventing patients from speeding up the count as they might be able to do when counting 1, 2, 3, etc.) Inability to count more than 10 numbers indicates a potentially significant decline in vital capacity, although we do not know if the correlation is monotonic, nonlinear, or exponential. Patients with oropharyngeal weakness have a weak cough, nasal voice, and problems handling oral secretions. Recruitment of accessory muscles can be visible on inspection, but a better means of discerning it is palpating the sternocleidomastoid muscles to identify contraction. The hallmark of neuromuscular respiratory failure is the presence of a paradoxical breathing pattern—an inward rather than the normal outward movement of the abdominal wall with each inspiration.

These are clinical manifestations of the failure of the breathing mechanics, which eventually leads to insufficient ventilation. Briefly, accessory muscles (other muscles attached to the ribcage) only partially compensate for the failure of the diaphragm (major component) and intercostal muscles (smaller component) to lift the ribcage. The abdominal muscles assist only with coughing and expiration. Poor lung expansion leads to reduced air flow and alveolar collapse. Atelectasis causes hypoxemia, and eventually hypoventilation results in hypercapnia. Aspiration due to coexisting oropharyngeal weakness may worsen gas exchange even more. The physiological compensatory response increases respiratory frequency but cannot increase tidal volumes.

Upon entering their rooms, physicians may see these patients visibly struggling to breathe, sitting up in bed, and maintaining only marginal pulse oximeter values (oxygen saturations in the low 90s) despite increasing oxygen requirements. Hypercapnia occurs later in acute cases but may be seen earlier in patients with exacerbated chronic neuromuscular disorders. Yet, a "normal $PaCO_2$" value in a tachypneic patient is actually abnormal and indicates that the patient is not "blowing off" CO_2. Some visibly restless, tachypneic patients do not sense distress and may even want to delay intubation. Waiting might be unsafe, and we greatly prefer proceeding with intubation electively rather than emergently.

Bedside spirometry gauges forced vital capacity and maximal inspiratory and expiratory pressures. Additionally, arterial blood gases and a chest X-ray should complement the physical examination in the initial evaluation of these patients. We coach patients carefully before spirometry testing, and make sure they can satisfactorily seal the mouthpiece of the spirometer with their lips before moving forward with the test. When the results are worse than expected—based on the physical exam and the blood gases—poor technique, insufficient mouth sealing, and suboptimal effort are the most frequent explanations. We have found that mask spirometry is better for getting reliable data on patients with facial diplegia.

When this initial assessment confirms the diagnosis of neuromuscular respiratory failure, the next steps are deciding whether the patient needs mechanical ventilation and determining the most probable cause of the weakness. Both priorities are closely related. The urgency of action and the type of mechanical ventilation (invasive or noninvasive) to be chosen depend on the type of neuromuscular disorder being treated. Establishing the neuromuscular diagnosis not only is crucial to selecting optimal treatment but also carries major prognostic implications. Patients with acute neuromuscular respiratory failure of unclear cause after extensive evaluations—a situation we encounter in more than 10% of all cases admitted to the intensive care unit (ICU) with acute neuromuscular respiratory failure—rarely

> **BOX 9.1 Clinical Findings That Predict Rapid Worsening and Need for Intubation in Patients With Acute Neuromuscular Respiratory Weakness**
>
> Pooling secretions due to oropharyngeal weakness
>
> Increased work of breathing and restlessness
>
> Rapidly progressive muscle weakness
>
> Increasing oxygen requirements
>
> Aspiration or major atelectasis on chest X-ray
>
> Evidence of respiratory infection
>
> Failure to improve with BiPAP[a]
>
> [a] BiPAP is not recommended for patients worsening from Guillain-Barré syndrome.

recover well despite aggressive respiratory treatment. Clinical pointers helpful to decide whether a patient needs ventilatory assistance are shown in Box 9.1.

GBS and myasthenic crisis are the most common causes of acute neuromuscular respiratory failure. Although these two immunological disorders are similar in some respects, their ideal respiratory management differs substantially. Patients with GBS can worsen very quickly; when they do, they often have manifestations of dysautonomia, such as rapid swings in blood pressure and cardiac arrhythmias. Also, if ventilatory impairment occurs, their course toward full-blown respiratory failure is unstoppable. GBS patients should be intubated without delay before reaching their nadir because they may develop sudden respiratory arrest. Spirometry results can be confidently used to guide the timing of elective intubation in GBS (Table 9.1).

When patients worsen from myasthenia gravis, the presentation differs from that of GBS. One study in 250 cases of myasthenic crisis found that the crisis itself is often the first manifestation of myasthenia gravis. Patients tend to be older and male. Comorbidities are high. Although patients with myasthenic crisis often require intubation, they greatly benefit from noninvasive ventilatory support with bilevel positive airway pressure (BiPAP) if it is started early. Before respiratory muscles fail, patients with myasthenia gravis may develop progressive but still reversible fatigability. When

TABLE 9.1 Bedside Respiratory Tests Predicting Need for Mechanical Ventilation in GBS

Parameter	Normal Value	Critical Value[a]
Forced vital capacity	40–70 mL/kg	20 mL/kg
Maximal inspiratory pressure	Men: > –100 cmH$_2$O Women: > –70 cmH$_2$O	–30 cmH$_2$O
Maximal expiratory pressure	Men: >200 cmH$_2$O Women: >140 cmH$_2$O	40 cmH$_2$O

[a] Best remembered as the 20-30-40 rule.

aided by BiPAP, these muscles can sustain adequate ventilation longer, thus allowing time for immunomodulatory therapy to become effective. If started on time, BiPAP can avert intubation and prevent its pulmonary complications (atelectasis and pneumonia) but only if a rapid effect of plasma exchange (not intravenous immunoglobulin) treatment can be achieved. Thus, one should not wait too long to start BiPAP; once patients become hypercapnic (an indication that the ventilatory muscles have already failed), noninvasive ventilation is unlikely to be successful. Although bedside spirometry results are often measured in a myasthenic crisis, they are less reliable indicators of the need for mechanical ventilation than in GBS.

Other disorders causing respiratory failure include amyotrophic lateral sclerosis (ALS) and congenital myopathies. Severe chronic myopathies eventually will involve the oropharyngeal musculature and diaphragmatic function; common examples are the major dystrophies (Duchenne, limb-girdle) and metabolic myopathies such as X-linked myotubular myopathy, centronuclear myopathies, acid maltase deficiency, or Pompe disease. (In hereditary myopathy with early respiratory failure, respiratory weakness is the predominant feature along with disproportionate—but sometimes mild—distal weakness.) When a chronic myopathy causes acute respiratory failure requiring endotracheal intubation and invasive ventilation, there is a high likelihood of successfully weaning off the ventilator (with or without tracheostomy) and returning to the previous level of function. The reason is that there has been some intercurrent infection.

Neuromuscular respiratory failure and aspiration pneumonia are common reasons for hospitalizations, including emergency ICU admissions, in ALS. ALS patients intubated for acute respiratory failure, with or without an established diagnosis, rarely achieve independence from the ventilator. All these patients need long-term ventilatory support, and the degree of respiratory support increases with time.

Our patient had an axonal type of GBS. We intubated her immediately that morning, and in a matter of hours, she progressed and was completely paralyzed by her disease. During her ICU admission, she developed various manifestations of severe dysautonomia including a brief period of asystole during tracheal suctioning, sudden hypertensive surges, and hypotensive plunges. Despite the extreme severity of her disease at nadir, she recovered full function within the following year.

Decision-making in acute neuromuscular respiratory failure requires good judgment. In myasthenia gravis, early use of BiPAP may prevent the need for intubation and prolonged mechanical ventilation. In GBS, neuromuscular respiratory failure may progress rapidly, become difficult to manage, or even lead to a fatal outcome if physicians hesitate to intubate. The options for triage to the ICU are not disease but symptom based and are summarized in Figure 9.1. Remember the five Ds; dysphagia,

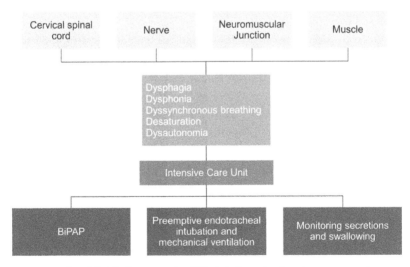

FIGURE 9.1 Key clinical findings prompting ICU admission and options for management.

dysphonia, dyssynchronous breathing, desaturation, and dysautonomia. Each of them spells trouble; the presence of more than one indicates real danger.

KEY POINTS TO REMEMBER

- Paradoxical breathing is the most characteristic sign of advanced neuromuscular respiratory failure, but there are subtler, earlier signs.
- Identifying the neuromuscular cause of the ventilatory failure is essential to formulate the best plan for respiratory management.
- Patients with GBS should be intubated electively when they develop their first signs of ventilatory failure (i.e., before hypoxemia and certainly before hypercapnia).
- Patients with myasthenic crisis are best treated with noninvasive ventilation (BiPAP) if this support is initiated before the development of hypercapnia.

Further Reading

Birch, T. B. "Neuromuscular Disorders in the Intensive Care Unit." [In eng]. *Continuum (Minneap Minn)* 27, no. 5 (Oct 1 2021): 1344–64. https://doi.org/10.1212/con.00000 00000001004.

Cabrera Serrano, M., and A. A. Rabinstein. "Causes and Outcomes of Acute Neuromuscular Respiratory Failure." [In eng]. *Arch Neurol* 67, no. 9 (Sep 2010): 1089–94. https://doi.org/10.1001/archneurol.2010.207.

Cabrera Serrano, M., and A. A. Rabinstein. "Usefulness of Pulmonary Function Tests and Blood Gases in Acute Neuromuscular Respiratory Failure." [In eng]. *Eur J Neurol* 19, no. 3 (Mar 2012): 452–56. https://doi.org/10.1111/j.1468-1331.2011.03539.x.

Cheng, Y., K. Liu, C. Li, et al. "Risk Factors for Mechanical Ventilation in Patients With Guillain-Barré Syndrome." [In eng]. *Neurocrit Care* 37, no. 1 (Aug 2022): 121–28. https://doi.org/10.1007/s12028-022-01457-8.

Gross, M., E. F. M. Wijdicks, M. Damian, and O. Summ, eds. *Clinical Neurorespiratory Medicine*. Cambridge University Press; 2025.

Hawkes MA, Wijdicks EFM. Improving Outcome in Severe Myasthenia Gravis and Guillain-Barré Syndrome [In eng]. *Semin Neurol*. 2024 Jun;44(3):263-270. doi: 10.1055/s-0044-1785509. Epub 2024 Apr 1.

Kramer, C. L., M. McCullough, and E. F. Wijdicks. "Teaching Video Neuroimages: How to Unmask Respiratory Strength Confounded by Facial Diplegia." [In eng]. *Neurology* 84, no. 8 (Feb 24 2015): e57–58. https://doi.org/10.1212/wnl.0000000000001296.

Lawn, N. D., D. D. Fletcher, R. D. Henderson, et al. "Anticipating Mechanical Ventilation in Guillain-Barré Syndrome." [In eng]. *Arch Neurol* 58, no. 6 (Jun 2001): 893–98. https://doi.org/10.1001/archneur.58.6.893.

McKenzie, E.D., Kromm, J.A., Mobach, T., Solverson, K., Waite, J., Rabinstein, A. A. "Risk Stratification and Management of Acute Respiratory Failure in Patients With Neuromuscular Disease." *Crit Care Med.* 2024 Nov 1;52(11):1781–1789. doi: 10.1097/CCM.0000000000006417. Epub 2024 Sep 19. PMID: 39297721.

Neumann, B., K. Angstwurm, P. Mergenthaler, et al. "Myasthenic Crisis Demanding Mechanical Ventilation: A Multicenter Analysis of 250 Cases." [In eng]. *Neurology* 94, no. 3 (Jan 21 2020): e299–313. https://doi.org/10.1212/wnl.0000000000008688.

Patel, N., K. Chong, and A. Baydur. "Methods and Applications in Respiratory Physiology: Respiratory Mechanics, Drive and Muscle Function in Neuromuscular and Chest Wall Disorders." [In eng]. *Front Physiol* 13 (2022): 838414. https://doi.org/10.3389/fphys.2022.838414.

Seneviratne, J., J. Mandrekar, E. F. Wijdicks, and A. A. Rabinstein. "Noninvasive Ventilation in Myasthenic Crisis." [In eng]. *Arch Neurol* 65, no. 1 (Jan 2008): 54–58. https://doi.org/10.1001/archneurol.2007.1.

Singh, T. D., and E. F. M. Wijdicks. "Neuromuscular Respiratory Failure." [In eng]. *Neurol Clin* 39, no. 2 (May 2021): 333–53. https://doi.org/10.1016/j.ncl.2021.01.010.

van Doorn, P. A., P. Y. K. Van den Bergh, R. D. M. Hadden, et al. "European Academy of Neurology/Peripheral Nerve Society Guideline on Diagnosis and Treatment of Guillain-Barré Syndrome." [In eng]. *J Peripher Nerv Syst* 28, no. 4 (Dec 2023): 535–63. doi:10.1111/jns.12594.

Walgaard, C., H. F. Lingsma, L. Ruts, et al. "Prediction of Respiratory Insufficiency in Guillain-Barré Syndrome." [In eng]. *Ann Neurol* 67, no. 6 (Jun 2010): 781–87. https://doi.org/10.1002/ana.21976.

Wijdicks, E. F. M. "The Neurology of Acutely Failing Respiratory Mechanics." [In eng]. *Ann Neurol* 81, no. 4 (Apr 2017): 485–94. https://doi.org/10.1002/ana.24908.

10 Life-Threatening Complications of Intravenous Thrombolysis

An 82-year-old woman with a history of hypertension was brought to the emergency department 45 minutes after acute onset of dysarthria and left hemiparesis. Her home medications included lisinopril, metoprolol, and hydrochlorothiazide. We examined her in the emergency department and found that her National Institutes of Health Stroke Scale (NIHSS) score was 7, with deficits consisting of moderate weakness of the left lower facial muscles, dysarthria, and pyramidal-distribution weakness of the left upper extremity.

After no contraindications to thrombolysis were identified, she received intravenous (IV) recombinant tissue plasminogen activator (rt-PA) (0.9 mg/kg) and was admitted to the neuroscience intensive care unit. Upon arrival, her nurse notes that the patient has developed swelling of the lips and tongue, asymmetrically worse on the left, which seems to be worsening.

What do you do now?

Orolingual angioedema, if rapidly progressive, can cause severe upper airway obstruction, even to the point that the patient cannot be intubated. It is one of the causes of a "can't intubate, can't ventilate" situation, and a major complication of IV thrombolysis. Orolingual angioedema affects 1% to 5% of patients treated with IV rt-PA for stroke, but severe presentations are uncommon. The risk is increased in patients taking angiotensin-converting enzyme (ACE) inhibitors—as in our patient—because of higher baseline accumulation of bradykinin levels. Most fascinating is that the angioedema is commonly asymmetric with a more prominent appearance on the affected side (contralateral to supratentorial brain ischemia). This may be the result of infarction of the insular cortex with resultant autonomic dysfunction and vasomotor changes. The risk of angioedema is probably similar with rt-PA and tenecteplase.

We should all get a bit apprehensive when lip swelling appears soon after thrombolysis administration. Fortunately, in most cases, the angioedema is self-limited and not severe. However, because the clinical course is difficult to predict and the consequences can be dire, a short course of empiric medical therapy with antihistamines and corticosteroids is justified in most cases. When to intubate and when to wait is the next pressing question, but nobody really knows. It has been suggested that the anatomic location of edema may help to predict the risk of progression to the point of requiring endotracheal intubation. Thus, if the angioedema is limited exclusively to the anterior tongue and lips, intubation will not be required. Patients with edema affecting the larynx and hypopharynx are obviously at highest risk, while those with involvement of the palate and oropharynx are at intermediate risk. In any event, without being too particular, a skilled physician should perform early flexible fiberoptic airway inspection and intubation for symptomatic patients or those with edema extending beyond the lips.

Our patient was treated with 50 mg IV diphenhydramine and 10 mg IV dexamethasone, and the edema plateaued and gradually resolved. We were able to avoid intubation because the edema did not involve the oropharynx, but we remained at the bedside and felt uneasy about it all the way. In rapidly evolving cases some pharmacists have recommended a C1 esterase inhibitor (Berinert) at a dose of 20 units/kg, administered as an intravenous piggyback, which was rounded to a complete vial for a total dose of 2,500 units. Icatibant, a bradykinin B2 receptor antagonist, administered as a

30 mg subcutaneous dose is another valid alternative. These agents may produce more rapid resolution of angioedema.

A swollen tongue after IV thrombolysis can also be caused by another rare complication: a lingual hematoma. Traumatic injury to the lingual artery could be caused by a tongue bite, but that may suggest the patient had a seizure mimicking a stroke. This is a rare complication with only a few reported cases, but we have seen it. One case had severe hemorrhage from the lingual artery and was successfully treated with ligation of a branch of the left lingual artery.

Adrenal bleeding with hemodynamic collapse has also been linked to IV thrombolysis, but most reported cases were related to administration for myocardial infarction or massive pulmonary emboli and not ischemic stroke.

The more common complication of IV thrombolysis is intracranial hemorrhage (ICH). Most studies are in patients with ischemic stroke, but devastating ICH can occur in patients treated with rt-PA infusions for peripheral arterial occlusive disease in the management of acute limb ischemia. The risk is lower when IV thrombolysis is given for myocardial infarction, but it still exists.

Hemorrhage may occur in an infarcted brain and not necessarily become symptomatic. Most studies have concentrated on symptomatic intracranial hemorrhage (sICH). The definition of sICH has varied among different studies. In the 1995 National Institute of Neurological Disorders and Stroke (NINDS) trial, sICH, defined as ICH in the setting of any neurological decline, occurred in 6.4% of patients receiving rt-PA. In the European Cooperative Acute Stroke Study (ECASS-2) trial, sICH was defined as any radiological evidence of ICH associated with an increase in the NIHSS score of at least 4 points. In the registry Safe Implementation of Thrombolysis in Stroke-Monitoring Study (SITS-MOST), the radiological criterion was restricted to parenchymal hematomas. The ECASS-2 and SITS-MOST definitions have been shown to be the most clinically relevant as manifested by the repercussions of the sICH on functional disability at 3 months. Patients at highest risk for sICH are the elderly and those with severe neurological deficits (higher NIHSS score) and large areas of brain ischemia. Thus, patients at highest risk are individuals already facing a poor prognosis and high likelihood of disability if they would go without treatment. Other features that predict sICH are hyperglycemia, longer time to thrombolysis, higher systolic blood pressure at presentation, high NIHSS score, worse prestroke modified Rankin scale, and lower platelet count.

Most cases of sICH occur within the infarcted tissue and are caused by reperfusion injury. However, we have also seen sICH in the opposite hemisphere from where the stroke was located (Figure 10.1). Preexisting cerebral amyloid angiopathy may be the predisposing condition in many of these cases not related to reperfusion.

The 90-day mortality rate for patients with sICH after thrombolysis is high, ranging from 75% to 92%. In most cases, sICH happens early—either during the infusion or within hours after its completion. Neurological worsening and new severe headache with nausea and vomiting early after IV thrombolysis are symptoms very suggestive of this serious complication.

The decision to "reverse" the thrombolytic effect of the thrombolytic agent is not straightforward. Radiological factors to consider are the size and location of the hemorrhage, presence and severity of mass effect, and intraventricular hemorrhage. We have seen small regions of asymptomatic hemorrhage after the thrombolysis enlarges and becomes symptomatic in the absence of reversal (Figure 10.2).

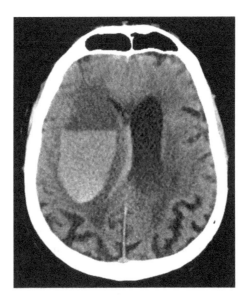

FIGURE 10.1 Large spontaneous hemorrhage in the opposite hemisphere several hours after IV tissue plasminogen activator administration in an 86-year-old patient with severe aphasia.

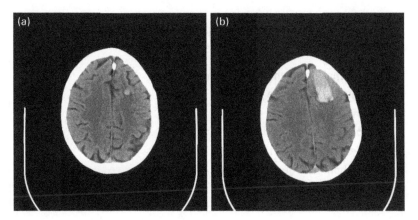

FIGURE 10.2 (A) Noncontrast CT scan shows a small asymptomatic intracranial hemorrhage in the left frontal lobe. (B) CT repeated 24 hours later shows interval enlargement of the left frontal lobe hemorrhage, which had become symptomatic.

There are no evidence-based or universally accepted treatment algorithms for these situations. It goes without saying to stop infusion of the thrombolytic immediately if a hemorrhage is suspected. Complete blood count, fibrinogen level, coagulation parameters, and blood type and screen should be obtained. We give 1 gram of tranexamic acid immediately, usually adding 10 U of cryoprecipitate; some clinicians only consider administering cryoprecipitate when the fibrinogen level is low (cryoprecipitate 0.15 U/kg if fibrinogen <150 or 200 mg/dL). Surgical evacuation of a hematoma is an option for large or threatening hemorrhages, considering the patient's overall medical condition and rehabilitation potential. The major and minor complications of IV thrombolysis are summarized in Box 10.1.

IV thrombolysis has changed the outcome of all types of ischemic strokes including those caused by large-vessel occlusions (Chapter 11). IV thrombolysis increases the odds of a good outcome by 11% to 13% in absolute terms and by 30% in relative terms even including patients with sICH. There are clear contraindications for its use that should be strictly respected. However, providing information about potential side effects to those who must give consent has only very rarely resulted in refusal of the drug. Lastly, some data suggest that the risk of sICH is lower with tenecteplase than with tissue plasminogen activator, and this possible safety advantage might further increase the use of tenecteplase for acute stroke reperfusion

> **BOX 10.1 Major and Minor Complications of IV Thrombolysis**
>
> **Major**
>
> Parenchymal intracranial hemorrhage
>
> Orolingual angioedema
>
> Anaphylactoid reaction
>
> Gastrointestinal hemorrhage
>
> Retroperitoneal hemorrhage
>
> Adrenal hemorrhage
>
> **Minor**
>
> Petechial hemorrhage in cerebral infarction
>
> Skin ecchymosis
>
> Bleeding at arterial and venous puncture sites[a]
>
> Hematuria
>
> ---
>
> [a] Arterial bleeding at a compressible site such as femoral or brachial artery. May become serious requiring a vascular surgeon.

in the future. Tenecteplase has higher rates of excellent functional outcome when compared with TPA and it is certainly superior for patients presenting with large vessel occlusion.

KEY POINTS TO REMEMBER

- A swollen tongue after IV thrombolysis may obstruct the airway rapidly due to orolingual angioedema or, less commonly, a lingual hematoma.
- Patients taking ACE inhibitors and patients with insular cortex infarction may be at higher risk of angioedema after IV thrombolysis.
- If angioedema is emerging, empiric treatment with IV corticosteroids and antihistamines should be started and the airway should be closely monitored. Rapid administration of icatibant or C1 esterase inhibitor may be very useful.
- Suspect acute hemorrhage in any patient who is receiving or has received IV thrombolysis when there is sudden headache or rapid neurological worsening.

- Stop the infusion of IV thrombolytic immediately when a hemorrhage is suspected; get a computed tomography scan; and if hemorrhage is confirmed and symptomatic, administer an antifibrinolytic drug and consider cryoprecipitate.

Further Reading

Asuzu, D., K. Nyström, H. Amin, et al. "Turn: A Simple Predictor of Symptomatic Intracerebral Hemorrhage After IV Thrombolysis." [In eng]. *Neurocrit Care* 23, no. 2 (Oct 2015): 166–71. https://doi.org/10.1007/s12028-015-0131-z.

Engelter, S. T., F. Fluri, C. Buitrago-Téllez, et al. "Life-Threatening Orolingual Angioedema During Thrombolysis in Acute Ischemic Stroke." [In eng]. *J Neurol* 252, no. 10 (Oct 2005): 1167–70. https://doi.org/10.1007/s00415-005-0789-9.

Fröhlich, K., K. Macha, S. T. Gerner, et al. "Angioedema in Stroke Patients with Thrombolysis." *Stroke* 50, no. 7 (2019): 1682–87. https://doi.org/doi:10.1161/STROKEAHA.119.025260. https://www.ahajournals.org/doi/abs/10.1161/STROKEAHA.119.025260.

Fugate, J. E., E. A. Kalimullah, and E. F. Wijdicks. "Angioedema After tPA: What Neurointensivists Should Know." [In eng]. *Neurocrit Care* 16, no. 3 (Jun 2012): 440–43. https://doi.org/10.1007/s12028-012-9678-0.

Hill, M. D., T. Lye, H. Moss, et al. "Hemi-Orolingual Angioedema and ACE Inhibition After Alteplase Treatment of Stroke." [In eng]. *Neurology* 60, no. 9 (May 13 2003): 1525–27. https://doi.org/10.1212/01.wnl.0000058840.66596.1a.

Huang J, Zheng H, Zhu X, Zhang K, Ping X. Tenecteplase versus alteplase for the treatment of acute ischemic stroke: a meta-analysis of randomized controlled trials [In eng]. *Ann Med.* 2024 Dec;56(1):2320285. doi: 10.1080/07853890.2024.2320285. Epub 2024 Mar 5.

Palaiodimou L, Katsanos AH, Turc G, Asimakopoulos AG, Mavridis D, Schellinger PD, Theodorou A, Lemmens R, Sacco S, Safouris A, Katan M, Sarraj A, Fischer U, Tsivgoulis G. Tenecteplase vs Alteplase in Acute Ischemic Stroke Within 4.5 Hours: A Systematic Review and Meta-Analysis of Randomized Trials. *Neurology.* 2024 Nov 12;103(9):e209903. doi: 10.1212/WNL.0000000000209903. Epub 2024 Oct 16.

Pitts, J. K., D. M. Burns, and K. R. Patellos. "Tenecteplase-associated Orolingual Angioedema: A Case Report and Literature Review." [In eng]. *Am J Health Syst Pharm* 81, no. 9 (Apr 19 2024): e220–e225.

Powers, W. J., A. A. Rabinstein, T. Ackerson, et al. "Guidelines for the Early Management of Patients With Acute Ischemic Stroke: 2019 Update to the 2018 Guidelines for the Early Management of Acute Ischemic Stroke: A Guideline for Healthcare Professionals From the American Heart Association/American Stroke Association." [In eng]. *Stroke* 50, no. 12 (): e344–418. https://doi.org/10.1161/str.0000000000000211.

Rao, N. M., S. R. Levine, J. A. Gornbein, and J. L. Saver. "Defining Clinically Relevant Cerebral Hemorrhage After Thrombolytic Therapy for Stroke: Analysis of the National Institute of Neurological Disorders and Stroke Tissue-Type Plasminogen Activator Trials." [In eng]. *Stroke* 45, no. 9 (Sep 2014): 2728–33. https://doi.org/10.1161/strokeaha.114.005135.

Seet, R. C., and A. A. Rabinstein. "Symptomatic Intracranial Hemorrhage Following Intravenous Thrombolysis for Acute Ischemic Stroke: A Critical Review of Case Definitions." [In eng]. *Cerebrovasc Dis* 34, no. 2 (2012): 106–14. https://doi.org/10.1159/000339675.

Warach, S. J., A. Ranta, J. Kim, et al. "Symptomatic Intracranial Hemorrhage With Tenecteplase vs Alteplase in Patients With Acute Ischemic Stroke: The Comparative Effectiveness of Routine Tenecteplase vs Alteplase in Acute Ischemic Stroke (Certain) Collaboration." [In eng]. *JAMA Neurol* 80, no. 7 (Jul 1 2023): 732–38. https://doi.org/10.1001/jamaneurol.2023.1449.

Wrenn, K. "Tissue Plasminogen Activator-Associated Lingual Artery Hemorrhage." [In eng]. *Ann Emerg Med* 19, no. 10 (Oct 1990): 1184–86. https://doi.org/10.1016/s0196-0644(05)81526-4.

11 When to Retrieve a Clot in Acute Stroke

A 62-year-old man with a history of hypertension, diabetes mellitus type 2, and atrial fibrillation presents to the emergency department after a sudden onset of speech difficulties and right-sided weakness. Neurological examination demonstrates global aphasia, left gaze preference, right hemianopia, right hemiplegia, and profound sensory loss (National Institutes of Health Stroke Scale score of 23). He is vomiting and intubated for airway protection. Computed tomography (CT) scan shows no acute parenchymal abnormalities (Alberta Stroke Program Early CT score [ASPECTS] 10), but there is a hyperdensity at the top of the left intracranial internal carotid artery (ICA) (Figure 11.1). A CT angiogram confirms the presence of an occluding clot in the left supraclinoid ICA and middle cerebral artery (MCA) with good collateral flow distant to the occlusion (Figure 11.2). He is treated with 0.25 mg/kg of intravenous (IV) tenecteplase 72 minutes after symptom onset.

What do you do now?

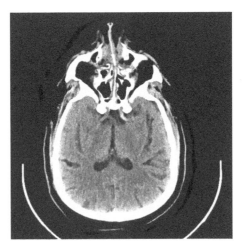

FIGURE 11.1 CT scan without contrast with no evidence of early ischemic changes but showing a hyperdense left ICA sign.

Mechanical thrombectomy for recanalization and reperfusion of large cerebral artery occlusions causing disabling strokes is one of the most effective emergency treatments available in medicine. Multiple randomized controlled trials have conclusively demonstrated that

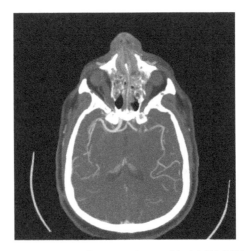

FIGURE 11.2 CT angiogram showing a flow gap at the top of the left ICA /MCA consistent with an occluding thrombus. Note good flow through collateral vessels distal to the site of occlusion.

endovascular reestablishment of flow improves the outcome of acute stroke patients with large intracranial vessel occlusions in carefully selected candidates with a timely intervention. The benefit is substantial: endovascular intervention in selected patients increases the relative proportion of patients regaining functional independence by 60% to 80% compared to those treated with IV thrombolysis alone. Between 40% and 70% of patients in these trials who were treated with endovascular intervention achieved functional independence at 90 days, and one more patient will regain independent function for every three to seven patients treated. These remarkably positive results are now possible because of the high rates of recanalization that can be achieved by using retrievable stents or direct aspiration catheters. These devices enable reopening of the occluded vessel (i.e., recanalization) in over 80% of cases. Rates of near-complete reperfusion are similarly high. Reperfusion is usually classified using the modified Thrombolysis in Cerebral Infarction (mTICI) score, which measures the extent of capillary blush around the previously occluded large vessel—a score of 3 meaning filling of the entire territory, and 2b signifying filling of more than 50% of the territory. However, other conditions are necessary for favorable outcomes to occur (Boxes 11.1 and 11.2).

First, patients must have good functional reserve to "bounce back" from the stroke (good brain resilience). The great majority of patients treated with embolectomy will have residual deficits and will need comprehensive neurorehabilitation. Frail, cognitively impaired patients as well as those of advanced age or with extensive medical comorbidities most often do not recover well from the stroke even if the intervention is successful. However, age is a less

---

BOX 11.1 Conditions to Be Met by Candidates for Endovascular Recanalization Therapy for Acute Ischemic Stroke

Disabling neurological deficits

Large intracranial vessel occlusion

Absence of large territorial established infarction (more than 12–24 hours after last known normal)

Good prestroke level of function

Good rehabilitation potential

> **BOX 11.2 Worse Prognosis After Acute Endovascular Stroke Therapy**
>
> Lack of recanalization or persistent distal occlusion with poor reperfusion
>
> Major initial stroke severity
>
> Large area of diffusion restriction and FLAIR changes on MRI or black hypodensity on CT.
>
> Absence of large radiological penumbra before the intervention
>
> Poor collateral arterial supply
>
> Internal carotid artery occlusion
>
> Postprocedural intracranial hemorrhage
>
> *Older age*
>
> *Major comorbidities*
>
> *Atrial fibrillation*
>
> *Admission hyperglycemia*
>
> Probable associations are in italics.

defining factor: octogenarians in good functional condition can recover well after successful thrombectomy, and we have even treated some nonagenarians with good prestroke function. Second, the intervention must be timely. Reperfusion should be achieved as rapidly as possible (optimally within 6 hours from symptom onset), and it is ideal for the time between noncontrast CT and groin puncture not to exceed 60 minutes. Third, the benefit has only been proven thus far for proximal vessel occlusions; these include middle cerebral artery (MCA) occlusions in the M1 and proximal M2 segments, supraclinoid ICA occlusions, and vertebrobasilar occlusions. Fourth, the patient should not have a large, established infarction before the intervention. Yet, that means not seeing a large hypodense (black) area on the head CT or hyperintensity on fluid-attenuated inversion recovery (FLAIR) magnetic resonance imaging (MRI). More recent clinical trials have shown that even patients with a large core defined by early ischemic changes (i.e., low ASPECTS scores) can benefit from successful thrombectomy. We are also seeing severe reperfusion injury (massive edema or hemorrhage) with immediate worse outcomes. We have not clearly defined which patient with a large infarction remains eligible and the decision is made after an explanation to the family.

The best imaging selection for mechanical thrombectomy remains controversial. Options to determine the core include careful review of the noncontrast CT scan for early signs of ischemia (trials consistently relied on the use of the ASPECTS score to standardize these assessments), evaluation of the CT angiogram for grading of the collateral flow, use of CT perfusion scans (the core defined by critically reduced cerebral blood flow or reduced cerebral blood volume), and performance of an MRI with diffusion-weighted imaging (DWI). CT perfusion and especially MRI with DWI are more reliable methods to visualize the core. CT perfusion and the addition of perfusion-weighted imaging to the MRI protocol can also provide convincing information on the amount of tissue at risk (ischemic penumbra). Using CT perfusion may identify patients more likely to benefit, but it rarely changes the decision whether to proceed with thrombectomy in most instances, especially within the first 6 hours from stroke onset. The concern that CT perfusion may overestimate the size of the core and minimize the potential benefit of recanalization to some patients is shared by more than a few stroke clinicians, including us. Furthermore, trial results supporting the value of mechanical thrombectomy for patients with large cores further question the utility of CT perfusion. Core evaluation by DWI is more accurate but much less practical.

In our practice, we adjust the imaging selection to the individual situation. When a patient presents early and has a CT scan with normal parenchyma and a hyperdense MCA or ICA sign, we proceed directly to embolectomy without any additional imaging. In all other patients with disabling deficits, we obtain a CT angiogram to confirm the site of the occlusion and evaluate the collateral circulation. We still add CT perfusion to our initial imaging assessment in patients who present beyond the 6-hour window with ischemic changes on CT and suboptimal or poor collaterals on CT angiogram. We also use information from CT perfusion to estimate the volumes of ischemic core and penumbra in suboptimal candidates who are unlikely to recover if they have a sizable stroke despite the intervention. In other words, we try to figure out if saving the penumbra will result in meaningful improvement (see Chapter 12.)

The majority of the patients enrolled in recent endovascular trials received IV recombinant tissue plasminogen activator (rt-PA) before enrollment. Although few patients had recanalized with rt-PA when catheter angiography was done, the thrombolytic drug may improve the chances of endovascular recanalization or the degree of reperfusion after recanalization. Furthermore, in multiple trials, direct thrombectomy has failed to meet the criterion of noninferiority when compared with the standard of combined therapy (IV thrombolysis bridging to mechanical thrombectomy). Also, tenecteplase achieved higher rates of recanalization than rt-PA in patients with proximal arterial occlusions. Thus, we gave IV tenecteplase as quickly as possible and then move to endovascular intervention without delay (i.e., not waiting to see if the patient gets better, but rather assuming that recanalization will not occur and that the patient will need embolectomy).

The risks of symptomatic intracranial hemorrhage and other manifestations of reperfusion injury (such as accelerated brain edema) have been conspicuously low (6% or less) in all the trials of mechanical thrombectomy, even when performed between 6 and 24 hours from the last known normal and including patients with early hypodensitty on CT. That said, parenchymal hematomas were quite frequent (more than 30% of cases) after thrombecomy in the trials enrolling patients with large ischemic core and the low rate of symptomatic intracranial hemorrhage in these trials may be in part explained by a ceiling effect of the NIHSS (score could not go much higher when already high at onset).

The indications for mechanical thrombectomy have expanded over the last few years to include extended time window, basilar occlusion, and large cores. We do not know whether patients with mild deficits despite large-vessel occlusion and those with disabling deficits from occlusions of middle-size arteries will benefit from the intervention. These situations represent the most difficult decisions in our daily practice.

At present it is uncertain if there is any advantage between doing the procedure under general anesthesia, conscious sedation, or just local anesthesia. Local preferences define practice in this regard. In our neuroradiology suite we only use local anesthesia when at all possible. The management of blood pressure after successful reperfusion is a topic of active research. At present, trials evaluating more aggressive treatment of hypertension have not shown any benefit, and this strategy may actually be harmful. Greater blood pressure variability correlates with worse outcomes after acute stroke reperfusion. Therefore, our current practice is not to lower the blood pressure after successful endovascular reperfusion unless the systolic is above 180 mmHg.

Our patient was an ideal candidate for endovascular reperfusion therapy. He had severe deficits from a large intracranial vessel occlusion that was unlikely to recanalize with IV tenecteplase alone; we could treat him early; and he had good potential for recovery because of excellent prestroke function, younger age, absence of early ischemic changes on the CT scan, and good collateral circulation on CT angiogram. After obtaining consent from the family, the patient was emergently taken to the angiography suite, where he underwent successful treatment with a retrievable stent (Figure 11.3). Full recanalization and reperfusion (TICI score 3) were achieved 2 hours after symptom onset.

The patient evolved very favorably. Within hours in the neuroICU he was starting to communicate and could lift his right arm. At 24 hours, his neurological deficits were minimal. His follow-up CT scan at 24 hours also showed a small area of hypodensity in the left basal ganglia (Figure 11.4). He was discharged from the hospital with a normal neurological examination. While such a dramatic improvement with complete recovery is not always achieved, good functional recovery with mild residual symptoms is now more common and represents another example of a very favorable outcome for a patient who presented with a severely disabling stroke.

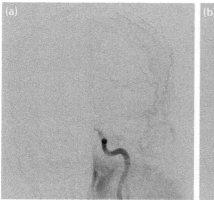 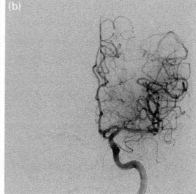

FIGURE 11.3 (A) Digital subtraction angiogram (left carotid injection) confirming occlusion of the supraclinoid left ICA. (B) Full recanalization and reperfusion (TICI 3) after treatment with a stent retriever.

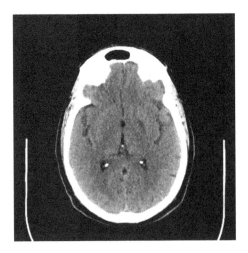

FIGURE 11.4 Follow-up CT scan 24 hours after stroke onset showing only a small hypodensity in the left basal ganglia.

But considering everything, no more than 15% to 20% of patients with acute stroke may be currently eligible for endovascular treatment. These are the patients with the most severe and potentially disabling strokes. Endovascular intervention in selected patients with proximal cerebral occlusions can make the difference between permanent incapacity (and death from swelling) and a return to active life. Thus, no efforts should be spared to provide this opportunity to patients with severe stroke. Seeing a patient moving a previously paralyzed arm or recovering the ability to speak after reperfusion is rewarding. We have seen this degree of dramatic improvement hours later in the neurosciences ICU many times. We are still astonished to see major stroke syndromes (25 for NIHSS aficionados) vanish on the neuroendovascular table. Few treatments in medicine offer such formidable benefit.

KEY POINTS TO REMEMBER

- Embolectomy (in combination with IV thrombolysis) is very effective for patients with severe stroke from large intracranial vessel occlusion.

- Rapid and complete reperfusion is the main determinant of a favorable outcome.
- Indications for mechanical thrombectomy continue to expand, but we still have difficulty to decide if thrombectomy should be pursued in patients with large-vessel occlusion but mild deficits and patients with disabling deficits from middle-size-vessel occlusions.
- The optimal radiological method for embolectomy selection of candidates has not been defined.
- Endovascular reperfusion should not be offered to the wrong patient: if a patient was doing poorly before a large stroke, we cannot anticipate a benefit even if successful reperfusion is achieved.

Further Reading

Alberts, M. J., T. Shang, and A. Magadan. "Endovascular Therapy for Acute Ischemic Stroke: Dawn of a New Era." *JAMA Neurol* 72 (2015): 1101–3. https://doi.org/10.1001/jamaneurol.2015.1743.

Campbell, B. C. V., G. A. Donnan, K. R. Lees, et al. "Endovascular Stent Thrombectomy: The New Standard of Care for Large Vessel Ischaemic Stroke." [In eng]. *Lancet Neurol* 14, no. 8 (Aug 2015): 846–54. https://doi.org/10.1016/s1474-4422(15)00140-4.

Chen, H., J. S. Lee, P. Michel, B. Yan, and S. Chaturvedi. "Endovascular Stroke Thrombectomy for Patients With Large Ischemic Core: A Review." [In eng]. *JAMA Neurol* (Aug 12 2024). doi:10.1001/jamaneurol.2024.2500. Epub ahead of print. PMID: 39133467.

Ghozy, S., A. Mortezaei, M. Elfil, et al. "Intensive vs Conventional Blood Pressure Control After Thrombectomy in Acute Ischemic Stroke: A Systematic Review and Meta-Analysis." [In eng]. *JAMA Netw Open* 7, no. 2 (Feb 5 2024): e240179. doi:10.1001/jamanetworkopen.2024.0179. PMID: 38386320; PMCID: PMC10884884.

Goyal, M., B. K. Menon, W. H. van Zwam, et al. "Endovascular Thrombectomy After Large-Vessel Ischaemic Stroke: A Meta-Analysis of Individual Patient Data From Five Randomised Trials." [In eng]. *Lancet* 387, no. 10029 (Apr 23 2016): 1723–31. https://doi.org/10.1016/s0140-6736(16)00163-x.

Jadhav, A. P., S. M. Desai, and T. G. Jovin. "Indications for Mechanical Thrombectomy for Acute Ischemic Stroke: Current Guidelines and Beyond." [In eng]. *Neurology* 97, no. 20 Suppl 2 (Nov 16 2021): S126–36. https://doi.org/10.1212/wnl.0000000000012801.

Jovin, T. G., R. G. Nogueira, M. G. Lansberg, et al. "Thrombectomy for Anterior Circulation Stroke Beyond 6 H From Time Last Known Well (Aurora): A Systematic Review and Individual Patient Data Meta-Analysis." [In eng]. *Lancet* 399, no. 10321 (Jan 15 2022): 249–58. https://doi.org/10.1016/s0140-6736(21)01341-6.

Kobeissi, H., G. Adusumilli, S. Ghozy, et al. "Endovascular Thrombectomy for Ischemic Stroke With Large Core Volume: An Updated, Post-Tesla Systematic Review and Meta-Analysis of the Randomized Trials." [In eng]. *Interv Neuroradiol* (Jun 28 2023): 15910199231185738. doi:10.1177/15910199231185738. Epub ahead of print. PMID: 37376869.

McDonough, R. V., J. M. Ospel, B. C. V. Campbell, et al. "Functional Outcomes of Patients ≥85 Years With Acute Ischemic Stroke Following EVT: A Hermes Substudy." [In eng]. *Stroke* 53, no. 7 (Jul 2022): 2220–26. https://doi.org/10.1161/strokeaha.121.037770.

Powers, W. J., A. A. Rabinstein, T. Ackerson, et al. "Guidelines for the Early Management of Patients With Acute Ischemic Stroke: 2019 Update to the 2018 Guidelines for the Early Management of Acute Ischemic Stroke: A Guideline for Healthcare Professionals From the American Heart Association/American Stroke Association." *Stroke* 50, no. 12 (2019): e344–418. https://www.ahajournals.org/doi/abs/10.1161/STR.0000000000000211.

Ravipati, S., A. Amjad, K. Zulfiqar, et al. "Endovascular Thrombectomy for Acute Ischemic Stroke with a Large Infarct Area: An Updated Systematic Review and Meta-Analysis of Randomized Controlled Trials." [In eng]. *J Stroke Cerebrovasc Dis* 33, no. 8 (Aug 2024): 107818. doi:10.1016/j.jstrokecerebrovasdis.2024.107818.

12 A "Wake-Up" Major Stroke

A 75-year-old man with history of multiple vascular risk factors (hypertension, hyperlipidemia, diabetes mellitus type 2, and obesity) woke up with inability to speak and right-sided weakness. He felt fine when he went to bed the night before, 7 hours earlier. In the emergency department, he was aphasic and had a right visual field deficit, right hemiparesis, and right hemisensory loss. His National Institutes of Health Stroke Scale (NIHSS) score was 16. Head computed tomography (CT) showed possible early ischemic changes in the left caudate, putamen, insula, and frontal lobe (Alberta Stroke Program Early CT score [ASPECTS] 6) (Figure 12.1). Head CT angiogram showed a proximal left middle cerebral branch (M2) occlusion with a fair number of collaterals.

What do you do now?

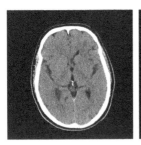 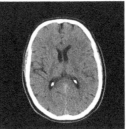 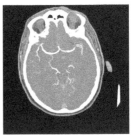

FIGURE 12.1 Left and middle image: CT of the brain shows early contour changes in the left caudate and putamen and left insular cortex and early hypodensity in the left frontal lobe. Right image: CT angiogram of the brain demonstrates occlusion of the proximal left anterior M2 branch of the middle cerebral artery (arrow).

By now we are all convinced that the outcome of major acute ischemic stroke has greatly improved with mechanical thrombectomy. Multiple randomized controlled trials unequivocally proved that clot retrieval and reperfusion potentially is a remarkably effective treatment for patients with anticipated disabling deficits caused by a proximal intracranial artery occlusion (commonly known as large-vessel occlusion [LVO]). Yet, all randomized controlled trials primarily included patients presenting early, and more specifically, within the first 6 hours after symptom onset. Patients with "wake-up strokes," for whom the "last known normal" time was often many hours before noticing a deficit, were excluded from those initial trials because of concern about excessive risk of reperfusion hemorrhage. Yet, many of these patients present with no established ischemic infarction on head CT.

The stroke community felt these patients were potentially missing out, certainly when the CT scan did not show a large area of established infarction and while the patient still had major symptoms. This suggested that the stroke may have awakened the patient or occurred close to awakening. Typically, CT scans need several hours to show changes even when a major cerebral artery is occluded.

Two randomized controlled trials specifically addressed whether mechanical thrombectomy could also be effective in patients with disabling deficits from LVO presenting hours from absent neurologic symptoms. Patients enrolled in these trials often had wake-up strokes, but not exclusively, because a delay in seeking help may occur even with significant symptoms.

Some patients cannot alert someone else that they are in trouble, and this commonly occurs with nondominant right-sided hemispheric stroke, when the patient is unaware of left hemibody neglect. Similarly when there is severe aphasia. The DAWN trial used a clinical-radiological mismatch criterion for enrollment (i.e., severe deficits with smaller-than-predicted infarct volume on diffusion-weighted magnetic resonance imaging [MRI] or CT perfusion) and included patients up to 24 hours from the time they were without symptoms. The Endovascular Therapy Following Imaging Evaluation for Ischemic Stroke (DEFUSE-3) trial relied exclusively on radiological criteria to determine eligibility (i.e., mismatch between infarct core and potentially salvageable ischemic penumbra by CT perfusion or magnetic resonance perfusion) and enrolled patients up to 16 hours from time of last known normal. Both clinical trials showed that mechanical thrombectomy remarkably improved outcomes with minimal risk of hemorrhagic complications due to reperfusion. In these extended therapeutic window trials, nearly half of patients treated with mechanical thrombectomy were independent at 90 days (despite presenting with an overall high NIHSS score of 16–17). The number necessary to treat for one additional patient to achieve functional independence at 90 days was between three and four, which is remarkably good.

It is less clear whether mechanical thrombectomy is still beneficial in patients not meeting the criteria used for randomization in DAWN or DEFUSE-3. Yet, some evidence from observational studies indicates that patients without large infarctions on a head CT and with good collateral flow on CT angiogram may benefit from mechanical thrombectomy even if not selected by automated perfusion imaging. Therefore, we do not think that CT perfusion or magnetic resonance diffusion/perfusion is absolutely needed prior to proceeding with endovascular therapy in patients with severe wake-up strokes from an LVO. The decision to press ahead with an urgent cerebral angiogram by a neurointerventional team could potentially be made on a patient with markedly disabling deficits, a plain CT showing no major stroke, and a CT angiogram displaying a large-vessel occlusion and good collaterals.

Recent trials have shown benefit from thrombectomy in patients with large ischemic core (ASPECTS < 6 or large cores [generally > 70 mL] on CTP or DWI) and presenting up to 24 hours from last known well and this included "wake-up" strokes. However, most of the patients enrolled in these clinical trials had stroke symptoms less than 12 hours from "last known normal" and stroke during waking up from sleep represented was seen in a minority of cases.

It is different with intravenous thrombolysis. Its benefit for patients with a wake-up stroke (and other patients presenting beyond 4.5 hours after last known well) is much more limited. Some clinical trials can guide us. The Efficacy and Safety of MRI-Based Thrombolysis in Wake-Up Stroke (WAKE-UP) trial showed that intravenous alteplase may be modestly beneficial in patients with mild to moderate strokes who have MRI diffusion-weighted imaging (DWI)–fluid-attenuated inversion recovery (FLAIR) mismatch (i.e., abnormal signal seen on DWI but not on FLAIR, also suggesting salvageable brain tissue) and can be treated within 4.5 hours from when the symptoms were first noted. This trial was designed to identify patients with wake-up stroke who could have had relatively recent stroke onset (indicated by the DWI-FLAIR mismatch). Although we can never know for sure, there is a collective understanding that some patients (perhaps more than we think) may wake up soon after stroke rather than sleep through the night with a major deficit. Another trial Tenecteplase in wake-up ischemic stroke (TWIST) randomized patients presenting with wake-up stroke to receive intravenous Tenecteplase or placebo within 4.5 hours of awakening but using only noncontract head CT for patient selection. Tenecteplase was not associated with better functional outcomes at 90 days, though the risk of symptomatic intracranial hemorrhage was not significantly different between the two groups. Similarly, the Thrombolysis in Imaging Eligible, Late Window Patients to Assess the Efficacy and Safety of Tenecteplase (TIMELESS) trial compared Tenecteplase with placebo and between 4.5 and 24 hours from last known normal in patients with radiologically documented large vessel occlusion and ischemic penumbra. No benefit from thrombolysis on functional outcomes was found; the rate of symptomatic intracranial hemorrhage was higher with 3.2% in the thrombolysis group versus 2.3% in patients without thrombolysis (of note is that 77% of patients in this trial were also treated with mechanical thrombectomy). In patients with large vessel occlusion and salvageable tissue who cannot be treated with mechanical thrombectomy, the Tenecteplase Reperfusion Therapy in Acute Ischemic Cerebrovascular

Events–III (TRACE III) trial showed that Tenecteplase can be beneficial in the extended time window. There are other data suggesting benefit from intravenous thrombolysis between 4.5 and 9 hours of last known well using CT perfusion scans for patient selection regardless of whether a large vessel occlusion is present. This is an emerging therapeutic avenue but often with a population treated with multiple modalities making its interpretation difficult. At this point, we think that intravenous thrombolysis beyond the usual therapeutic window of 4.5 hours should only be considered for patients carefully selected by either MRI or CT perfusion.

Our patient had a head CT perfusion that demonstrated a core of 19 mL in the left frontal region with a much larger volume of ischemic penumbra extending throughout most of the rest of the left middle cerebral artery territory (Figure 12.2).

We took the patient to the neurointerventional suite and were able to achieve prompt recanalization with complete reperfusion (Figure 12.3) despite a sizable left frontal infarction on follow-up MRI (Figure 12.4). The patient experienced major functional recovery and had only mild deficits at 3 months.

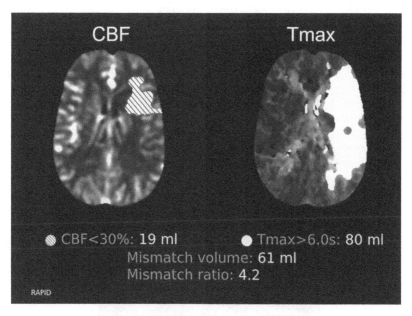

FIGURE 12.2 A black-and-white drawing of the CT perfusion results (note the mismatch in the white areas and calculations). CBF, cerebral blood flow; Tmax, time to maximum.

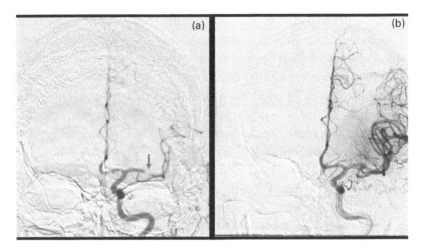

FIGURE 12.3 Catheter cerebral angiogram showing the initial occlusion of the dominant left M2 branch (A) with complete recanalization after mechanical thrombectomy (B).

The evidence from well executed trials and growing clinical experience is convincing. Once we see an LVO, we need to find credible arguments *not* to attempt recanalization. The default should be treating, if at all possible. Some guidance is provided in Figure 12.5.

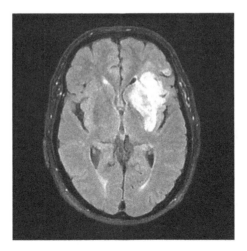

FIGURE 12.4 Brain MRI the following day shows the area of infarction.

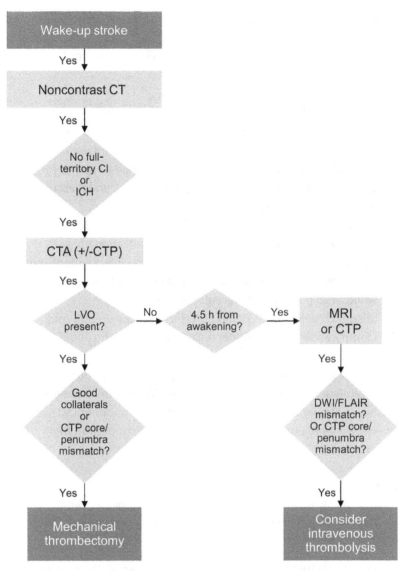

FIGURE 12.5 A proposed algorithm for the emergency evaluation and management of wake-up stroke. CI, cerebral infarct; CTA, computed tomography angiogram; CTP, computed tomography perfusion; DWI, diffusion-weighted imaging; FLAIR, fluid-attenuated inversion recovery; ICH, intracranial hemorrhage; LVO, large-vessel occlusion; MRI, magnetic resonance imaging.

We both remember the days before intravenous thrombolysis and mechanical thrombectomy. Ischemic stroke back then often resulted in living with a potential severe disability. Look where we are now!

KEY POINTS TO REMEMBER

- When the patient presents with a disabling wake-up stroke and the head CT does not show an established infarction, CT angiogram should be emergently obtained to search for a large cerebral vessel occlusion. When found, endovascular thrombectomy should follow.
- When a stroke is seen on plain CT, CT perfusion or MRI diffusion/perfusion could assist in better selection of candidates most likely to benefit from these interventions, but these advanced imaging modalities are not critical to decide whether to pursue endovascular therapy.
- Mismatch between DWI and FLAIR sequences on MRI may identify patients with milder wake-up strokes who could benefit from intravenous thrombolysis.
- Perfusion imaging may help identify patients without established infarction on noncontract CT who might benefit from intravenous thrombolysis beyond 4.5 hours of last known well, but there is no firm evidence supporting this practice.

Further Reading

Albers, G. W., M. Jumaa, B. Purdon, et al.; TIMELESS Investigators. "Tenecteplase for Stroke at 4.5 to 24 Hours with Perfusion-Imaging Selection." [In eng]. *N Engl J Med* 390, no. 8 (Feb 22 2024): 701–11.

Campbell, B. C. V., H. Ma, P. A. Ringleb, et al. "Extending Thrombolysis to 4·5-9 H and Wake-Up Stroke Using Perfusion Imaging: A Systematic Review and Meta-Analysis of Individual Patient Data." [In eng]. *Lancet* 394, no. 10193 (Jul 13 2019): 139–47. https://doi.org/10.1016/s0140-6736(19)31053-0.

Chen, H., J. S. Lee, P. Michel, B. Yan, and S. Chaturvedi. "Endovascular Stroke Thrombectomy for Patients With Large Ischemic Core: A Review." [In eng]. *JAMA Neurol* (Aug 12 2024). doi:10.1001/jamaneurol.2024.2500. Epub ahead of print. PMID: 39133467.

Dittrich, T. D., P. B. Sporns, L. F. Kriemler, et al. "Mechanical Thrombectomy Versus Best Medical Treatment in the Late Time Window in Non-Defuse-Non-Dawn Patients: A Multicenter Cohort Study." [In eng]. *Stroke* 54, no. 3 (Mar 2023): 722–30. https://doi.org/10.1161/strokeaha.122.039793.

Nogueira, R. G., A. P. Jadhav, D. C. Haussen, et al. "Thrombectomy 6 to 24 Hours After Stroke With a Mismatch Between Deficit and Infarct." [In eng]. *N Engl J Med* 378, no. 1 (Jan 4 2018): 11–21. https://doi.org/10.1056/NEJMoa1706442.

Roaldsen, M. B., A. Eltoft, T. Wilsgaard, et al. "Safety and Efficacy of Tenecteplase in Patients With Wake-Up Stroke Assessed by Non-Contrast CT (TWIST): A Multicentre, Open-Label, Randomised Controlled Trial." [In eng]. *Lancet Neurol* 22, no. 2 (Feb 2023): 117–26. https://doi.org/10.1016/s1474-4422(22)00484-7.

Thomalla, G., C. Z. Simonsen, F. Boutitie, et al. "MRI-Guided Thrombolysis for Stroke With Unknown Time of Onset." [In eng]. *N Engl J Med* 379, no. 7 (Aug 16 2018): 611–22. https://doi.org/10.1056/NEJMoa1804355.

Xiong, Y., B. C. V. Campbell, L. H. Schwamm, et al. "Tenecteplase for Ischemic Stroke at 4.5 to 24 Hours Without Thrombectomy." [In eng]. *N Engl J Med* 391, no. 3 (2024): 203–12.

13 Recognizing an Acute Embolus to the Basilar Artery

A 71-year-old male with a heavy smoking history and untreated hypertension was brought to the emergency department after vomiting and later being found collapsed on the ground. A bystander initiated cardiopulmonary resuscitation (CPR). Upon emergency medical service arrival, there was pulseless electrical activity arrest. He attained restoration of systemic circulation after three rounds of CPR and 1 mg intravenous (IV) epinephrine. He remained unresponsive and, upon arrival to the emergency department, had a blood pressure of 249/149 mmHg and heart rate of 114 beats per minute. His pupils were anisocoric (and questionably reactive), and corneal reflexes were absent. A spontaneous horizontal-rotary nystagmus was found. Cough to suctioning was present, and he had spontaneous extensor motor responses. Computed tomography (CT) of the head was read as "normal" but, upon further scrutiny, was concerning for a hyperdense basilar artery reflecting presence of an embolus (Figure 13.1). CT angiogram of the head and neck demonstrated a complete basilar artery occlusion at the vertebrobasilar junction (Figure 13.2A).

What do you do now?

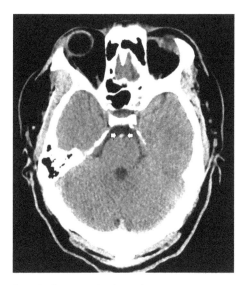

FIGURE 13.1 Hyperdense basilar artery sign (arrows).

The decision when an acute embolus has occluded the basilar artery primarily must be to take the patient to a radiology suite and have a neurointerventionalist retrieve the clot—no matter how much time has passed since the onset of symptoms. We have no choice. We really don't. We have known for years that without this intervention, the outcome in

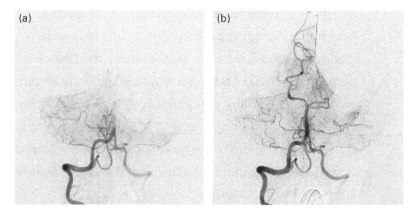

FIGURE 13.2 (A) Acute embolus situated at the junction of posterior cerebral arteries and thalamus perforators (top of the basilar). (B) Restoration of basilar artery flow after endovascular retrieval of the clot. Persistent right posterior cerebral artery occlusion.

> **BOX 13.1 Unfavorable Predictors in Patients with Basilar Artery Occlusion Treated With Endovascular Clot Retrieval**
>
> *Clinical predictors*
>
> Coma
>
> Fixed pupils and absent corneal reflex
>
> Oropharyngeal symptoms at onset
>
> Ictus to treatment >72 hours
>
> *Radiological predictors*
>
> Long clot trajectory
>
> Midbasilar and top of the basilar clot location
>
> Pretreatment MRI involvement of pons and thalami
>
> Pretreatment multiterritorial involvement on perfusion CT

acute basilar artery occlusion is miserably poor (up to 80% mortality and severe morbidity) and that all attempts at restoring flow must be considered. While poor predictors have been identified, they rarely stop anyone from proceeding (Box 13.1). Basically, this is one of the disorders for which the term "Hail Mary pass" entered medical argot.

Therefore, our patient emergently underwent mechanical embolectomy with successful recanalization of the basilar artery (Figure 13.2B). Unfortunately, there was persistent occlusion of the right posterior cerebral artery. Multiple attempts at recanalization were unsuccessful, and the patient was taken to the intensive care unit for further management. Magnetic resonance imaging (MRI) of the brain demonstrated extensive posterior circulation infarcts, mass effect with effacement of the basilar cisterns, and obstructive hydrocephalus (Figure 13.3). The family elected to pursue comfort measures after the patient failed to improve during the following days with persistent loss of upper brainstem reflexes strongly signifying poor prognosis.

Is this embarrassing confession time? With hindsight, we must ask whether this use of enormous resources was warranted. Could we not have recognized earlier that this perhaps was a futile attempt? To answer these questions, we need to review the clinical trajectory and manifestations of acute occlusion of the basilar artery.

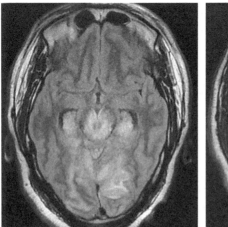 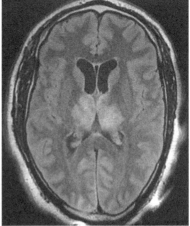

FIGURE 13.3 MRI hyperintensities in thalamus, brainstem, and occipital lobe.

We know that acute occlusions of the middle cerebral artery often suddenly present with a major deficit—but not always. Some patients improve only to worsen presumably when the collateral circulation fails. This pattern of fluctuation is far more common in occlusions of the vertebrobasilar artery and symptoms, and signs may appear and vanish. These signs are ataxia, diplopia, dysphagia, and dysarthria. Hemiparesis may come and go on either side, or both. Not being deceived by fluctuations and seemingly major improvement of clinical signs becomes important in decisions on endovascular treatment for acute stroke (Figure 13.4).

Any clot can break up spontaneously and lead to full resolution of deficits, but that is not too common. Therefore, there is an emerging consensus that it is better to retrieve the clot occluding a large vessel if the clinical features have been severe and are still disabling. Past experiences have taught us to anticipate later worsening. Moreover, complete return to normal is not common and, obviously, may be determined by the thoroughness of the examination particularly in posterior circulation disease (testing sitting upright, stance and gait, eye findings, and swallowing). Abnormal eye findings in acute basilar artery occlusion are often diagnostic. (We find none of these clinical symptoms graded in the National Institutes of Health Stroke Scale.) Some possibly seen neuro-ophthalmologic signs include (1) a lesion of the medial longitudinal fasciculus that produces an

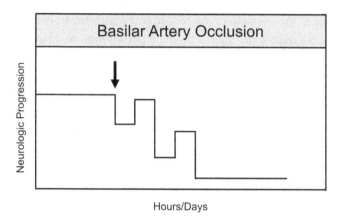

FIGURE 13.4 Possible clinical trajectory in acute basilar artery occlusion. Note the marked fluctuation, and even back to normal, before the next bout.

internuclear ophthalmoplegia consisting of abnormal ipsilateral adduction and more profound nystagmus in the abducting eye; (2) one-and-a-half syndrome, consisting of one immobile eye in the horizontal plane and preservation of abduction alone in the other eye; (3) ocular bobbing, a type of vertical nystagmus frequently found in patients with extensive pontine ischemia and recognizable by brisk conjugate, downward eye movement, followed by slow correction to baseline midposition; (4) bilateral ptosis due to involvement of the sympathetic fibers in the pontine tegmentum, or unilateral ptosis due to ischemia to the third-nerve nucleus; and (5) skew deviation, with eyes positioned out of their normal vertical axis. Pupils are abnormal and often anisocoric. Pinpoint pupils indicate a lesion in the pons and mid-size position pupils localize to the mesencephalon.

When hemiparesis occurs, the most affected side may alternate from left to right in the first hours. Hemiplegia falsely suggesting hemispheric involvement is present in 40% of patients seen early in the course of the disorder. Initial occlusion of the paramedian penetrating arteries may produce hemiparesis and horizontal gaze palsy in association with normal speech, swallowing, and level of consciousness (Foville syndrome). However, acute basilar artery occlusion may be presenting with acute coma with no obvious lateralization signs, and this presentation is a reason it is so often missed as a (treatable) stroke.

Top of the basilar artery syndrome is a constellation of signs and symptoms caused by an obstructing distal embolus. The strategic location of the clot at the juncture of the basilar artery with the posterior cerebral arteries and thalamic perforators produces, in addition to infarction in the mesencephalon, extensive areas of infarction in thalamic nuclei, medial temporal lobes, and occipital lobes unless prompt reperfusion occurs. At presentation, patients have an impaired, fluctuating level of consciousness from ischemia to the bilateral paramedian rostral brainstem or thalamic nuclei. In contrast to clot occlusion in the anterior circulation, an embolus to the basilar artery may propagate, grow, and knock out perforators one by one.

Many neurointensivists, who have repeatedly observed quite dramatic improvement in a substantial number of patients, were disappointed with the initial results of the randomized trial Endovascular Treatment versus Standard Medical Treatment for Vertebrobasilar Artery Occlusion (BEST) but continued to offer endovascular clot retrieval. Two randomized trials ((Endovascular Treatment for Acute Basilar Artery Occlusion (ATTENTION) and Basilar Artery Occlusion Chinese Endovascular Trial (BAOCHE) found a clear benefit of endovascular therapy over best medical care alone with reduction of poor outcome (a modified Rankin scale score of 4–6) by 23% and 22% among patients presenting with severe deficits that was sustained at the one-year mark. Others found that basilar artery occlusion without vertebral artery stenosis or occlusion (tandem lesion) correlated with shorter procedural time, higher rates of successful recanalization (85%), and a more favorable clinical outcome. Good outcome can be expected in patients with a slowly progressive clinical course, limited neurologic deficits, short segmental abnormalities, and good collateral flow on cerebral angiography. Thus, endovascular clot retrieval offers the potential for major improvement. When patients present within 4.5 hours of last known well, IV thrombolysis should also be administered.

Some investigators have tried to develop better selection criteria for patients with basilar artery occlusion. The European guidelines can be consulted, but the level of evidence for many recommendations is categorized as "very low". For example, increased clot length (threshold undefined) independently predicts unfavorable clinical outcome, and most patients with complete or partial recanalization have clots less than 10 mm in length. The odds of unsuccessful recanalization supposedly increase 1.06 for each additional 1 mm of thrombus length. In considering perfusion imaging prior to intervention, one study quantified hypoperfusion using a new score named the critical area perfusion score (CAPS). It quantifies severe hypoperfusion (T_{max} >10) in the cerebellum (1 point per hemisphere), pons (2 points), and midbrain and/or thalamus (2 points). When patients were divided into favorable (CAPS ≤3) and unfavorable (CAPS >3) groups, cerebral perfusion imaging identified patients highly likely to benefit from reperfusion after endovascular treatment. Patients with a CAPS less than or equal to 3 had very favorable outcomes following successful endovascular treatment, unlike patients with CAPS greater than 3, who did poorly regardless of whether treatment achieved reperfusion. Yet, we rarely use CT perfusion for decision-making and we would still proceed despite abnormalities on CT scan unless there are bilateral swollen cerebellar and thalamic infarcts with loss of many brainstem reflexes.

Finally, albeit not too specific, a hyperdense basilar artery sign on noncontrast head CT is an often-overlooked, critical sign that requires vascular studies. In patients presenting with posterior circulation and stroke-like symptoms, this sign predicts basilar artery thrombosis.

The diagnosis of basilar artery occlusion is not easy and requires a focused approach that differs from other stroke presentations. This type of stroke is also very uncommon (<1% of all strokes) and, thus, remains unrecognized in certain patients until it is too late. Aphasia is a sensitive marker for large-vessel occlusion in the anterior circulation. Markers for occlusion in the basilar artery are much different and include (1) acute coma and extensor posturing with wide and narrow pupil combination, (2) hemiplegia followed by contralateral side hemiplegia and bulbar signs, and (3) locked-in syndrome. Remember that patients presenting with these symptoms initially have a normal CT scan, and immediately proceeding with a vascular study such as a CT angiogram should localize the occlusion in the basilar artery. So, the answer to the question whether we were too aggressive is a resounding no! There is no way we can reliably predict outcome before endovascular treatment. We can reliably predict outcome if we do not intervene—it is poor.

KEY POINTS TO REMEMBER

- In patients presenting with posterior-circulation, stroke-like symptoms, a hyperdense basilar-artery sign on noncontrast head CT predicts basilar artery thrombosis.
- Anisocoria, nystagmus, and loss of brainstem reflexes in an acutely comatose patient must lead to consideration of a basilar artery occlusion.
- Because outcomes are so poor without recanalization, acute reperfusion therapy should be attempted whenever possible.
- Severe brainstem involvement after recanalization determines outcome.
- Outcome can be predicted by the extent of CT perfusion abnormalities but more definitively by MRI.

Further Reading

Alemseged, F., T. N. Nguyen, S. B. Coutts, et al. "Endovascular Thrombectomy for Basilar Artery Occlusion: Translating Research Findings Into Clinical Practice." [In eng]. *Lancet Neurol* 22, no. 4 (Apr 2023): 330–37. https://doi.org/10.1016/s1474-4422(22)00483-5.

Baik, S. H., H. J. Park, J. H. Kim, et al. "Mechanical Thrombectomy in Subtypes of Basilar Artery Occlusion: Relationship to Recanalization Rate and Clinical Outcome." [In eng]. *Radiology* 291, no. 3 (Jun 2019): 730–37. https://doi.org/10.1148/radiol.2019181924.

Cereda, C. W., G. Bianco, M. Mlynash, et al. "Perfusion Imaging Predicts Favorable Outcomes After Basilar Artery Thrombectomy." [In eng]. *Ann Neurol* 91, no. 1 (Jan 2022): 23–32. https://doi.org/10.1002/ana.26272.

Hankey, G. J. "Endovascular Therapy for Acute Basilar Artery Occlusion." [In eng]. *Circulation* 146, no. 1 (Jul 5 2022): 18–20. https://doi.org/10.1161/circulation aha.122.060571.

Hawkes, M. A., E. Blaginykh, M. W. Ruff, et al. "Long-Term Mortality, Disability and Stroke Recurrence in Patients With Basilar Artery Occlusion." [In eng]. *Eur J Neurol* 27, no. 3 (Mar 2020): 579–85. https://doi.org/10.1111/ene.14126.

Jovin, T. G., C. Li, L. Wu, et al. "Trial of Thrombectomy 6 to 24 Hours After Stroke Due to Basilar-Artery Occlusion." [In eng]. *N Engl J Med* 387, no. 15 (Oct 13 2022): 1373–84. https://doi.org/10.1056/NEJMoa2207576.

Langezaal, L. C. M., E. J. R. J. van der Hoeven, F. J. A. Mont'Alverne, et al. "Endovascular Therapy for Stroke Due to Basilar-Artery Occlusion." [In eng].

N Engl J Med 384, no. 20 (May 20 2021): 1910–20. https://doi.org/10.1056/NEJMoa 2030297.

Li, R., C. Tao, J. Sun, C. Zhang, et al.; ATTENTION Investigators. "Endovascular vs Medical Management of Acute Basilar Artery Occlusion: A Secondary Analysis of a Randomized Clinical Trial." [In eng]. *JAMA Neurol* (Aug 26 2024): e242652. doi:10.1001/jamaneurol.2024.2652. Epub ahead of print.

Liu, Z., and D. S. Liebeskind. "Basilar Artery Occlusion and Emerging Treatments." [In eng]. *Semin Neurol* 41, no. 1 (Feb 2021): 39–45. https://doi.org/10.1055/s-0040-1722638.

Strbian, D., G. Tsivgoulis, J. Ospel, et al. "European Stroke Organization (ESO) and European Society for Minimally Invasive Neurological Therapy (ESMINT) Guideline on Acute Management of Basilar Artery Occlusion." [In eng]. *J Neurointerv Surg* 16, no. 9 (Aug 14 2024): e7. doi:10.1136/jnis-2024-022053.

Tao, C., R. G. Nogueira, Y. Zhu, et al. "Trial of Endovascular Treatment of Acute Basilar-Artery Occlusion." [In eng]. *N Engl J Med* 387, no. 15 (Oct 13 2022): 1361–72. https://doi.org/10.1056/NEJMoa2206317.

Yue, C., W. Deng, J. Liu, et al. "Endovascular Treatment in Patients With Coma That Developed Secondary to Acute Basilar Artery Occlusion." [In eng]. *J Neurosurg* (Mar 18 2022): 1–10. https://doi.org/10.3171/2022.1.Jns212967.

14 Timing of Hemicraniectomy in Swollen Ischemic Stroke

A 48-year-old man collapsed on the bathroom floor, where he was found by his wife. In an outside hospital, he was found to have profound aphasia and hemiplegia weakness. Computed tomography (CT) showed a left hyperdense middle cerebral artery sign, and CT angiography showed bilaterally occluded carotid arteries. He received intravenous thrombolysis. No endovascular intervention was available in the outside hospital, and on arrival, after considerable delay in transport, stroke was established and mature. On examination, he did not open his eyes to pain, was mute, and had minimally reactive 4-mm pupils, but corneal reflexes were intact. There was a forced eye deviation to the right. He localized to pain only on the right side. His left arm and leg were flaccid. He had an irregular breathing pattern but seemed to protect his airway well. He had atrial fibrillation but with a normal ventricular response, and blood pressure was consistently within normal range. A repeat CT scan showed an evolving infarct involving the right frontal, parietal, basal ganglia, and caudate nucleus areas (Figure 14.1).

What do you do now?

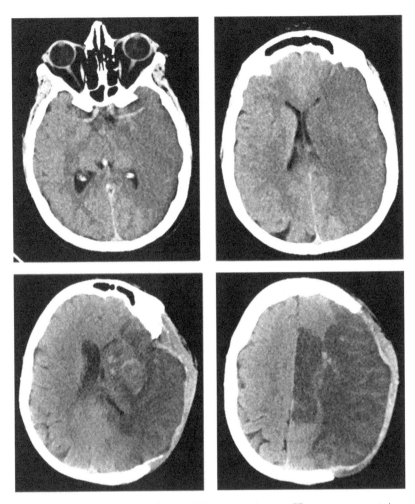

FIGURE 14.1 Serial CT scans from ictus to 3 days postcraniectomy. CT scans were repeated every few days, and note gradual progression even after decompression.

Neurosurgical treatment of a developing swollen hemispheric stroke is a difficult decision for sure. Doing nothing but knowing the patient will lapse into coma is a poor option in a relatively young, presumably healthy person. Further swelling of a major territorial infarct can be anticipated in acute carotid artery occlusion, and often these patients deteriorate beyond drowsiness. Multiple territorial infarcts can swell, increasing their volume. Medical management with osmotic agents is often ineffective when patients worsen quickly. Hemicraniectomy may result in a potentially meaningful recovery for some patients. Yet, preemptive removal of half the skull at the site of a newly developing hemispheric infarct (to create space for swelling) may be perceived as overly aggressive. Responsible physicians must consider expected quality of life, socioeconomic factors such as support from family members, age, comorbidities, and perhaps the patient's vigor (as understood by close family members). How the patient will handle a protracted, endlessly frustrating neurorehabilitation that may still lead to a permanent major disability is difficult to judge but is an important consideration.

What difference does it really make? Hemicraniectomy could shift patients from the "likely to die" category to the "severely disabled" category, and indeed, families may not fully appreciate the changed life ahead. Some will always choose severe disability over death, even after learning that a permanently bedridden state is a possible outcome. But there is also the potential for only moderate disability or even a return to functional independence (albeit uncommon). Recently published guidelines from the Neurocritical Care Society and American Heart Association both conclude that there is sufficient evidence to justify this neurosurgical intervention but only in a subset of young patients.

Comparing the "natural history" with the outcome of patients undergoing hemicraniectomy remains seriously flawed due to the possibility of less aggressive care in non–surgically treated patients. Thankfully, we have clinical trials. What do they teach us? In a pooled analysis of three prospective randomized trials of patients younger than 60 years with a large hemispheric infarct (i.e., occlusion of the middle cerebral artery or carotid artery occlusion), mortality was significantly reduced with hemicraniectomy compared to medical management (22% vs. 71%), and two of three trials showed improvement in the percentage of survivors with likely acceptable outcomes (defined as a modified Rankin scale [mRS] score ≤4). Among posthemicraniectomy survivors, the breakdown between severe disability and better outcomes is basically 50/50.

But what about older patients? A more recent trial focused on patients ≥60 years found mortality to be substantially decreased with hemicraniectomy (from 70% to 33%). Yet, outcomes assessed a year after decompressive surgery found no patients with mild disability (mRS ≤2). Very few patients (6% in the hemicraniectomy group compared to 5% in the control group) had moderate disability (mRS = 3); that is, they required help to function but could walk unassisted. About half of the patients fell into the worst mRS categories. These results should clearly discourage hemicraniectomy in most patients over 60 years old. Another recent finding is that hemorrhagic conversion of the infarct may worsen outcome, but this may simply be due to increased volume and increased brain tissue shift.

For many patients younger that 60 years old, decompressive hemicraniectomy is a life-saving procedure that creates a severely disabled state but with a 50% prospect of further, potentially substantial improvement. There are also good physiological arguments for decompressive surgery. Apart from preventing permanent brainstem injury from direct compression, reducing even marginally elevated intracranial pressure may improve cerebral blood flow and brain tissue oxygenation. These effects improve functional recovery in a proportion of survivors, as observed in randomized trials.

These are the critical questions: can we identify the best candidates for decompressive craniectomy, and what should trigger (early) surgery in patients with hemispheric infarcts? Should this large hemicraniectomy be offered to all patients regardless of level of consciousness, involvement of additional vascular territories, or hemispheric dominance? Does early magnetic resonance imaging (MRI) predict clinical deterioration or only radiological worsening? Most of these questions have no satisfactory answers, but we summarized some criteria in Box 14.1.

BOX 14.1 **Criteria for Decompressive Craniectomy in Swollen Hemispheric Stroke**

Age <60 years

Rehabilitation potential

Patient able to cope with severe handicap

No major comorbidity

Any clinical deterioration in consciousness and need for intubation

Anticipated or documented multiple territorial involvement

Early (<24 hours) evidence of mass effect on CT scan

If available, MRI diffusion-weighted imaging volume ($\geq$80 mL) within 6 hours

Optimal timing of surgery remains partially undefined, but surgery should be conducted within 48 hours of onset. While many neurosurgeons wait for clinical deterioration and some remain skeptical of the benefit to be gained from surgery, neurointensivists must take charge and decide when surgery is indicated. We determine that at the bedside but also by scrutinizing serial CT scans. Craniectomy should be sizable (at least 12 × 12 cm) and be combined with extensive durotomy. Removing additional bone from the squamous part of the temporal bone and the temporalis muscle is optional. Some neurosurgeons resect the temporal pole and perform a tentoriotomy, but the value of these particularly aggressive approaches is uncertain, to say the least. Hemicraniectomy is no simple solution; 1 in 10 patients on average require subsequent medical or surgical intervention because of cerebrospinal fluid leakage or infection. Seizures have been reported in one of three patients, and they are more common when the bone flap is put back in.

The main principle of neurocritical management is to avoid further brain injury. Therefore, attention should be directed toward maintaining adequate intravascular volume (hydrate with 0.9% saline, avoiding hypotonic solutions and excessively positive fluid balance), treating fever (using a cooling device if necessary), preventing aspiration pneumonitis (with broad-spectrum antibiotics until cultures are known), providing deep venous thrombosis prophylaxis (subcutaneous heparin three times a day or enoxaparin), and controlling blood pressure (systolic blood pressure <180 mmHg and diastolic <105 mmHg). Swallowing precautions are needed, and most patients will need nasogastric feeding.

Medical management of large, swollen, hemispheric strokes has been mostly disappointing. These infarctions are complicated by an unrelenting swelling that is usually unresponsive to "antiedema" therapy. (Regrettably, the sobriquet "malignant edema" with its closer connection to oncology has been used.) That said, mannitol and hypertonic saline have been inadequately evaluated for the treatment of ischemic brain edema, and clinical empirical experience is mixed, with patients improving clinically and others progressing to brainstem compression. Some clinicians found that need for osmotic therapy based on CT edema and worsening within 24 hours after presentation were predictive of failed medical therapy. Protracted, later-onset edema can be temporized with medical management. We often start a mannitol dose of 0.5 g/kg every 6 hours and infuse sufficient isotonic or hypertonic saline to compensate for the increased diuresis, thus reducing the risk of kidney injury from mannitol. The goal for serum osmolarity should be 310 to 320 mOsm/L. The gap between measured and calculated osmolality (osmolality = 2 Na + glucose/18 + blood urea nitrogen/2.8) should be monitored to ensure the safety of mannitol. Mannitol can be safely continued if the osmolar gap is less than 15 to 20, serum sodium is less than 160 mmol/L, or serum osmolarity is less than 320 mOsm/L (even higher if osmolar gap is <15–20). Using scheduled doses of hypertonic saline instead of mannitol is similarly reasonable. Hyperventilation in patients intubated for airway protection has not been studied systematically and may negatively impact cerebral oxygenation; thus, it is not recommended except for very brief periods. Adding hypothermia with cooling devices is likely ineffective.

What did we do? Our patient underwent decompressive hemicraniectomy and developed considerable swelling outside the skull but without clinical deterioration (Figure 14.1). In this case, one could certainly imagine tissue compression and shift caused by the swollen ischemic mass in a smaller confined space leading to profound, new clinical deterioration. Six months later, his functional outcome was not favorable despite being able to ambulate with a cane and tolerating oral intake. He was aphasic and had difficulty expressing his needs. He required assistance with bathing, toileting, and transfers from bed to chair. His 6-month outcome is less than satisfactory, and we do not know whether to expect more improvement over time. This is a common outcome after hemicraniectomy, and for outsiders it is hard to judge whether it represents an acceptable quality of life for the patient.

A judicious attitude toward aggressive treatment of these massive cerebral infarcts is necessary, but also knowing that neurosurgical intervention may be beneficial in some cases. Some patients are grateful for such aggressive treatment, but it is difficult to predict who they will be. Once families to decide to go ahead with decompressive craniectomy they may later have to face great financial and societal burden of a major stroke without affording functional recovery. Evidence from the National Inpatient Sample database showing increasing rates of craniectomy in the US may point to indiscriminate use. This is an incredibly difficult problem without a great solution. Think of the last time you went along with decompressive hemicraniectomy—did you think it was the right thing to do? We suggest you follow these patients for years to find out.

KEY POINTS TO REMEMBER

- Middle cerebral artery territory infarcts may be due to acute carotid artery occlusion, and such infarcts may become more extensive and lead to (rapid) swelling.
- Progressing hemispheric swelling occurs in 30% of patients with large-vessel occlusion.
- Medical management with osmotic agents can be temporizing but is often ineffective long term.
- Decompressive craniectomy should be considered in patients younger than 60 years of age, with mass effect on CT scan, and evidence of early neurological decline.
- Decompressive craniectomy in the elderly may reduce mortality, but neurological morbidity is considerable and an issue of enormous importance to address with proxy.

Further Reading

Brown, D. A., and E. F. Wijdicks. "Decompressive Craniectomy in Acute Brain Injury." [In eng]. *Handb Clin Neurol* 140 (2017): 299–318. https://doi.org/10.1016/b978-0-444-63600-3.00016-7.

Ellens, N. R., G. P. Albert, M. T. Bender, B. P. George, and D. C. McHugh. "Trends and Predictors of Decompressive Craniectomy in Acute Ischemic Stroke, 2011–2020." [In eng]. *J Stroke Cerebrovasc Dis* 33, no. 6 (Jun 2024): 107713. doi:10.1016/j.jstrokecerebrovasdis.2024.107713

Franco, A. C., T. Fernandes, A. R. Peralta, et al. "Frequency of Epileptic Seizures in Patients Undergoing Decompressive Craniectomy After Ischemic Stroke." [In eng]. *Seizure* 101 (Oct 2022): 60–66. https://doi.org/10.1016/j.seizure.2022.07.011.

Hernández-Durán, S., D. Mielke, V. Rohde, and C. von der Brelie. "Decompressive Craniectomy in Malignant Stroke After Hemorrhagic Transformation." [In eng]. *Stroke* 52, no. 8 (Aug 2021): e486–87. https://doi.org/10.1161/strokeaha.121.035072.

Huttner, H. B., and S. Schwab. "Malignant Middle Cerebral Artery Infarction: Clinical Characteristics, Treatment Strategies, and Future Perspectives." [In eng]. *Lancet Neurol* 8, no. 10 (Oct 2009): 949–58. https://doi.org/10.1016/s1474-4422(09)70224-8.

Jüttler, E., A. Unterberg, J. Woitzik, et al. "Hemicraniectomy in Older Patients with Extensive Middle-Cerebral-Artery Stroke." [In eng]. *N Engl J Med* 370, no. 12 (Mar 20 2014): 1091–100. https://doi.org/10.1056/NEJMoa1311367.

Kurland, D. B., A. Khaladj-Ghom, J. A. Stokum, et al. "Complications Associated With Decompressive Craniectomy: A Systematic Review." [In eng]. *Neurocrit Care* 23, no. 2 (Oct 2015): 292–304. https://doi.org/10.1007/s12028-015-0144-7.

Maramattom, B. V., M. M. Bahn, and E. F. Wijdicks. "Which Patient Fares Worse After Early Deterioration Due to Swelling From Hemispheric Stroke?" [In eng]. *Neurology* 63, no. 11 (Dec 14 2004): 2142–45. https://doi.org/10.1212/01.wnl.000 0145626.30318.8a.

Ong, C. J., S. G. Keyrouz, and M. N. Diringer. "The Role of Osmotic Therapy in Hemispheric Stroke." [In eng]. *Neurocrit Care* 23, no. 2 (Oct 2015): 285–91. https://doi.org/10.1007/s12028-015-0173-2.

Pilato, F., G. Pellegrino, R. Calandrelli, et al. "Decompressive Hemicraniectomy in Patients With Malignant Middle Cerebral Artery Infarction: A Real-World Study." [In eng]. *J Neurol Sci* 441 (Oct 15 2022): 120376. https://doi.org/10.1016/j.jns.2022.120376.

Rabinstein, A. A., N. Mueller-Kronast, B. V. Maramattom, et al. "Factors Predicting Prognosis After Decompressive Hemicraniectomy for Hemispheric Infarction." [In eng]. *Neurology* 67, no. 5 (Sep 12 2006): 891–93. https://doi.org/10.1212/01.wnl.0000233895.03152.66.

Sehweil, S. M. M., and Z. A. Goncharova. "How I Do It: Decompressive Hemicraniectomy Supplemented With Resection of the Temporal Pole and Tentoriotomy for Malignant Ischemic Infarction in the Territory Supplied by the Middle Cerebral Artery." [In eng]. *Acta Neurochir (Wien)* 164, no. 6 (Jun 2022): 1653–57. https://doi.org/10.1007/s00701-022-05152-7.

Shlobin, N. A., J. R. Clark, J. M. Campbell, et al. "Ethical Considerations in Surgical Decompression for Stroke." [In eng]. *Stroke* 53, no. 8 (Aug 2022): 2673–82. https://doi.org/10.1161/strokeaha.121.038493.

Thomalla, G., F. Hartmann, E. Juettler, et al. "Prediction of Malignant Middle Cerebral Artery Infarction by Magnetic Resonance Imaging Within 6 Hours of Symptom Onset: A Prospective Multicenter Observational Study." [In eng]. *Ann Neurol* 68, no. 4 (Oct 2010): 435–45. https://doi.org/10.1002/ana.22125.

Torbey, M. T., J. Bösel, D. H. Rhoney, et al. "Evidence-Based Guidelines for the Management of Large Hemispheric Infarction: A Statement for Health Care Professionals From the Neurocritical Care Society and the German Society for Neuro-Intensive Care and Emergency Medicine." [In eng]. *Neurocrit Care* 22, no. 1 (Feb 2015): 146–64. https://doi.org/10.1007/s12028-014-0085-6.

Vahedi, K., J. Hofmeijer, E. Juettler, et al. "Early Decompressive Surgery in Malignant Infarction of the Middle Cerebral Artery: A Pooled Analysis of Three Randomised Controlled Trials." [In eng]. *Lancet Neurol* 6, no. 3 (Mar 2007): 215–22. https://doi.org/10.1016/s1474-4422(07)70036-4.

Wijdicks, E. F. "Management of Massive Hemispheric Cerebral Infarct: Is There a Ray of Hope?" [In eng]. *Mayo Clin Proc* 75, no. 9 (Sep 2000): 945–52. https://doi.org/10.4065/75.9.945.

Wijdicks, E. F., K. N. Sheth, B. S. Carter, et al. "Recommendations for the Management of Cerebral and Cerebellar Infarction With Swelling: A Statement for Healthcare Professionals From the American Heart Association/American Stroke Association." [In eng]. *Stroke* 45, no. 4 (Apr 2014): 1222–38. https://doi.org/10.1161/01.str.0000441965.15164.d6.

15 Worsening Cerebral Venous Thrombosis Despite Anticoagulation

A 46-year-old woman was brought into the emergency department by her husband because she was behaving strange. On arrival, she was disoriented but without focal neurological deficits. Computed tomography (CT) of the brain showed unusual bilateral deep brain infarctions, which prompted us to consider a cerebral venous thrombosis. A magnetic resonance (MR) venogram confirmed occlusion of the left sigmoid and transverse sinus, the proximal portion of the superior sagittal sinus, and the deep venous system. A thrombophilia panel was sent, and a lower-extremity ultrasound was negative for deep venous thrombosis. Her intravaginal estrogen ring was removed.

She was started on intravenous (IV) heparin and was adequately hydrated. She remained stable for 24 hours before becoming progressively lethargic and slower to move the left side. She was mute but occasionally could follow one-step commands; at other times, she only could do so when aided by visual guidance (mimicking the examiner's movements). A repeat head CT showed hemorrhagic transformation of the thalamic infarctions (Figure 15.1).

What do you do now?

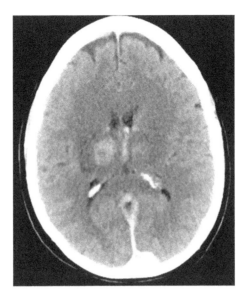

FIGURE 15.1 Noncontrast head CT scan shows hemorrhagic infarcts involving the bilateral thalami and basal ganglia. Compression of the ventricles results from edema of the thalami and right caudate head. The superficial hyperdensity along the left falx likely represents a thrombosed vein (cord sign).

Patients with a cerebral venous sinus thrombosis (CVST) usually present with gradual onset of an ultimately severe headache, a localizing deficit (weakness or aphasia), focal seizures, or all of the above—but not our patient. The diagnosis of CVST can mislead any clinician because it often begins insidiously, and then the findings on CT scan (if recognized) are a surprise. Bithalamic strokes are notorious for causing indistinct symptoms such as a poorly characterized "confusion," fluctuating alertness, and impaired vigilance and attention. Inability to retain experiences is commonly observed ("thalamic dementia"). This presentation is expected with involvement of the medial nuclei of the thalamus and is explained by damaged amygdalothalamic circuitry. Other clinical syndromes may indicate involvement of specific sinuses and veins. For example, the presence of orbital and unrelenting face pain, marked facial swelling, chemosis, proptosis, and oculomotor palsies points to a cavernous sinus syndrome. Involvement of the dominant transverse sinus may cause aphasia, and cortical vein thrombosis may result in sensorimotor deficits and focal seizures. When considering a diagnosis of CVST, it is important to ask about a personal or family history of venous thromboembolism, use of contraceptives or recent childbirth, ongoing or recent infections (e.g., otitis media, sinusitis, or mastoiditis), systemic inflammatory disease or malignancy (acute leukemias), recent traumatic brain injury (often minor and trivial), or excessive dehydration caused by combined vomiting and diarrhea. Of course, a normal head CT does not exclude CVST, and in fact, CT is normal in up to half of cases. Therefore, imaging of the cerebral veins by CT or MR venogram is critical.

Once the diagnosis has been confirmed, we screen patients for hypercoagulable states and then start anticoagulation without delay (Box 15.1). Small, randomized trials have shown that anticoagulation reduces the risk of death or disability by 13% when compared to placebo (without reaching statistical significance because of lack of power). There is sufficient pathophysiological rationale to anticoagulate patients with CVST to prevent thrombus propagation, facilitate recanalization of the

---

BOX 15.1 **Evaluation of Cerebral Venous Sinus Thrombosis**

Peripheral blood smear

Complete blood cell count with differential

Drug screen

Antithrombin III

Protein C activity and free protein S antigen

Prothrombin G20210A mutation

Factor V Leiden mutation

Heparin cofactor II

Fibrinogen

Lupus anticoagulant[a]

Beta-2 glycoprotein 1 antibodies[a]

Anticardiolipin antibodies[a]

Plasma homocysteine

Consider hemoglobin electrophoresis

Consider venous duplex of the lower extremities and MR pelvis

[a] Elevated titers during the acute phase should be later confirmed (after weeks or months) before concluding that the patient has antiphospholipid antibody syndrome.

occluded sinus, and improve venous outflow. Both American and European guidelines recommend anticoagulation for all patients with CVST unless contraindicated but without a clear definition of what should be those contraindications. Treatment is usually with IV heparin or subcutaneous low-molecular-weight heparin. This means that patients with venous infarctions and hemorrhagic conversion of infarctions of modest or small size should be anticoagulated. In two retrospective studies of patients with CVST complicated by moderate-sized hematomas, anticoagulation did not worsen outcomes. Increased hematoma size may even relate to progression of untreated thrombosis rather than effects of anticoagulation.

All patients with CSVT should be kept on oral anticoagulation for 3-6 months. There is now evidence that direct oral anticoagulants (DOACs) are effective for the treatment of CVST. The RESPECT-CVT trial (Comparing Efficacy and Safety of Dabigatran Etexilate with Warfarin in Patients with Cerebral Venous and Dural Sinus Thrombosis) randomized 120 patients with CVST to dabigatran versus warfarin and the two treatment groups showed no significant differences in efficacy and safety outcomes. A large, multicenter, international, retrospective, observational study Direct oral anticoagulant versus warfarin in the treatment of cerebral venous thrombosis (ACTION-CVT) found that direct oral anticoagulant treatment correlated with a similar risk of recurrence, death, and CVST recanalization rates, but a lower risk of major hemorrhage, than warfarin treatment. DOACs therefore may become an easier alternative to warfarin (no INR checks).

After anticoagulation is initiated, deterioration is still possible, and patients must be closely observed, particularly in the early days. Some reasons for decline are listed in Box 15.2.

Cerebral edema may be treated with osmotic therapy. In some patients, an enlarging hematoma may produce significant mass effect and brainstem compression, and craniotomy is indicated to evacuate the hematoma.

Seizures occur in 10% to 15% of patients with CVST and are typically focal. It is unknown whether patients with CVST benefit from prophylactic use of anti-seizure medication.

Thrombus propagation despite adequate anticoagulation with IV heparin or low-molecular-weight heparin calls for endovascular intervention. A recent systematic review found that 88% of 25 patients who received systemic thrombolysis for CVST achieved functional independence, but

> **BOX 15.2** **Causes of Deterioration in Cerebral Venous Sinus Thrombosis**
>
> Propagation of thrombus
>
> Venous infarction
>
> Hemorrhagic transformation of venous infarctions
>
> Brainstem compression from an enlarging hematoma
>
> Cerebral edema
>
> Raised intracranial pressure
>
> Seizures (convulsive or nonconvulsive)
>
> Pulmonary emboli

there were also three cases of serious intracranial hemorrhage including two deaths. In a review of 42 studies encompassing 185 patients with cerebral venous thrombosis treated with endovascular therapy, 84% had good outcomes, defined as a modified Rankin scale score of 0 to 2, and 12% died. A considerable number (86%) of these patients rapidly deteriorated while on heparin. This means that most physicians and neurointerventionalists attempt endovascular clot removal only when IV heparin "fails." But there are several caveats. We do not know how many patients are adequately anticoagulated before endovascular intervention is initiated. Moreover, it is legitimate to ask if watchful waiting is good enough or if we should just retrieve the clot at the very first opportunity. Procedure-related risks have been estimated at 10%, but these data come from observational studies using older (and less safe) suction devices, such as AngioJet; newer devices may be more effective. Moreover, in an evolving pathological process, procedure-related risks may be hard to prove, and certainly, postprocedure intracranial hematoma may be unrelated to the procedure itself. Nonetheless, endovascular treatment may benefit patients and there are early indications from prospective registries that we may need to consider endovascular interventions earlier in overall management.

Our patient deteriorated from hemorrhagic infarction in the right thalamus and worsening cerebral edema and underwent mechanical thrombectomy. The catheter was left in the posterior aspect of the superior sagittal sinus, and local thrombolysis was administered at a dose of

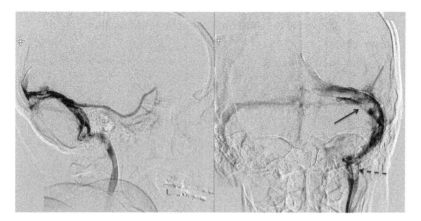

FIGURE 15.2 Lateral (left) and anterior-posterior (right) views of digital subtraction venography with injection of the left transverse sinus. A guiding catheter is present at the junction of the transverse and sigmoid sinuses. A microcatheter (arrow), for recombinant tissue plasminogen activator infusion, is present in the left transverse sinus and a micro-guidewire has been placed into the dorsal aspect of the superior sagittal sinus. Large filling defects are present within the transverse and sigmoid sinuses (arrow), indicating thrombus, which extends down to the jugular bulb and superior aspect of the jugular vein (dashed arrow).

recombinant tissue plasminogen activator of 0.5 mg/h for 24 hours (Figure 15.2). After catheter removal, she was continued on a heparin infusion and was treated with scheduled doses of mannitol for 48 hours with improved level of consciousness. Heparin was transitioned to warfarin, and she was ultimately discharged to inpatient rehabilitation. All other tests were negative so we assumed that CVST was caused by the intravaginal estrogen ring. Six months after hospital discharge, she was able to return to work with just minimal residual cognitive symptoms.

Outcomes correlate with time to diagnosis and initiation of anticoagulation. Coma at presentation, presence of an underlying systemic disease, and seizures are unrelated to outcome and should not preclude aggressive treatment. Overall outcomes are favorable, with an in-hospital mortality rate of 2% and a long-term death and dependency rate of 15%. Predictors of poor prognosis include central nervous system infection, hydrocephalus, and extensive parenchymal lesions, but there are exceptions. Cognition may be affected in a considerable proportion of patients. Still, individual prognosis is difficult to predict accurately, and overall outcomes are good with about two-thirds of patients recovering without sequelae.

A little perspective is in order. What remains most important is to recognize this entity; clinicians need to appreciate that some infarcts or hemorrhages might be venous in origin. Anticoagulation works well for most patients. We will probably see a shift toward earlier endovascular management when procedure-related risks decline further with safer devices—and more resources—make it easier to intervene. Remember that cerebral venous thrombosis is infrequent and even more infrequently severe. We see the worst cases in the intensive care unit, and these patients have been underrepresented in clinical trials. Therefore, more clinical experience (and ideally a clinical trial) is needed to support a shift to an early endovascular treatment.

KEY POINTS TO REMEMBER

- Neurologic deterioration in cerebral venous and dural sinus thrombosis can result from extension of thrombus, venous infarction, intracerebral hemorrhage, cerebral edema, and seizures.
- Hematoma evacuation may be needed in a patient deteriorating from brainstem compression.
- Endovascular intervention should be strongly considered in a patient deteriorating from clot propagation despite adequate IV heparinization or use of low-molecular-weight heparin.
- For secondary prevention, direct oral anticoagulants have a similar risk of recurrence but a lower risk of major hemorrhage than warfarin.

Further Reading

Abdalkader, M., F. Hui, M. R. Amans, et al. "Cerebral Venous Disorders: Diagnosis and Endovascular Management." [In eng]. J Neuroradiol. 2023 Nov;50(6):581–592. https://doi.org/10.1016/j.neurad.2023.06.002.

Bousser, M. G., and J. M. Ferro. "Cerebral Venous Thrombosis: An Update." [In eng]. *Lancet Neurol* 6, no. 2 (Feb 2007): 162–70. https://doi.org/10.1016/s1474-4422(07)70029-7.

Bücke, P., H. Henkes, J. Kaesmacher, et al. "Early Versus Late Initiation of Endovascular Therapy in Patients with Severe Cerebral Venous Sinus Thrombosis." [In eng]. *Neurocrit Care* (Jul 23 2024). doi:10.1007/s12028-024-02046-7.

Coutinho, J., S. F. de Bruijn, G. Deveber, and J. Stam. "Anticoagulation for Cerebral Venous Sinus Thrombosis." [In eng]. *Cochrane Database Syst Rev* 2011, no. 8 (Aug 10 2011): CD002005. https://doi.org/10.1002/14651858.CD002005.pub2.

Ferro, J. M., M. G. Bousser, P. Canhão, et al. "European Stroke Organization Guideline for the Diagnosis and Treatment of Cerebral Venous Thrombosis—Endorsed by the European Academy of Neurology." [In eng]. *Eur J Neurol* 24, no. 10 (Oct 2017): 1203–13. https://doi.org/10.1111/ene.13381.

Ferro, J. M., J. M. Coutinho, F. Dentali, et al. "Safety and Efficacy of Dabigatran Etexilate vs Dose-Adjusted Warfarin in Patients With Cerebral Venous Thrombosis: A Randomized Clinical Trial." [In eng]. *JAMA Neurol* 76, no. 12 (Dec 1 2019): 1457–65. https://doi.org/10.1001/jamaneurol.2019.2764.

Itoh, C.Y., E. F. M. Wijdicks, Cavernous Sinus Thrombosis; Then and Now. *Pract Neurol* Dec 22:pn-2024-004396. doi: 10.1136/pn-2024-004396. Online ahead of print.

Nasr, D. M., W. Brinjikji, H. J. Cloft, et al. "Mortality in Cerebral Venous Thrombosis: Results From the National Inpatient Sample Database." [In eng]. *Cerebrovasc Dis* 35, no. 1 (2013): 40–44. https://doi.org/10.1159/000343653.

Saposnik, G., F. Barinagarrementeria, R. D. Brown, Jr., et al. "Diagnosis and Management of Cerebral Venous Thrombosis: A Statement for Healthcare Professionals From the American Heart Association/American Stroke Association." [In eng]. *Stroke* 42, no. 4 (Apr 2011): 1158–92. https://doi.org/10.1161/STR.0b013e31820a8364.

Siddiqui, F. M., S. Dandapat, C. Banerjee, et al. "Mechanical Thrombectomy in Cerebral Venous Thrombosis: Systematic Review of 185 Cases." [In eng]. *Stroke* 46, no. 5 (May 2015): 1263–68. https://doi.org/10.1161/strokeaha.114.007465.

Viegas, L. D., E. Stolz, P. Canhão, and J. M. Ferro. "Systemic Thrombolysis for Cerebral Venous and Dural Sinus Thrombosis: A Systematic Review." [In eng]. *Cerebrovasc Dis* 37, no. 1 (2014): 43–50. https://doi.org/10.1159/000356840.

Zubkov, A.Y., R. D. McBane, R. D. Brown, and A. A. Rabinstein. "Brain Lesions in Cerebral Venous Sinus Thrombosis." [In eng]. *Stroke* 40, no. 4 (Apr 2009): 1509–11. https://doi.org/10.1161/strokeaha.108.529172.

16 Aneurysmal Subarachnoid Hemorrhage: From Good to Bad Grade

A 44-year-old woman presented to the emergency department after a thunderclap headache. Her neurological examination was normal (World Federation of Neurological Surgeons [WFNS] grade I). Head computed tomography (CT) scan revealed diffuse hemorrhage in the subarachnoid cisterns with some blood in the lateral ventricles, and were not enlarged (modified Fisher grade 4) (Figure 16.1A). She was admitted to our neurosciences intensive care unit for further care. Three hours later, she became increasingly drowsy (WFNS grade IV). Her blood pressure trended upward, and she developed sinus bradycardia. Her neurological examination still showed no focal deficits, but upward eye movements were limited. Repeat CT scan confirmed the clinically suspected hydrocephalus (Figure 16.1B).

What do you do now?

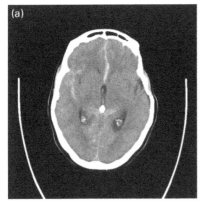 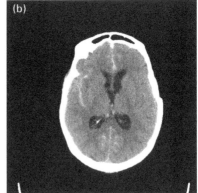

FIGURE 16.1 (A) Initial head CT scan shows SAH with aneurysmal pattern and some blood layering in the ventricles consistent with a modified Fisher scale grade 4. (B) Follow-up CT scan hours later shows hydrocephalus.

Patients with an aneurysmal subarachnoid hemorrhage (aSAH) often appear deceptively stable. They may "look great" only to decline into a much worse neurological state. The precise timing when neurological changes occur with hydrocephalus is sometimes difficult to pinpoint (as with cerebral vasospasm), but in other instances, changes are overwhelmingly clear (as with rebleeding). When caring for an aSAH patient with worsening neurological condition, the differential diagnosis depends on the time from aneurysm rupture. This is clearly demonstrated by this patient, who declined early, due to hydrocephalus, and later, as we will see, due to cerebral vasospasm.

The major risks to the patient on the first day after aneurysmal rupture are rebleeding and acute hydrocephalus. Rebleeding is hard to overlook because the clinical changes are often dramatic. The patient acutely becomes stuporous or comatose, and the altered consciousness is accompanied by new severe hypertension, tachypnea (or apnea), and tachycardia (or brief asystole). Motor responses change, and extensor posturing (mimicking a seizure to the untrained observer) may occur. In comatose patients with a poor-grade aSAH, rebleeding may cause loss of pupillary light reflexes and corneal reflexes, and even all brainstem reflexes. Rebleeding may also occur in a patient who just had a ventriculostomy placed and the nursing staff may see fresh red blood in the drainage bag.

As hydrocephalus develops, patients usually become progressively less interactive, then drowsier, and finally unresponsive. This progression may occur rapidly over several hours rather than suddenly (alarms do not go off), and patients may only be gradually sleepier throughout the day— not infrequently falsely attributed to a poor night's rest. The only physical sign may be limited vertical eye movements caused by the pressure of the expanded third ventricle over the tectum of the midbrain. Given the paucity of clinical clues, the recognition of acute hydrocephalus remains a challenge for physicians outside the neurosciences, and many do not appreciate the dilated ventricles on first or later CT scans.

Symptomatic hydrocephalus demands immediate cerebrospinal fluid diversion. We prefer ventriculostomy, but lumbar drainage is a reasonable alternative in patients without an obstructive intraventricular pattern. In fact, lumbar drainage might reduce the risk of delayed cerebral ischemia. One study found this difference in patients who often had the combination of ventriculostomy and lumbar drainage—a protocol used for the trial but rarely practiced. Level of drainage should be adjusted to ensure that the hydrocephalus is adequately treated. Practices vary in regard to the modality of ventricular drainage. We keep the ventriculostomy open, but others drain intermittently. A prospective trial is necessary to define which strategy is superior and how it could affect drain dependency and later ventriculoperitoneal shunting. It is a travesty that we still do not have a definitive answer for such a common problem.

The only effective way to prevent rebleeding is securing the ruptured aneurysm. However, there is no proof that ultra-early treatment of the aneurysm is beneficial. It is important to stabilize the patient to make sure the intervention (whether open neurosurgery or endovascular) can be done safely. There is no solid evidence to support the argument that aggressive treatment of hypertension reduces the risk of aneurysm rebleeding—and greater blood pressure variability, which can result from antihypertensive therapy, is associated with worse outcomes in aSAH. Hence, it may be safer to lower the blood pressure gradually, considering the blood pressure at presentation and the likelihood of increased intracranial pressure. Lastly, antifibrinolytics can no longer be recommended in aSAH. Long used to reduce the risk of rebleeding, we now know from a convincing ULtra-early Tranexamic Acid after subarachnoid hemorrhage (ULTRA) trial that intravenous tranexamic acid does not improve outcomes even if used early and briefly after aSAH onset, and it might in fact reduce the chances of excellent recovery (defined in this trial as modified Rankin score 0-2).

How did our patient do? She improved after placement of a ventriculostomy catheter. She underwent endovascular coiling of her ruptured anterior communicating artery aneurysm without complications. She remained well until post rupture day 5, when she became slightly confused. Mean blood flow velocities on transcranial Doppler (TCD) had increased by 30% compared with the previous day, with velocities in the 180 cm/s range. Now, on post rupture day 6, she is at times restless or drowsy. We now must seriously consider the development of delayed cerebral ischemia from cerebral vasospasm.

Cerebral vasospasm occurs days later, typically starting 3 to 5 days after the hemorrhage and reaching a peak around day 7 before resolving by days 10 to 12. Contrary to a common assumption of trainees, the first manifestation of cerebral vasospasm is not usually a focal deficit. Instead, diminished alertness and lucidity again tend to be the presenting symptoms of this complication. Patients developing cerebral vasospasm are often febrile and have developed hyponatremia, which are also factors that may diminish responsiveness. Consequently, the diagnosis of symptomatic cerebral vasospasm is far from straightforward, and good clinical judgment and experience are necessary to recognize it. We cannot use declining scores or scales because it is often that patients become withdrawn, silent and detached. Some patients are at higher risk for delayed cerebral ischemia from cerebral vasospasm after aSAH; these risk factors are listed in Box 16.1.

BOX 16.1 **Risk Factors for Development of Delayed Cerebral Ischemia After Aneurysmal Subarachnoid Hemorrhage**

Extensive clot in subarachnoid cisterns on admission CT scan[a]

Intraventricular hemorrhage on CT scan within first 24 hours[a]

Early age

Active smoking

Cocaine use

Poor clinical neurological examination at onset

[a] The modified Fisher scale can be used: grade 0, no subarachnoid hemorrhage (SAH) and no intraventricular hemorrhage (IVH); grade 1, thin SAH without IVH; grade 2, thin SAH with IVH; grade 3, thick SAH without IVH; grade 4, thick SAH with IVH.

TABLE 16.1 **Modalities for Diagnosis and Monitoring of Cerebral Vasospasm and Delayed Ischemic Damage**

Diagnostic Modality	Parameter Evaluated
Catheter angiography	Large-vessel spasm
Transcranial Doppler	Large-vessel spasm (circle of Willis)
CT angiography	Large-vessel spasm
CT perfusion	Cerebral perfusion
MR angiography	Large-vessel spasm
MRI with diffusion-weighted/ perfusion-weighted imaging	Cerebral perfusion and early ischemia
Continuous EEG	Alpha-delta ratio
Brain tissue O_2	Local brain oxygenation

Useful modalities for the screening of cerebral vasospasm and diagnosis of delayed cerebral ischemia are summarized in Table 16.1.

TCD is useful to monitor for cerebral vasospasm, especially when documenting trends from serial measurements. We suspect cerebral vasospasm when the mean blood flow velocity in the M1 segment of the middle cerebral artery exceeds 120 cm/s and consider it severe when this measurement is greater than 200 cm/s. Following the ratio of the flow velocities in the middle cerebral artery versus the cervical internal carotid artery (MCA/ICA ratio or Lindegaard ratio) is useful to differentiate vasospasm from hyperemia related to hypertension. (MCA velocities increase way beyond the ICA velocities in vasospasm; both velocities increase to a similar extent with hypertension.) A ratio greater than 3 is supportive of vasospasm, and a ratio greater than 6 is supportive of severe vasospasm.

We have increasingly used a combination of CT angiogram and CT perfusion in patients with suspected cerebral vasospasm. Conventional angiography is reserved for patients who are refractory to medical therapy and might be candidates for endovascular treatment. However, all these techniques have limitations. Cerebral vasospasm is primarily caused by endothelial dysfunction and involves primarily the microcirculation. TCD and angiograms are sensitive for the detection of vasospasm in the large arterial segments but much less accurate for more distal cerebral vasospasm. Thus, patients may develop ischemic lesions, particularly in deep brain regions, despite having normal or near-normal velocities on TCD and vessel diameters on cerebral angiogram. CT perfusion scans only partially overcome this limitation because their interpretation in practice relies on side-to-side comparison, which loses value in common cases of diffuse, bilateral cerebral vasospasm. CT perfusion may show hypoperfusion much more clearly in the cortex than in the deep white matter. Since ischemia can occur in the absence of documented vasospasm (either because we do not have the right tools to identify it or because mechanisms other than reductions in arterial luminal diameter are causing the ischemia), the term "delayed cerebral ischemia" is more appropriate than "symptomatic cerebral vasospasm."

Unsurprisingly, "good grade" patients with aSAH may rapidly become "poor grade" patients. The causes are well documented and need to be recognized and treated rapidly. Care by a resolute team of neuroscience nurses and skilled physicians with expertise in the management of aSAH is essential to reduce the morbidity of this disease. Our patient was treated with hemodynamic augmentation for a number of days and did well. Some do not and need a next tier of intervention.

The outcome experienced by our patient is far from uncommon in our experience. Patients who present with good-grade aSAH (WNFS I–II) and deteriorate within 24 hours but again reach a good grade after neurological and neurosurgical interventions can achieve a full or nearly full recovery. Adaptation and tenacity might be far greater than we think. We will return to the treatment of delayed cerebral ischemia and options available to the neurointerventionalist in Chapter 17.

KEY POINTS TO REMEMBER

- The causes of neurological decline in aSAH relate to the time from aneurysm rupture.
- During the first few hours consider rebleeding if the decline is rapid and profound and hydrocephalus if the patient drifts into stupor.

- Many patients with acute hydrocephalus after an aSAH benefit from a ventriculostomy, and many benefit can be seen within 12 hours.
- Cerebral vasospasm typically occurs after the third day from aneurysmal rupture. It often presents with subtle changes in attention before focal deficits are noted.
- TCD, CT perfusion, and cerebral angiogram are useful to monitor and document cerebral vasospasm, but the diagnosis of delayed cerebral ischemia remains primarily clinical.

Further Reading

Claassen, J., and S. Park. "Spontaneous Subarachnoid Haemorrhage." [In eng]. *Lancet* 400, no. 10355 (Sep 10 2022): 846–62. https://doi.org/10.1016/s0140-6736(22)00938-2.

Denneman, N., R. Post, B. A. Coert, R. van den Berg, D. Verbaan, and W. P. Vandertop. "Resilience After High-Grade Subarachnoid Hemorrhage: A Prospective Cohort Study on Quality of Life." [In eng]. *Neurosurgery* (Jun 24 2024). doi:10.1227/neu.0000000000003047.

Frontera, J. A., A. Fernandez, J. M. Schmidt, et al. "Clinical Response to Hypertensive Hypervolemic Therapy and Outcome After Subarachnoid Hemorrhage." [In eng]. *Neurosurgery* 66, no. 1 (Jan 2010): 35–41; discussion 41. https://doi.org/10.1227/01.Neu.0000359530.04529.07.

Hasan, D., M. Vermeulen, E. F. Wijdicks, et al. "Management Problems in Acute Hydrocephalus After Subarachnoid Hemorrhage." [In eng]. *Stroke* 20, no. 6 (Jun 1989): 747–53. https://doi.org/10.1161/01.str.20.6.747.

Hoh, B. L., N. U. Ko, S. Amin-Hanjani, et al. "2023 Guideline for the Management of Patients With Aneurysmal Subarachnoid Hemorrhage: A Guideline From the American Heart Association/American Stroke Association." [In eng]. *Stroke* 54, no. 7 (Jul 2023): e314–70. https://doi.org/10.1161/str.0000000000000436.

Macdonald, R. L. "Delayed Neurological Deterioration After Subarachnoid Hemorrhage." [In eng]. *Nat Rev Neurol* 10, no. 1 (Jan 2014): 44–58. https://doi.org/10.1038/nrneurol.2013.246.

Post, R., M. R. Germans, M. A. Tjerkstra, et al. "Ultra-Early Tranexamic Acid After Subarachnoid Hemorrhage (Ultra): A Randomised Controlled Trial." [In eng]. *Lancet* 397, no. 10269 (Jan 9 2021): 112–18. https://doi.org/10.1016/s0140-6736(20)32518-6.

Rabinstein, A. A., J. A. Friedman, S. D. Weigand, et al. "Predictors of Cerebral Infarction in Aneurysmal Subarachnoid Hemorrhage." [In eng]. *Stroke* 35, no. 8 (Aug 2004): 1862–66. https://doi.org/10.1161/01.STR.0000133132.76983.8e.

Rabinstein, A. A., and G. Lanzino. "Aneurysmal Subarachnoid Hemorrhage: Unanswered Questions." [In eng]. *Neurosurg Clin N Am* 29, no. 2 (Apr 2018): 255–62. https://doi.org/10.1016/j.nec.2018.01.001.

Rabinstein, A. A., G. Lanzino, and E. F. Wijdicks. "Multidisciplinary Management and Emerging Therapeutic Strategies in Aneurysmal Subarachnoid Haemorrhage." [In eng]. *Lancet Neurol* 9, no. 5 (May 2010): 504–19. https://doi.org/10.1016/s1474-4422(10)70087-9.

Treggiari, M. M., A. A. Rabinstein, K. M. Busl, et al. "Guidelines for the Neurocritical Care Management of Aneurysmal Subarachnoid Hemorrhage." [In eng]. *Neurocrit Care* 39, no. 1 (Aug 2023): 1–28. https://doi.org/10.1007/s12028-023-01713-5.

Wolf, S., D. Mielke, C. Barner, et al. "Effectiveness of Lumbar Cerebrospinal Fluid Drain Among Patients With Aneurysmal Subarachnoid Hemorrhage: A Randomized Clinical Trial." [In eng]. *JAMA Neurol* 80, no. 8 (2023): 833–42. https://doi.org/10.1001/jamaneurol.2023.1792.

17 Delayed Cerebral Ischemia in Aneurysmal Subarachnoid Hemorrhage

A 65-year-old woman suffered a fall and was taken to a local emergency department. Upon arrival, she was alert but disoriented and had no focal weakness. Computed tomography (CT) scan showed acute subarachnoid hemorrhage filling the basal cisterns, particularly prominent in the anterior interhemispheric fissure. An anterior communicating artery aneurysm found during cerebral angiography was successfully treated with coil embolization. She was monitored closely in the neuroscience intensive care unit, receiving intravenous (IV) fluids and oral nimodipine. Five days after admission, she became drowsy and developed worsening confusion and inattention. On examination she has new visual loss, fever (38.5°C), and an increase in blood pressure to 161/91 mmHg. A CT angiogram shows interval development of diffuse severe vasospasm involving both supraclinoid internal carotid arteries, the bilateral proximal anterior and middle cerebral arteries, and the basilar artery. She is started on IV norepinephrine to increase systolic blood pressure to 200 mmHg, but she does not improve.

What do you do now?

ere, we go into more depth and discuss management and indications for endovascular intervention in delayed cerebral ischemia after a ruptured aneurysm. Let us again review what is common knowledge. Delayed cerebral vasospasm and ischemia after aneurysmal subarachnoid hemorrhage (aSAH) is called "delayed" because this potentially disabling complication typically occurs after 3 days of the aneurysmal rupture and does not fully resolve for 1 to 2 weeks. Most patients with aSAH will develop angiographic vasospasm, yet only about half of them will develop clearly referable ischemic symptoms. Further, the degree of narrowing does not always correlate with the risk of ischemia and infarction. Some patients with severe large-vessel vasospasm never develop symptoms, while others with more modest spasm may develop infarctions. The clinical recognition of delayed cerebral ischemia has remained a bane for neurointensivists and neurosurgeons, and no set of clinical criteria will suffice. New focal findings, such as new brainstem findings, speech impediment, or hemiparesis, are not too common. Subtle cognitive or behavioral changes, such as disinhibition or sleepiness, are the most frequent manifestations of vasospasm (which is global more often than focal), but they are often difficult to recognize because of their lack of specificity.

Once cerebral vasospasm is established, ischemia can rapidly progress in a downward spiral despite treatment, and there has been considerable interest to find a way to prevent the arterial narrowing from developing in the first place. Many drug therapies seemed promising when studied in animal models or in preliminary trials, but almost none have ultimately proven to improve clinical outcomes. For example, statins were studied with variable results in single-center randomized trials, but in a large, international, multicenter, double-blinded, randomized trial (Simvastatin in aneurysmal subarachnoid haemorrhage [STASH]) there was no short-term or long-term benefit of simvastatin (40 mg) compared to placebo. Similarly, while clazosentan, an endothelin-1 receptor antagonist, reduced the incidence of angiographic vasospasm in a phase IIb trial (Clazosentan to Overcome Neurological Ischemia and Infarction Occurring After Subarachnoid Hemorrhage [CONSCIOUS]-1), it did not improve clinical outcomes in aSAH patients who were clipped (CONSCIOUS-2) or coiled (CONSCIOUS-3), despite improving angiographic measures of vasospasm. The lack of benefit from clazosentan was confirmed in another phase 3 trial (REACT) in which the drug did not reduce the rates of delayed cerebral ischemia. IV magnesium sulfate is yet another disappointment; the Magnesium for Aneurysmal Subarachnoid Hemorrhage (MASH)-2 trial showed no difference in outcomes for patients treated with magnesium sulfate compared to patients treated with placebo. The only intervention widely accepted in current clinical practice that has been shown to have a positive effect on outcomes related to SAH-associated vasospasm is oral nimodipine, given 60 mg every 4 hours. This is based on results from four randomized controlled trials, which showed that nimodipine prevented cerebral infarctions and improved neurological outcomes—albeit modestly—when compared to placebo. Yet it has not been shown to prevent angiographic vasospasm, which has raised questions regarding the mechanism responsible for the improved outcomes.

Some postulated that mechanically dilating blood vessels preemptively might prevent the complications from vasospasm and thus improve outcomes. One phase II multicenter randomized study of 170 patients evaluated this concept but did not find a statistically significant improvement in clinical outcomes with preemptive balloon angioplasty. Derring-do dilatation of smaller arteries at the beginning of the study resulted in fatal vessel perforations and required a revision of the protocol. Although endovascular therapy for medically refractory vasospasm was needed twice as often in the control group as in the preemptive balloon angioplasty group, this hazardous approach cannot be justified in practice without proof of clear benefit in functional outcomes. Exposing all patients to the risk of aggressive invasive treatment only to save up to half from the same treatment later is not a sound approach.

We should just improve perfusion through vasospastic arteries, large and small. It has been suggested that early placement of a lumbar drain for cerebrospinal fluid (CSF) diversion in patients with aSAH reduces symptomatic vasospasm by reducing the blood factors that trigger the mechanisms of vasospasm and by lowering intracranial pressure. Some trials evaluating early implementation of lumbar drainage showed improved outcomes with the interventions, while others have not. The EARLY DRAIN trial even compared the effect of both ventriculostomy and early lumbar drain, which as alluded to previously is a very uncommon practice. Larger well-designed prospective randomized studies are needed to validate new treatment strategies. Decisions are often at random and based on consultants' preferences. We have seen too many "protocols du jour."

For the clinician, the question remains: once cerebral vasospasm is demonstrated, how is it best handled? If the patient is asymptomatic, the focus should be on maintaining a neutral fluid balance, correcting electrolyte disturbances, and ordering full bedrest if cerebral vasospasm is severe. The concept of how to best administer IV fluids in these patients has changed over the years. We know that hypovolemia is detrimental to a patient with diffuse vasospasm because it can reduce blood flow through already narrowed vessels. Given that cerebral salt wasting is such a common phenomenon in aSAH, patients are particularly prone to hypovolemia, and any lost fluid and salt must be repleted carefully. On the other hand, markedly positive fluid balances can also be harmful. A positive fluid balance has been associated with worse outcomes in patients with aSAH. Although this can be due to an increase in cardiopulmonary complications, there may be an independent effect as well.

When we suspect a patient with delayed cerebral ischemia, we initiate hemodynamic augmentation therapy. The former approach of the "triple H" (hypervolemia, hypertension, hemodilution) has fallen out of favor, for good reasons. Hypervolemia is not sufficient to produce a sustained increase in cerebral blood flow and perfusion. Furthermore, it can impair brain oxygenation and it is the main cause of cardiopulmonary complications in these patients. More than that, there is no benefit of additional (liberal) blood transfusions (transfusion at a hemoglobin level of ≤10 g per deciliter) when compared with a restrictive strategy (transfusion at a hemoglobin level of ≤8 g per deciliter). Hemodilution, if excessive, can compromise oxygen-carrying capacity and result in insufficient brain oxygen delivery.

We rely mostly on inducing hypertension after ensuring a normovolemic state. Most frequently we use norepinephrine (rarely phenylephrine in patients who are tachycardic), and we aim to increase the mean arterial pressure by 20% to 25% as the first step. If symptoms persist, we keep raising the blood pressure, sometimes reaching mean arterial pressures of 140 mmHg. When induced hypertension fails to yield clinical improvement or in some patients who cannot tolerate this medical treatment (e.g., apical ballooning syndrome), IV milrinone is a valid alternative. Milrinone has inotropic properties and also can induce cerebral vasodilatation. The main problem with its use is that it can drop the systemic blood pressure because of peripheral vasodilatory effects, and therefore one must be ready to provide more vasopressor support. When medical treatments are ineffective or deemed contraindicated (e.g., advanced ischemic cardiomyopathy), we promptly pursue endovascular therapies. While the precise timing of when to proceed with endovascular rescue therapy remains a matter of debate, the goal should be to intervene without delay. Treatment options commonly include intra-arterial infusion of a calcium channel blocker (some practices use intra-arterial milrinone instead) for diffuse and distal vasospasm (Table 17.1 and Figure 17.1) and, less commonly, balloon angioplasty for proximal segments of large-vessel spasm (Figure 17.2).

Calcium channel antagonists such as verapamil, nimodipine, and nicardipine are the preferred agents for intra-arterial therapy. The main limitation of these drugs is a short duration of action. Intra-arterial verapamil antagonizes voltage-gated calcium channels in the arterial wall smooth muscle cells, resulting in vasodilatation. Optimal dosing is not known with certainty; some suggest limiting the total dose to 10 mg into each vascular territory but using up to 20 mg per territory is not uncommon. There are

TABLE 17.1 **Intra-Arterial Medication Options to Treat Cerebral Vasospasm**

Drug	Mechanism of Action	Half- Life (hours)	Suggested Dosing	Side Effects
Nimodipine	Dihydropyridine calcium channel blocker	8–9	1–3 mg at 25% dilution over 10–30 minutes; maximum 5 mg	Increased ICP Decreased BP
Verapamil	L-type calcium channel inhibitor	6–10	1–2 mg over 2 minutes, up to 10–20 mg per vascular territory	Increased ICP Decreased BP
Nicardipine	Dihydropyridine calcium channel blocker	14–16	0.2–0.5 mg/ mL; up to 20 mg per vascular territory	Increased ICP Decreased BP
Milrinone	Phosphodiesterase inhibitor	2–2.5	10–20 mg per vascular territory	Increased ICP Decreased BP

BP, blood pressure; ICP, intracranial pressure.

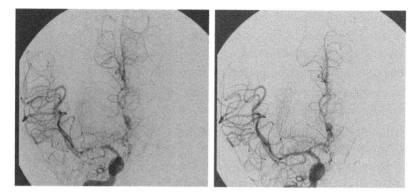

FIGURE 17.1 Digital subtraction catheter angiography shows moderate vasospasm of the right supraclinoid internal carotid artery and severe vasospasm of the right proximal middle cerebral and anterior cerebral arteries (left) with improvement in caliber after administration of intra-arterial verapamil (right).

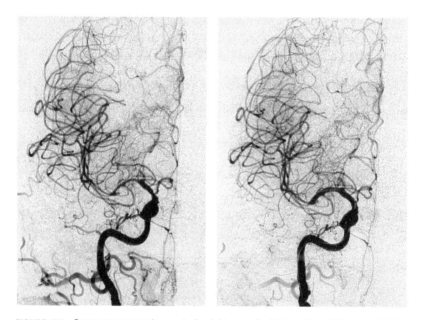

FIGURE 17.2 Severe vasospasm is seen in the right supraclinoid internal carotid artery and right M1 segment of the middle cerebral artery (left) with improvement after balloon angioplasty.

only a few case series supporting its efficacy. Intra-arterial nimodipine has also been reported to result in clinical improvement and has a slightly longer half-life. Nimodipine can be infused intra-arterially, and like the other agents the optimal dosing is unknown. Nicardipine is an alternative agent with an even longer half-life of nearly 16 hours. Intra-arterial milrinone is used in some institutions either alone or combined with a calcium channel blocker in recalcitrant cases. Complications from these agents are low but can include increased intracranial pressure, due to increased cerebral blood volume, and a drop in systemic blood pressure.

Transluminal balloon angioplasty is a more effective treatment of proximal large-vessel vasospasm but cannot be used to treat vasospasm affecting the distal cerebrovascular circulation. Angioplasty stretches the blood vessel wall, fragmenting the collagen matrix and tunica media and impairing vessel contractility. One study of 50 patients treated with angioplasty showed sustained neurological improvement within 72 hours in 61% of patients. Thus, this effect may also be transient, though it is more durable than treatment with intra-arterial calcium channel blockers alone. The intracranial arteries most amenable to angioplasty are the vertebral, basilar, and supraclinoid internal carotid arteries and M1 segments of the middle cerebral artery. Smaller-diameter vessels carry a higher risk of vessel rupture. Arterial dissection, reperfusion injury, and thromboembolic events are other possible complications. Procedural complications occur in about 2% of procedures.

Following an endovascular procedure, we keep the patient on hemodynamic augmentation and strict bedrest, avoid intravascular volume contraction, and continue to follow the neurological examination very closely. We respond to any hypotension and fever quickly. In our experience, patients with refractory vasospasm who require several sessions of intra-arterial endovascular treatment have gone on to have cerebral infarction and poor functional outcome despite aggressive treatment. Clinical results are much more favorable when the situation can be controlled with just one or two trips to the angiographic suite. Advanced age and poor clinical state at SAH ictus are independent predictors of poor outcome.

Our patient was taken for emergent cerebral angiography after her symptoms failed to improve with induced hypertension. She had both clinical and radiographic improvement following endovascular treatment with intra-arterial verapamil (Figure 17.1), but she worsened the following day. Repeat angiogram showed more severe vasospasm that was treated with balloon angioplasty and repeat intra-arterial verapamil (Figure 17.2). A third session of intra-arterial verapamil was necessary 2 days later. Ultimately she improved clinically but suffered brain infarctions at the junction of the right parietal and occipital lobes.

Three months after discharge to a skilled nursing facility, she transitioned to assisted living. She ambulated with a walker and had persistent partial visual field loss and intermittent confusion. This patient demonstrates how cerebral ischemia from symptomatic cerebral vasospasm can be a major source of long-standing disability. Previous failed attempts at finding effective measures may feel discouraging, but prevention and treatment must remain a focus of research.

KEY POINTS TO REMEMBER

- Whenever delayed cerebral ischemia is suspected, the first step is to ensure that the patient is not hypovolemic.
- We are not certain if these practices still exist, but prophylactic endovascular therapy carries risk of vascular complications and has not been shown to improve functional outcomes. Therefore, it is not an advisable approach.
- Induced hypertension is the most useful initial medical treatment to reverse symptoms of delayed cerebral ischemia. Milrinone may also help.
- Endovascular therapy is necessary when symptoms are refractory, or the patient has poor cardiopulmonary reserve and cannot tolerate hemodynamic augmentation.
- Intra-arterial infusion of calcium channel antagonists is effective to improve vasospasm in most patients, but the effect may be short-lived.
- Balloon angioplasty is the most effective treatment for proximal large-artery vasospasm and has a more durable effect but cannot treat vasospasm of the distal circulation.

Further Reading

English, S. W., Delaney, A. Fergusson, D. A. et al., for the SAHARA Trial Investigators on behalf of the Canadian Critical Care Trials Group Liberal or Restrictive Transfusion Strategy in Aneurysmal Subarachnoid Hemorrhage. *N Eng J Med* published on line December 9 2024. DOI: 10.1056

Guenego, A., R. Fahed, A. Rouchaud, et al. "Diagnosis and Endovascular Management of Vasospasm After Aneurysmal Subarachnoid Hemorrhage— Survey of Real-Life Practices." [In eng]. *J Neurointerv Surg* 16, no. 7 (Jun 17 2024): 677–83. https://doi.org/10.1136/jnis-2023-020544.

Hoh, B. L., N. U. Ko, S. Amin-Hanjani, et al. "2023 Guideline for the Management of Patients With Aneurysmal Subarachnoid Hemorrhage: A Guideline From the American Heart Association/American Stroke Association." [In eng]. *Stroke* 54, no. 7 (2023): e314–70. https://doi.org/doi:10.1161/STR.0000000000000436. https://www.ahajournals.org/doi/abs/10.1161/STR.0000000000000436.

Jun, P., N. U. Ko, J. D. English, et al. "Endovascular Treatment of Medically Refractory Cerebral Vasospasm Following Aneurysmal Subarachnoid Hemorrhage." [In eng]. *AJNR Am J Neuroradiol* 31, no. 10 (Nov 2010): 1911–16. https://doi.org/10.3174/ajnr.A2183.

Kissoon, N. R., J. N. Mandrekar, J. E. Fugate, et al. "Positive Fluid Balance Is Associated With Poor Outcomes in Subarachnoid Hemorrhage." [In eng]. *J Stroke Cerebrovasc Dis* 24, no. 10 (Oct 2015): 2245–51. https://doi.org/10.1016/j.jstrokecerebrovasdis.2015.05.027.

Pandey, A. S., A. E. Elias, N. Chaudhary, et al. "Endovascular Treatment of Cerebral Vasospasm: Vasodilators and Angioplasty." [In eng]. *Neuroimaging Clin N Am* 23, no. 4 (Nov 2013): 593–604. https://doi.org/10.1016/j.nic.2013.03.008.

Panni, P., J. E. Fugate, A. A. Rabinstein, and G. Lanzino. "Lumbar Drainage and Delayed Cerebral Ischemia in Aneurysmal Subarachnoid Hemorrhage: A Systematic Review." [In eng]. *J Neurosurg Sci* 61, no. 6 (Dec 2017): 665–72. https://doi.org/10.23736/s0390-5616.16.03151-9.

Rabinstein, A. A., J. A. Friedman, D. A. Nichols, et al. "Predictors of Outcome After Endovascular Treatment of Cerebral Vasospasm." [In eng]. *AJNR Am J Neuroradiol* 25, no. 10 (Nov–Dec 2004): 1778–82.

Shah, V. A., L. F. Gonzalez, and J. I. Suarez. "Therapies for Delayed Cerebral Ischemia in Aneurysmal Subarachnoid Hemorrhage." [In eng]. *Neurocrit Care* 39, no. 1 (Aug 2023): 36–50. https://doi.org/10.1007/s12028-023-01747-9./

Treggiari, M. M., A. A. Rabinstein, K. M. Busl, et al. "Guidelines for the Neurocritical Care Management of Aneurysmal Subarachnoid Hemorrhage." [In eng]. *Neurocrit Care* 39, no. 1 (Aug 2023): 1–28. doi:10.1007/s12028-023-01713-5.

Zwienenberg-Lee, M., J. Hartman, N. Rudisill, et al. "Effect of Prophylactic Transluminal Balloon Angioplasty on Cerebral Vasospasm and Outcome in Patients With Fisher Grade III Subarachnoid Hemorrhage: Results of a Phase II Multicenter, Randomized, Clinical Trial." [In eng]. *Stroke* 39, no. 6 (Jun 2008): 1759–65. https://doi.org/10.1161/strokeaha.107.502666.

18 Nonaneurysmal Subarachnoid Hemorrhage Turning Aneurysmal

A 44-year-old female presented with an acute thunderclap-type severe headache and had briefly lost consciousness without other clinical manifestations. She became agitated in the emergency department and did not seem to protect her airway and required brief intubation. The computed tomography (CT) scan showed unilateral filling of the entire perimesencephalic cistern and a small clot in the third ventricle (Figure 18.1). The CT pattern was consistent with a more benign variant of subarachnoid hemorrhage, also know as perimesencephalic (pretruncal) nonaneurysmal hemorrhage. The cerebral angiogram showed indistinct caliber changes in the superior cerebellar artery. Magnetic resonance imaging (MRI) of the brain vessels was normal, but the second cerebral angiogram revealed unexpectedly the development of a dissecting aneurysm of the superior cerebellar artery.

What do you do now?

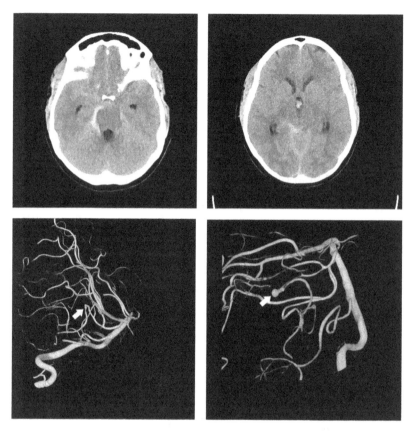

FIGURE 18.1 Upper row: CT scan of the brain shows a large blood clot in the right perimesencephalic cistern and small clot in the third ventricle. There is early hydrocephalus. Lower row: 3D views: left image shows irregularity (arrow) in the superior cerebellar artery day 1 posthemorrhage; right image day 6 posthemorrhage shows a newly formed aneurysm (arrow).

In most patients with a subarachnoid hemorrhage (SAH) in the basal cisterns, we can locate the ruptured aneurysm. In 1 in 10 patients, we find none. With no aneurysm on cerebral angiography, the distribution of hemorrhage becomes even more important, and we now know that we either have an aneurysmal pattern (many filled cisterns and fissures) or a very localized hemorrhage in the prepontine or perimesencephalic cisterns.

An SAH with such a localized pattern was characterized by the SAH Study Group from the Erasmus University in Rotterdam, the Netherlands, in

1985, and this perimesencephalic SAH variant was further characterized in a larger series of patients. The main observation has remained unchallenged. Patients invariably present clinically in a good-grade SAH and are seldom affected by it. Once a cerebral angiogram has excluded a posterior circulation aneurysm, rebleeding does not occur; cerebral vasospasm, if it occurs at all, can be in the basilar artery or diffusely spread throughout the cerebral circulation but generally does not lead to cerebral infarction. A few patients require a ventriculostomy due to CSF flow interruption—not at the cortex (where we find no blood) but in front of the brainstem when CSF moves upward with a pulsatile motion. Outcomes are typically excelllent.

MRI in later studies found that the hemorrhage fills the premedullary cistern and only secondarily affects the perimesencephalic region; thus, an alternative descriptive term, "pretruncal nonaneurysmal SAH," was suggested. (*Truncus cerebri* is Latin for brainstem.) This is not a simple semantic issue because we were concerned that these perimesencephalic hemorrhages could represent other entities.

This patient greatly surprised us because the supposedly ("classic") nonaneurysmal perimesencephalic SAH became aneurysmal on subsequent cerebral angiogram and even after MRI of the brain vessels. How could this have happened? Certainly, it was a worrisome development. Should we have done more cerebral angiograms in our prior patients, which had given us reassurance for so many years? in so many patient? Looking back at the first 3D digital subtraction angiography (DSA), we see irregularity, but so many 3D DSA studies have that indistinct finding.

It made us reflect on this a bit more. Are there perhaps two patterns of these hemorrhages without an aneurysm? The nearly exclusive localization of blood unilaterally in the perimesencephalic or ambient cistern is a distinctive feature here. The other, more typical distribution we see is pretruncal (before the truncus cerebri or brainstem) and therefore the term pretruncal nonaneurysmal subarachnoid hemorrhage is more accurate (Figure 18.2).

Intraventricular blood can appear due to CSF circulation, but it is unusual for pretruncal SAH. Equally problematic is the patient's thunderclap headache. Often these hemorrhages do not start like a split-second headache and have a more gradual onset. Loss of consciousness, which prompted

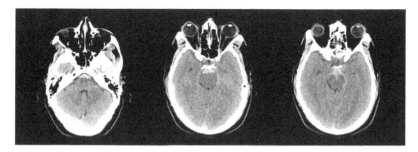

FIGURE 18.2 A more typical example of this variant. Note the hemorrhage is more concentrated in front of the brainstem with some extension into the ambient cistern (pretruncal).

the emergency department to intubate her, is even more unusual because the presentation is typically benign (we have found that loss of consciousness at onset is a reliable predictor that the bleeding is aneurysmal). This would of course point toward a ruptured aneurysm we initially failed to find. It is a stroke of luck we found it on the second angiogram.

This pretruncal variant of SAH has generated interest over the years. Multiple observations have been published; each claimed to have found the cause of a nonaneurysmal perimesencephalic hemorrhage. Most suggestions involved venous anomalies and arterial dissections. Candidate vessels for rupture are determined by which cistern has the largest amount of blood. However, a clear distinction cannot always be made. The ambient cistern is located lateral to the midbrain and posterior to the thalamus. It contains several blood vessels (posterior cerebral artery, superior cerebellar artery, and basal vein of Rosenthal) in addition to the trochlear nerve. The prepontine cistern is situated between the pons and the clivus. Generally, cranial nerves are not found in the prepontine cistern, but occasionally the sixth nerve courses in the prepontine cistern. The basilar artery traverses through this cistern and gives rise to the anterior inferior cerebellar artery and superior cerebellar cistern. The cistern also includes the anterior pontomesencephalic vein.

We and others have speculated that dissections (blister formation) are the main culprit. Arguments for this explanation include (1) small hemorrhage compatible with a dissection; (2) common-wall irregularity on some studies, often misinterpreted as early vasospasm; and (3) occasional presence of infarcts in the pons. However, more recently, a 3D cerebral angiogram showed small basilar artery outpouches that may appear and then disappear. Thrombosis and recanalization may explain the radiologic findings of reappearance of a small aneurysm after follow-up angiogram.

Other studies have repeatedly shown abnormal venous drainage patterns in patients with perimesencephalic nonaneurysmal hemorrhage, but in patients examined, venous structures in the interpeduncular or prepontine cisterns are without abnormalities except for an occasionally engorged anterior pontomesencephalic vein or an anomalous anastomotic cisternal vein. Some autopsy studies have found ruptured pontine perforating arteries, but a CT correlate has not been published, and no patient with a nonaneurysmal perimesencephalic hemorrhage has come to autopsy soon after the initial hemorrhage. In a patient with a pretruncal clot, we even found a CSF leak on an MRI in the cervical spine, which was done after the MRI showed unexpected descent of aqueduct and cerebellar tonsils (brain sagging). The mechanism here is different and likely involves venous engorgement from brain sagging and bleeding.

The discovery of a separate entity in a population of patients with "angiographic-negative SAH" means that neurologists and neurosurgeons now must specifically distinguish between three patterns—"perimesencephalic," "aneurysmal," and "nonaneurysmal/nonperimesencephalic"—basically distributed in the sulci. Sulcal hemorrhage (exclusively over the cerebral convexity) has another set of differential diagnoses, including trauma (most common), diffuse intravascular coagulation with consumptive thrombocytopenia, cerebral amyloid angiopathy, septic emboli, vascular malformation, cerebral venous thrombosis, and vasculitis (least common).

The widespread practice is that patients with an aneurysmal-pattern SAH have a cerebral angiogram as soon as feasible (except those presenting in an extremely poor condition or at very advanced age). When the first cerebral angiogram is negative (i.e., showing no aneurysm), a second and even a third cerebral angiogram is performed to definitively exclude a ruptured aneurysm. The yield of a revealed aneurysm in these repeated studies is relatively high, up to 11% in our series and more than 20% of cases in others. For many neurosurgeons, concerns remain even when patients have had repetitively negative cerebral angiograms. However, studies have emphasized a much better outcome in the nonaneurysm variant. One theory is that the aneurysm destroyed itself during rupture and the artery healed naturally. Regardless, rebleed rates in these patients are exceptionally low (but not zero).

The quandary is whether to be suspicious that an aneurysm has been missed or might form again a few days later. Given our example showing predominant perimesencephalic cistern involvement, you would think so. But can we make a reasonable argument to stop after a satisfactory 3D cerebral angiogram in other nonaneurysmal patterns, such as the isolated prepontine variant? When the presentation is benign (especially if the headache is not thunderclap), the answer is probably yes. In any event, we should carefully question patients about the quality of their headaches. If they worsen when sitting up (orthostatic headache), do an MRI of the brain. If there is unambiguous evidence of brain sagging, a spine MRI can identify or rule out a CSF leak. When brain sagging is absent (and we suspect this in many), we may be justified to hold off on further tests. As a result of improved imaging technology (and increased detection), decisions in these variants have become a lot more complicated and perhaps our threshold for a second cerebral angiogram should be lower. Are you still confused on what to do exactly? You should be!

KEY POINTS TO REMEMBER

- Failure to demonstrate a ruptured aneurysm depends on imaging mode (3D cerebral angiogram vs. CT angiogram) and distribution of bleeding pattern on CT scan.
- The clinical course is favorable but complicated with increased risk for diffuse cerebral vasospasm and acute obstructive hydrocephalus, which may need interventions.
- There is a low likelihood that a repeat cerebral angiogram will show an aneurysm later. If it does, re-review of the first study often identifies an arterial irregularity.
- Repeat cerebral angiogram may show the emergence of a dissecting aneurysm that may disappear when left untreated.
- MRI of the brain may be additionally needed to exclude brain sagging as a triggering cause.

Further Reading

Huttner, H. B., M. Hartmann, M. Köhrmann, et al. "Repeated Digital Subtraction Angiography After Perimesencephalic Subarachnoid Hemorrhage?" [In eng]. *J Neuroradiol* 33, no. 2 (Apr 2006): 87–89. https://doi.org/10.1016/s0150-9861(06)77236-4.

Mensing, L. A., M. D. I. Vergouwen, K. G. Laban, et al. "Perimesencephalic Hemorrhage: A Review of Epidemiology, Risk Factors, Presumed Cause, Clinical Course, and Outcome." [In eng]. *Stroke* 49, no. 6 (Jun 2018): 1363–70. https://doi.org/10.1161/strokeaha.117.019843.

Ossuna, M., M. A. Zanini, and P. T. Hamamoto Filho. "Nonaneurysmal Perimesencephalic Subarachnoid Hemorrhage Associated with an Anomalous Anastomotic Cisternal Vein." [In eng]. *World Neurosurg* 189 (Jun 18 2024): 201–2. doi:10.1016/j.wneu.2024.06.070.

Ringelstein, A., O. Mueller, O. Timochenko, et al. "Reangiographie nach perimesenzephaler Subarachnoidalblutung. [Reangiography After Perimesencephalic Subarachnoid Hemorrhage]." [In ger]. *Nervenarzt* 84, no. 6 (Jun 2013): 715–19. https://doi.org/10.1007/s00115-013-3803-y.

Rinkel, G. J., E. F. Wijdicks, M. Vermeulen, et al. "The Clinical Course of Perimesencephalic Nonaneurysmal Subarachnoid Hemorrhage." [In eng]. *Ann Neurol* 29, no. 5 (May 1991): 463–68. https://doi.org/10.1002/ana.410290503.

Rinkel, G. J., E. F. Wijdicks, M. Vermeulen, et al. "Nonaneurysmal Perimesencephalic Subarachnoid Hemorrhage: CT and MR Patterns That Differ From Aneurysmal Rupture." [In eng]. *AJNR Am J Neuroradiol* 12, no. 5 (Sep–Oct 1991): 829–34.

Roman-Filip, I., V. Morosanu, Z. Bajko, C. Roman-Filip, and R. I. Balasa. "Non-Aneurysmal Perimesencephalic Subarachnoid Hemorrhage: A Literature Review." [In eng]. *Diagnostics* 13 (2023): 1195. doi:10.3390/diagnostics13061195.

Rouchaud, A., V. T. Lehman, M. H. Murad, et al. "Nonaneurysmal Perimesencephalic Hemorrhage Is Associated with Deep Cerebral Venous Drainage Anomalies: A Systematic Literature Review and Meta-Analysis." [In eng]. *AJNR Am J Neuroradiol* 37, no. 9 (Sep 2016): 1657–63. doi:10.3174/ajnr.A4806.

Scheitler, K. M., C. L. Nesvick, and E. F. Wijdicks. "Pretruncal Subarachnoid Hemorrhage in a Patient With Cerebrospinal Fluid Leak." [In eng]. *Neurocrit Care* 34, no. 1 (Feb 2021): 350–53. https://doi.org/10.1007/s12028-020-01030-1.

Schievink, W. I., E. F. Wijdicks, and R. F. Spetzler. "Diffuse Vasospasm After Pretruncal Nonaneurysmal Subarachnoid Hemorrhage." [In eng]. *AJNR Am J Neuroradiol* 21, no. 3 (Mar 2000): 521–23.

van Gijn, J., K. J. van Dongen, M. Vermeulen, and A. Hijdra. "Perimesencephalic Hemorrhage: A Nonaneurysmal and Benign Form of Subarachnoid Hemorrhage." [In eng]. *Neurology* 35, no. 4 (Apr 1985): 493–97. https://doi.org/10.1212/wnl.35.4.493.

White, J. B., E. F. Wijdicks, H. J. Cloft, and D. F. Kallmes. "Vanishing Aneurysm in Pretruncal Nonaneurysmal Subarachnoid Hemorrhage." [In eng]. *Neurology* 71, no. 17 (Oct 21 2008): 1375–77. https://doi.org/10.1212/01.wnl.0000327 684.85469.b2.

Wijdicks, E. F., W. I. Schievink, and G. M. Miller. "Pretruncal Nonaneurysmal Subarachnoid Hemorrhage." [In eng]. *Mayo Clin Proc* 73, no. 8 (Aug 1998): 745–52. https://doi.org/10.4065/73.8.745.

Wijdicks, E. F. M., S. Braksick, and L. Rinaldo. "Perimesencephalic Hemorrhage from A Superior Cerebellar Artery Dissection." *Ann Neurol* 94, no. 6 (Dec 2023): 1164–5. doi:10.1002/ana.26779. Epub 2023 Sep 14.

19 Options in Acute Spinal Cord Compression Due to Cancer

A seemingly healthy 70-year-old man with no major medical history presents with a 3-week history of dull back pain. The pain is nagging, not shooting, and unassociated with tingling or electrical shock–like sensations. He denies sensory symptoms or urinary retention. His wife tells us that he has noted some leg weakness and has had frequent falls. When specifically asked, she also mentions that he has had a 20-pound weight loss. His neurological examination confirms that he can walk but also reveals proximal leg muscle weakness (Medical Research Council grade 4/5). No sensory level is found. He has hyperreflexia with clonus. There is pain to percussion at the thoracic spine level. Computed tomography (CT) and magnetic resonance imaging (MRI) show destructive lesions in the left superior pubic ramus and multiple other lesions in the spine. The largest lesion at T7 involves the posterior body pedicle with epidural extension and spinal cord displacement. His prostate-specific antigen (PSA) level is over 400 ng/mL. He has a fair amount of pain but does not think his leg weakness is worsening. His wife disagrees.

What do you do now?

Cancer can take a profound turn for the worse with spinal cord compression. Spinal cord compression may be the presenting symptom of metastatic disease—estimated in one of four patients—as it was in our patient. Common causes of compression are breast, prostate, renal, and lung cancers as well as non-Hodgkin lymphoma and myeloma. All too often, patients wait until damage is irreversible. Such a serious presentation requires a careful assessment of treatment options, and there are a few. One of the first decisions is to break down the lesion's place in the spine (Figure 19.1) and outside the spine and how the mass encroaches on the spinal cord.

The oncological prognosis generally guides decisions to proceed with surgical decompression. This is not as straightforward as it seems, and the likelihood of a patient with pretreatment motor dysfunction being able to recover ambulation is uncertain. However, a patient who can walk at the

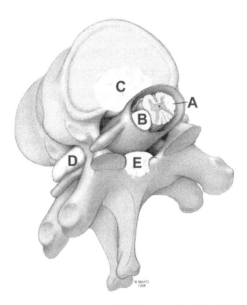

FIGURE 19.1 Several metastatic lesions capable of compressing the spinal cord. Localization of metastatic lesions in compartments inside the spinal canal: intramedullary process (A); leptomeningeal process (B); process in vertebral body extending into the epidural space (C); paravertebral process (D); and epidural process (E).

(Modified from Byrne TN. Spinal cord compression from epidural metastases. *N Engl J Med* 1992;327:614. With permission of the Massachusetts Medical Society.)

time of the intervention will probably continue to walk, and patients with slow-onset motor deficits typically have a better outcome than patients with a more rapid onset. Life expectancy prediction, in general, is difficult, but scoring systems are helpful. One example is the Tokuhashi score (Table 19.1). Several elements take life expectancy into account; in this scoring system, the primary site of the neoplasm and the neurological deficit are the most important predictors of survival.

In this patient, our main priority was assessing the degree of metastatic epidural compression of the spinal cord. The potential instability of the spine is unquestionably troubling. MRI can be graded by the Bilsky grading scale (Table 19.2), which specifically looks at instability (vertebral body collapse and posterolateral involvement of the spinal elements such as facet, pedicle, or costovertebral joint fracture). Others have used The Spinal Instability Neoplastic Score (SINS) to evaluate spinal instability due to a neoplastic process again focusing on spine location, mechanical or postural pain, presence of lytic lesions, spinal alignment, vertebral body involvement and whether located posteriorly. None of these scales or scores correlate well with surgical outcome.

There are several medical and surgical approaches to this clinical problem (Box 19.1). All patients receive corticosteroids immediately. It is uncertain whether to use a high-dose dexamethasone (100 mg/d) or a moderate dose (16 mg/d). Most physicians prefer an initial high dose in rapidly worsening patients.

The next priority is to determine whether the patient is a surgical candidate. In patients with pain only, stable neurological findings, and a radiosensitive tumor, radiotherapy is the first option. Criteria favoring operative management include rapidly progressing motor deficit, instability of the spine on MRI scan, medically intractable pain, and incomplete neurological injury. Some algorithms also include complete sensory and motor paraplegia over 24 hours as a reason to proceed with surgery. However, most patients receive external-beam radiotherapy, which requires a total of 30 Gy in 10 fractions. Radiotherapy is not considered in radio-resistant tumors, such as renal cell carcinoma. If the tumor is not radiosensitive, vertebroplasty or kyphoplasty with or without open stabilization surgery is an option.

Pain treatment is essential not only before but also during and after radiotherapy. There are many options for adequate pain management.

TABLE 19.1 **Tokuhashi Revised Scoring System for Preoperative Prognosis of Metastatic Spinal Tumors**

Parameter	Score
General condition	
Poor (PS 10%–40%)	0
Moderate (PS 50%–70%)	1
Good (PS 80%–100%)	2
No. of extraspinal metastases	
>3	0
1–2	1
0	2
No. of vertebral body metastases	
>3	0
2	1
1	2
Metastases to the major internal organs	
Nonremovable	0
Removable	1
None	2
Primary site of cancer	
Lung, stomach, bladder, bone, esophagus, pancreas	0
Liver, gallbladder, unidentified	1
Others	2
Kidney, uterus	3
Rectum	4
Thyroid, breast, prostate, carcinoid	5
Palsy or myelopathy	
Complete	0
Incomplete	1
None	2

The lower the score, the worse the prognosis. Those patients scoring from 0 to 8 have a prognosis of less than 6 months to live; a score of 9 to 11, between 6 and 12 months; and a score of 12 to 15, more than a year.

PS, performance status.

Adapted from Tokuhashi et al. *Spine* 2005; 30(19): 2186–91. Used with permission of Wolters Kluwer Health, Inc.

TABLE 19.2 MRI Bilsky Grading Scale

Bilsky 0	Tumor that is confined to the bone (i.e., without epidural involvement)
Bilsky 1a	Tumor with epidural involvement but without indentation of the thecal sac
Bilsky 1b	Tumor with epidural involvement and indentation of the thecal sac but without spinal cord contact
Bilsky 1c	Tumor with epidural involvement and spinal cord contact without cord compression
Bilsky 2	Tumor with epidural involvement and compression of the spinal cord but without obliteration of the surrounding CSF spaces
Bilsky 3	Tumor with epidural involvement and severe compression of the spinal cord with complete obliteration of the surrounding CSF spaces

A typical approach is using transdermal patches of fentanyl that can be changed every 3 to 4 days; oxycodone, 10 to 20 mg every 2 hours as needed; or hydromorphone, 4 mg every 4 hours. These generally provide good pain palliation. For patients with significant neuropathic pain (that may come

---

BOX 19.1 Treatment Options in Acute Spinal Cord Compression From Cancer

Assess surgical options
  Tokuhashi score
  Good surgical candidate?
  Instability?
Assess radiotherapy option
  Radiosensitive?
  Degree of spinal cord compression?
Assess options to minimize effect of tumor
  Corticosteroids
  Opioids
  Bisphosphonates
  Chemotherapy

later), gabapentin, 100 mg twice a day and 300 mg at bedtime, is a good starting dose; the medication could be titrated to a target between 1800 and 3600 mg/d. Bone pain adjuvants are necessary as well, and these include zoledronic acid, 4 mg intravenously every 3 to 4 weeks, or pamidronate, 90 mg intravenously every 3 to 4 weeks. Many patients will need bladder catheterization, and most can learn self-catheterization. Bowel regimen is also provided with bisacodyl or glycerin suppository daily, and docusate plus senna.

How did we manage our patient? His Tokuhashi revised score was 10, thus predicting a 6- to 12-month life expectancy. The patient underwent an orchidectomy that resulted in a good response, based on his PSA level. He was reluctant to undergo surgery and favored radiotherapy first. He was scheduled to undergo two to five radiation cycles, but unfortunately, he became paraplegic quite rapidly after three sessions of radiation. This resulted in immediate decompressive surgery, but the paraplegia persisted. Despite this motor deficit, he remained relatively functional and lived for another 4 years.

This case aptly illustrates the difficulty of choosing radiotherapy over surgery. This patient's decision to postpone surgery seemed justified due to his advanced age and the absence of any major neurological deficit. The sudden appearance of paraplegia may have had a vascular cause, as ischemic myelopathy is not uncommon in this situation. It is uncertain whether earlier epidural decompression would have prevented it. Overall, even with 45 to 50 Gy, delivered in 2 Gy/d fractions, external-beam radiation therapy carries a very low risk of radiation myelopathy (0.03%–0.2%), and rarely this complication does occur within the first 6 months after radiotherapy. Life-expectancy prediction after epidural spine compression is difficult and remains a gross estimation. This is particularly true in patients with metastatic prostate cancer who have a good response to castration, since they may have an extended period of survival with reasonable quality of life.

Outcome depends on the type and spread of the tumor, age and functional condition of the patient, severity of presentation, and location of the lesion. Compression occurs mostly in the thoracic segments with a much lower incidence in the lower spine. Not infrequently (up to a third of cases), imaging of the entire spine reveals multiple levels of compression. Survival can be short and measured in months when multiple segments are involved, but rehabilitation physicians have found that preservation of mobility is the main driver of outcome.

> **KEY POINTS TO REMEMBER**
>
> - Outcome after metastatic epidural cord compression is dependent on the type of tumor, radiosensitivity, rapidity of progression of neurological symptoms, and instability of the spine.
> - Aggressive surgical management is not indicated if there is pain only and no major neurological deficit.
> - Aggressive pain management with opioids and corticosteroids may provide adequate palliation.
> - The treatment modality that is best for the patient is determined based on the severity and acuity of the neurological deficit, nature of the tumor, instability of the spine, and general performance status and life expectancy of the patient.

Further Reading

Bobinski, L., J. Axelsson, J. Melhus, J. Åkerstedt, and J. Wänman. "The Spinal Instability Neoplastic Score Correlates with Epidural Spinal Cord Compression — A Retrospective Cohort of 256 Surgically Treated Patients with Spinal Metastases." [In eng]. *BMC Musculoskelet Disord* 25, no. 1 (Aug 15 2024): 644. doi:10.1186/s12891-024-07756-9.

Graber, J. J., and C. P. Nolan. "Myelopathies in Patients With Cancer." [In eng]. *Arch Neurol* 67, no. 3 (Mar 2010): 298–304. https://doi.org/10.1001/archneurol.2010.20.

Kuah, T., B. A. Vellayappan, A. Makmur, et al. "State-of-the-Art Imaging Techniques in Metastatic Spinal Cord Compression." [In eng]. *Cancers (Basel)* 14, no. 13 (Jul 5 2022): 3289. doi:10.3390/cancers14133289. PMID: 35805059.

O'Phelan, K. H., E. B. Bunney, S. D. Weingart, and W. S. Smith. "Emergency Neurological Life Support: Spinal Cord Compression (SCC)." [In eng]. *Neurocrit Care* 17, no. Suppl 1 (Sep 2012): S96–101. https://doi.org/10.1007/s12 028-012-9756-3.

Ong, W. L., S. Wong, H. Soliman, et al. "Radiation Myelopathy Following Stereotactic Body Radiation Therapy for Spine Metastases." [In eng]. *J Neurooncol* 159, no. 1 (Aug 2022): 23–31. https://doi.org/10.1007/s11060-022-04037-0.

Quraishi, N. A., Z. L. Gokaslan, and S. Boriani. "The Surgical Management of Metastatic Epidural Compression of the Spinal Cord." [In eng]. *J Bone Joint Surg Br* 92, no. 8 (Aug 2010): 1054–60. https://doi.org/10.1302/0301-620x.92b8.22296.

Ribas, E. S., and D. Schiff. "Spinal Cord Compression." [In eng]. *Curr Treat Options Neurol* 14, no. 4 (Aug 2012): 391–401. https://doi.org/10.1007/s11940-012-0176-7.

Ropper, A. E., and A. H. Ropper. "Acute Spinal Cord Compression." [In eng]. *N Engl J Med* 376, no. 14 (Apr 6 2017): 1358–69. https://doi.org/10.1056/NEJMra1516539.

Switlyk, M. D., U. Kongsgaard, S. Skjeldal, et al. "Prognostic Factors in Patients With Symptomatic Spinal Metastases and Normal Neurological Function." [In eng]. *Clin Oncol (R Coll Radiol)* 27, no. 4 (Apr 2015): 213–21. https://doi.org/10.1016/j.clon.2015.01.002.

Tokuhashi, Y., H. Matsuzaki, H. Oda, et al. "A Revised Scoring System for Preoperative Evaluation of Metastatic Spine Tumor Prognosis." [In eng]. *Spine (Phila Pa 1976)* 30, no. 19 (Oct 1 2005): 2186–91. https://doi.org/10.1097/01.brs.0000180 401.06919.a5.

20 Unanticipated Paraplegia After Aortic Repair

A 58-year-old man with hypertension, diabetes mellitus, and hyperlipidemia underwent a complex cardiovascular surgery with aortic valve and root replacement, modified total aortic arch replacement, and endovascular stent graft placement in the distal thoracic aorta. The surgery lasted 10 hours. Multimodal intraoperative neurophysiologic monitoring did not identify significant somatosensory evoked potential changes (defined as a ≥50% decrease in the cortical amplitude or a ≥10% prolongation of latency from baseline values). But unexpectedly, he could not move his legs following the surgery. We were called emergently to evaluate him in the surgical intensive care unit. On examination, we found a flaccid paraplegia and a sensory level to pinprick at the thoracic level (T10), below which he had no sensation to pinprick. His systemic blood pressure was 92/60 mmHg.

What do you do now?

With no warning signs during intraoperative monitoring, this was a surprise. What can be done now? Can any intervention ameliorate acute spinal cord ischemia and improve paraplegia?

Spinal cord infarction (SCI) or ischemia is a rare cause of myelopathy that usually affects adults in their 50s to 70s. Sudden flaccid paraplegia or quadriplegia, areflexia, loss of sensation to pain and temperature, and autonomic dysfunction (urinary retention and later ileus) are all key features, and the diagnosis is primarily clinical. Magnetic resonance imaging (MRI) of the thoracic and lumbar spine is the diagnostic modality of choice if SCI is suspected. (A high-quality computed tomography [CT] scan of the spine may exclude epidural hematoma, but it can fail to do so.) If the infarct is established, T2-weighted and fluid-attenuated inversion recovery sequences may show hyperintense signal within the cord (possibly in an "owl eyes" pattern on axial slices because of ventral gray matter vulnerability, shown in Figure 20.1). However, if hyperacute, the images may be unremarkable due to limited sensitivity of diffusion-weighted imaging, primarily related to its image distortion and artifact.

The neurological examination is diagnostic. Involvement of the corticospinal, pyramidal, and spinothalamic tracts and anterior horns results in flaccid paraplegia and absent sensation to pinprick, hot and cold, and light touch. Although the anatomic location of the watershed-perfusion

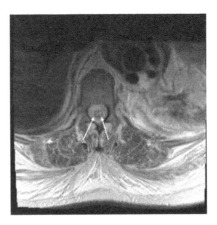

FIGURE 20.1 Axial T2-weighted MRI of the lower thoracic spinal cord shows characteristic hyperintense signal abnormalities in the ventral gray matter bilaterally (arrows, "owl's eyes") indicative of spinal cord infarction.

area suggests the midthoracic region as the most common sensory-level site, the sensory level is most frequently noted around T10. Proprioception and vibratory sense should be spared because the posterior column is not perfused by the anterior spinal artery, which is the vessel most commonly responsible for SCI. However, these sensory modalities may appear impaired on early examination, and in such instances, appropriate imaging may help to exclude spinal cord compression from an epidural hematoma. Subsequent examinations typically confirm that the patient appropriately perceives vibration and position. We must check for rectal sphincter tone, which may be lost. Flaccid-type paraplegia may occur, but the flexor reflex may manifest as (often violent) spasms once the spinal shock phase passes. Early hypotension from spinal shock is common.

The most common setting in which SCI occurs is as a complication of open or endovascular thoracoabdominal aortic surgery. Risk factors for SCI include a larger extent of aortic involvement, longer cross-clamp time, longer duration of operation, preoperative renal failure, previous aortic surgery, cardiovascular risk factors (e.g., hypertension, diabetes mellitus), and perioperative hypotension. However, few patients have spinal cord injury after major surgery, and the prevalence, with traditional surgery or endovascular repair, has remained stable for both interventions at about 2% to 3%. One study found older age (>65 years), prior neurologic disease, hyperlipidemia, coronary heart disease, heart failure, poor renal function, less than 6 months since last aortic repair, chronic anticoagulant use, preoperative thrombocytopenia and coagulopathy, and anatomic location of aneurysm caudal to T11 as risk factors for SCI after all types of aortic repair. In other words, SCI after thoracoabdominal surgery mostly occurs in patients with significant co-morbidity.

Several mechanisms can contribute to SCI in the perioperative period. First, clamping of the proximal thoracoabdominal aorta during the procedure temporarily interrupts blood supply to the spinal cord. Second, some segmental arteries arising from the aorta or subclavian artery supplying the spinal cord are permanently interrupted during the surgery. A combination of these two mechanisms may occur (e.g., clamping-related ischemic injury followed by marginal postoperative blood supply secondary to vessel sacrifice), and unstable hemodynamics can exacerbate the injury. Spinal cord ischemia is also a major complication of thoracic endovascular aortic repair (TEVAR) and fenestrated-branched endovascular aortic repair (F-BEVAR). Many surgeons prefer intra-operative monitoring of spinal function, which allows real time feedback, but it comes with high costs and uncertainty about its ability to detect and reduce spinal cord injury. Neuromonitoring with motor and sensory evoked potentials detect perioperative changes in spinal cord function but there are major discrepancies between changes with neuromonitoring and actual later post-operative spinal cord infarction, suggesting that monitoring is far from flawless.

How can we further minimize the risk of this debilitating complication? Most cardiovascular surgeons use hypothermia during extensive aortic procedures to slow the metabolism of spinal cord neurons, which prolongs the safe ischemic interval by a factor of 2.3 for every 10°C drop in temperature. Another intervention is placing a catheter in the lumbar subarachnoid space to drain cerebrospinal fluid (CSF) during and after the procedure. A randomized controlled trial evaluating the use of CSF drainage during and after open aortic surgery found that approximately 12% of patients without lumbar drainage developed postoperative paraparesis/paraplegia compared to only 3% of patients with lumbar drains. The study can be criticized, however, because the percentage in the untreated group was unusually high. In that study, drainage was continuous at 10 mmHg. Others advocate intermittent drainage (e.g., 10 mL drained every 2–4 hours) and a target lumbar CSF pressure of 10 to 12 mmHg (or 8–10 mmHg in the event of active or refractory signs of ischemia). If no neurological deficits occur, it is safe to remove the lumbar drain on the second postoperative day

Lumbar drain placement is a major procedure and requires procedural skill to avoid serious mishaps. Catheter-related morbidity is low (~4%), but lumbar drain–associated adverse events include lumbar epidural or subdural hematoma, catheter fracture, CSF leak, meningitis, and remote cerebellar or cerebral hemorrhage due to CSF hypotension and brain sagging. To minimize these risks, we remove the drain as soon as no longer necessary, and avoid excessive CSF drainage and anticoagulation.

Increasing mean arterial pressure (MAP) can also increase spinal cord perfusion. We must avoid lingering perioperative hypotension in patients who have undergone extensive aortic surgery. If they develop signs of post-operative SCI, we routinely induce hypertension by raising the MAP in increments of 10 to 20 mmHg to 85 to 90 mmHg in addition to lumbar CSF drainage. While perioperative lumbar drainage is not standard in all major institutions, it is a viable treatment option for acute SCI.

Although a few vascular surgeons use high-dose corticosteroids, there is no proven benefit of corticosteroids in resolving spinal cord ischemia or mitigating ischemic reperfusion insult. Additionally, high-dose corticosteroids are associated with adverse effects including hyperglycemia, gastric ulcer, greater risk of infection, and poor healing of the surgical incision. Therefore, we see no reason to use corticosteroids in the management of SCI.

Box 20.1 shows a stepwise approach when confronting acute spinal cord ischemia after vascular repair irrespective of ischemic findings on MRI.

How do patients ultimately fare? SCI can cause severe disability and even death from complications of immobilization. However, patients can potentially achieve substantial functional improvement over time. A main driver of prognosis is the severity of the neurological deficits at nadir. Unsurprisingly, patients with complete or nearly complete motor and sensory loss have worse long-term outcomes than those with a more benign clinical presentation. However, even some patients with severe deficits at onset may achieve substantial recovery. Factors associated with poorer prognosis include older age, female gender, and more extensive ischemic changes on MRI. In our experience of 115 patients with SCI with mean follow-up of 3 years, the mortality rate was 23%. Of 74 wheelchair-bound patients at the time of discharge, 41% were ambulatory at their last follow-up. At dismissal, 83 patients had indwelling urinary catheters due to persistent bladder

---

BOX 20.1 **Management Options for Postoperative Acute Spinal Cord Ischemia**

Increase MAP with vasopressors to 85–90 mmHg

Place lumbar drain, drain 10 mL, and maintain CSF pressure at 10 mmHg to a limit of drainage every hour, i.e., no more than 20 mL/h

Gradually reduce dose of vasopressors after 48 hours

When off vasopressors and tolerated well, wean lumbar drain by increasing height of lumbar drainage 5 mmHg every 12 hours and cap before 20 mmHg

CSF, cerebrospinal fluid; MAP, mean arterial pressure.

dysfunction, but at last follow-up, 33% of these patients were catheter-free. Others have reported similar experiences.

What happened to our patient? He was treated with hemodynamic augmentation with intravenous norepinephrine infusion and emergent lumbar CSF drainage. After these interventions, he regained the ability to move his legs to some extent. He was weaned from the vasopressor after 2 days, and the lumbar drain was removed on day 3, once his examination was stable. He was discharged to a rehabilitation unit, wheelchair dependent, but a year later, he was able to walk with a walker.

Overall, this dramatic postoperative complication is actually sometimes treatable with blood pressure augmentation and placement of a lumbar drain. Patients may improve over time, some more than we would have thought possible. However, we may sometimes be forced to accept permanent spinal cord injury as a clinical outcome to be managed with spine neurorehabilitation.

KEY POINTS TO REMEMBER

- Spinal cord ischemia occurs most commonly as a result of major aortic repair.
- Most patients with spinal cord ischemia present with acute flaccid weakness, absent sensation below a specific sensory level, and sphincter dysfunction.
- Treatment is to increase spinal cord perfusion with a combination of CSF drainage and augmentation of blood pressure targeted to a MAP of 85 to 90 mmHg.
- Spinal cord infarction is often disabling initially, but some patients with incomplete injury will still achieve a favorable functional outcome.

Further Reading

Behzadi, F., J. E. Simon, T. J. Zielke, et al. "Risk Factors Associated With Spinal Cord Ischemia During Aortic Aneurysm Repair." [In eng]. *Ann Vasc Surg* 91 (Apr 2023): 36–49. https://doi.org/10.1016/j.avsg.2022.12.079.

Coselli, J. S., S. A. LeMaire, C. Köksoy, et al. "Cerebrospinal Fluid Drainage Reduces Paraplegia After Thoracoabdominal Aortic Aneurysm Repair: Results of a

Randomized Clinical Trial." [In eng]. *J Vasc Surg* 35, no. 4 (Apr 2002): 631–39. https://doi.org/10.1067/mva.2002.122024.

Hanson, S. R., F. Romi, T. Rekand, and H. Naess. "Long-Term Outcome After Spinal Cord Infarctions." [In eng]. *Acta Neurol Scand* 131, no. 4 (Apr 2015): 253–57. https://doi.org/10.1111/ane.12343.

Kawaharada, N., K. Morishita, Y. Kurimoto, et al. "Spinal Cord Ischemia After Elective Endovascular Stent-Graft Repair of the Thoracic Aorta." [In eng]. *Eur J Cardiothorac Surg* 31, no. 6 (Jun 2007): 998–1003; discussion 1003. https://doi.org/10.1016/j.ejcts.2007.01.069.

Khan, N. R., Z. Smalley, C. L. Nesvick, et al. "The Use of Lumbar Drains in Preventing Spinal Cord Injury Following Thoracoabdominal Aortic Aneurysm Repair: An Updated Systematic Review and Meta-Analysis." [In eng]. *J Neurosurg Spine* 25, no. 3 (Sep 2016): 383–93. https://doi.org/10.3171/2016.1.Spine151199.

Lambrechts, M. J., T. Z. Issa, and A. S. Hilibrand. "Updates in the Early Management of Acute Spinal Cord Injury." *J Am Acad Orthop Surg* 31, no. 17 (Sep 1 2023): e619–32. https://doi.org/10.5435/JAAOS-D-23-0028.

Masson, C., J. P. Pruvo, J. F. Meder, et al. "Spinal Cord Infarction: Clinical and Magnetic Resonance Imaging Findings and Short Term Outcome." [In eng]. *J Neurol Neurosurg Psychiatry* 75, no. 10 (Oct 2004): 1431–35. https://doi.org/10.1136/jnnp.2003.031724.

Rabinstein, A. A. "Vascular Myelopathies." [In eng]. *Continuum (Minneap Minn)* 21, no. 1 Spinal Cord Disorders (Feb 2015): 67–83. https://doi.org/10.1212/01.CON.0000461085.79241.e0.

Robertson, C. E., R. D. Brown, Jr., E. F. Wijdicks, and A. A. Rabinstein. "Recovery After Spinal Cord Infarcts: Long-Term Outcome in 115 Patients." [In eng]. *Neurology* 78, no. 2 (Jan 10 2012): 114–21. https://doi.org/10.1212/WNL.0b013e31823efc93.

Spratt, J. R., K. L. Walker, T. J. Wallen, et al. "Safety of Cerebrospinal Fluid Drainage for Spinal Cord Ischemia Prevention in Thoracic Endovascular Aortic Repair." [In eng]. *JTCVS Tech* 14 (Aug 2022): 9–28. https://doi.org/10.1016/j.xjtc.2022.05.001.

Suarez-Pierre, A., X. Zhou, J. E. Gonzalez, et al. "Association of Preoperative Spinal Drain Placement With Spinal Cord Ischemia Among Patients Undergoing Thoracic and Thoracoabdominal Endovascular Aortic Repair." [In eng]. *J Vasc Surg* 70, no. 2 (Aug 2019): 393–403. https://doi.org/10.1016/j.jvs.2018.10.112.

Thet, M. S., M. D'Oria, D. Sef, T. Klokocovnik, A. Y. Oo, and S. Lepidi. "Neuromonitoring during Endovascular Thoracoabdominal Aortic Aneurysm Repair: A Systematic Review." [In eng]. *Ann Vasc Surg* 109 (Jul 14 2024): 206–15. doi:10.1016/j.avsg.2024.06.012.

21 When Status Epilepticus Cannot Be Controlled

A 42-year-old woman with a history of epilepsy was brought to our emergency department after three witnessed generalized tonic-clonic seizures. Her epilepsy was a result of prior traumatic brain injury. Recently the dose of valproic acid had been reduced. The paramedics decided to intubate her prior to transportation due to concerns about the patency of her airway. We are called into the emergency department to evaluate the patient after she has another generalized tonic-clonic seizure upon our arrival. The seizure lasts 90 seconds, and the patient remains unconscious at its conclusion. Her husband informs us that she has not been alert since the first seizure happened. She is intubated and mechanically ventilated with good oxygenation, afebrile, and mildly tachycardic and hypertensive. She has no neck stiffness and no lateralizing signs on motor examination. We lift her eyelids and notice nystagmoid-like movements of her eyes.

What do you do now?

Successful treatment of status epilepticus (SE) begins with the recognition that it is a neurological emergency. If you do not treat it early, SE becomes more refractory over time. This is due to downregulation in the gamma-aminobutyric acid (GABA) receptors and upregulation of glutamate receptors. These changes result in resistance to GABA agonists, such as benzodiazepines. Also, long-lasting SE increases the risk of complications including permanent neuronal damage and dropout. At its extreme, super-refractory SE develops (defined as status that cannot be permanently aborted within 24 hours).

We must ask ourselves the following questions. First, how do you recognize refractory SE? In patients with continuous generalized convulsions, the diagnosis of SE is self-evident (although it still requires differentiation from functional SE). But all too often, there is delay to diagnose SE in patients with rapidly repetitive seizures. These patients must be treated for SE if they do not recover full alertness between seizures. The diagnosis is also missed too frequently when the clinical manifestations are subtle (e.g., in cases of focal SE with impaired consciousness, previously known as complex partial SE) and when patients are comatose (in whom the only clinical manifestation, if any, may be nystagmoid eye movements or minimal flickering of a finger or a toe). Generalized convulsive SE becomes nonconvulsive over time, and electroencephalographic (EEG) recording is often needed to find a close correlation between subtle movements and ictal discharges.

Second, how do you treat SE when it becomes refractory? A staged approach is common and priorities often change leading some experts to think it might be better to combine treatments early. Knowing potent anesthetic agents will be used (and with variable half-lives) such an approach requires careful evaluation ideally in prospective trials. When we use combinations we carefully adjust dosages to avoid toxicity and try to minimize agents once the seizures have been under control for 12–24 hours. Even the suspicion of SE indicates immediate initiation of antiepileptic treatment. Benzodiazepines are the first-line therapy—intravenous lorazepam being the preferred choice because of its rapid onset of action and longer duration of antiepileptic effect—and should be given while emergently assessing airway patency, adequacy of ventilation and oxygenation, and circulatory status. In all cases, a capillary glucose level should be measured to exclude hypoglycemia. Draw blood to measure serum electrolytes, lactic acid, creatine kinase, complete cell count, and arterial gases. If seizures stop and the patient awakens, further escalation is not likely. But if the seizures do not stop, you need to move to the next line of therapy (fosphenytoin, valproic acid, or levetiracetam) without delay. In fact, treatment of SE is best optimized by following a clear protocol progressing from one line of therapy to the next until seizures stop. The dose should be adequate, and failure to prescribe the right dose is a common error. Always check whether the patient has received an appropriate dose of each drug (e.g., lorazepam, 0.1 mg/kg; fosphenytoin, 20 mg/kg; valproic acid, 40 mg/kg; levetiracetam, 60 mg/kg) before concluding it failed. Intravenous loading of fosphenytoin, valproic acid, and levetiracetam were similarly efficacious for control of SE in the Established Status Epilepticus Treatment Trial (ESETT), but none of the options were very effective. In this trial, only between 45% and 47% of patients had no recurrent clinical seizures and improvement of consciousness by 60 minutes of administration of any of the three drugs.

SE should be considered refractory after failure of two antiepileptic agents. In our practice, the diagnosis of refractory generalized SE means starting a continuous infusion of an anesthetic agent. This decision demands endotracheal intubation for mechanical ventilation and continuous EEG monitoring. Instead, in cases of focal SE (with or without impaired cognition), we try one or two more anticonvulsants (including phenobarbital) before using anesthetics because there is less evidence that uncontrolled focal seizures produce irreversible brain damage, at least in the short term. Furthermore, studies have shown that the use of anesthetics is associated with poor outcome in refractory SE, and we think that this finding should call for caution when considering anesthetics for focal SE. For the same reasons, we try to avoid intubation and anesthetic drugs in patients with epilepsia partialis continua.

Among anesthetic agents, we favor midazolam because of its better safety profile (Table 21.1). Midazolam can abort SE in high doses. We start with a bolus of 0.2 mg/kg body weight and an infusion of 0.2 mg/kg/h. However, we rapidly increase the infusion dose until we achieve suppression of the seizures and have reached doses as high as 5 mg/kg/h in the most recalcitrant cases. Tachyphylaxis develops quickly with benzodiazepines in general and midazolam in particular. This phenomenon may demand using

TABLE 21.1 Therapeutic Options for Refractory Status Epilepticus

Drug	Dose	Infusion Rate	Major Side Effects
Lorazepam	0.1 mg/kg	2 mg/min	Sedation Respiratory depression
Diazepam	0.2 mg/kg	5 mg/min	Sedation Respiratory depression
Fosphenytoin	20 mg/kg	150 mg/min	Hypotension Cardiac arrhythmia
Valproic acid	40 mg/kg	Over 10–15 minutes	Severe encephalopathy if high ammonia or mitochondrial disorder
Levetiracetam	60 mg/kg	Over 5–15 minutes	Sedation
Lacosamide	400 mg	Over 5 minutes	Sedation Atrioventricular block
Midazolam	0.2 mg/kg	0.2 to 5 mg/kg/h[a]	Sedation Hypotension Respiratory depression
Propofol	2 mg/kg	40 to 100 mcg/kg/min	Sedation Hypotension Respiratory depression Propofol infusion syndrome[b]
Ketamine	1 mg/kg	0.5 to 7 mg/kg/h	Hypotension/hypertension Raised intracranial pressure[c] Respiratory depression
Pentobarbital	5–10 mg/kg	1–5 mg/kg/h	Prolonged sedation Hypotension Respiratory depression Myocardial depression Infections (pneumonia) Liver dysfunction Ileus Metabolic acidosis (due to propylene glycol drug carrier)

[a] Much higher doses may be needed (and can be tolerated) in selected cases.

[b] Life-threatening risk with prolonged infusion of high doses of the drug; contraindicated in children.

[c] Uncommon in our experience.

even higher doses if the infusion needs to be maintained over time. Most patients tolerate these high doses, although support with vasopressor drugs often becomes necessary.

Propofol is a highly effective antiepileptic, but in our experience it can be dangerous in the doses necessary to control refractory SE (often >100 µg/kg/min). The main risk is the development of propofol infusion syndrome. This syndrome is manifested by lactic acidosis, rhabdomyolysis, myocardial failure, and, when most severe, total cardiovascular collapse and cardiac arrest. ECMO may be needed. In our experience, even careful monitoring of metabolic changes (serial lactic acid, arterial blood gases, and creatine kinase levels) may fail to recognize the beginning of a fatal form of this complication. Therefore, we rarely use propofol for the treatment of SE, and when we do, we strictly avoid infusing large doses. More than 80 µg/kg/min or 3 mg/kg/h for longer than 48 hours should be avoided. Propofol is contraindicated in patients with a diagnosis or strong suspicion of mitochondrial disorder and in patients on a ketogenic diet.

We rely frequently on the addition of ketamine when midazolam or propofol does not control the SE. When used early and in adequate doses, ketamine can be quite effective in aborting seizures. The side effect profile of ketamine is favorable; it does not cause profound hypotension (in fact, hypertension may occur) or induce prolonged coma. Increased intracranial pressure is much less frequent than commonly believed. We do not wait too long before trying ketamine because its efficacy is much lower when used as a late rescue treatment.

Continuous infusion of barbiturates, such as pentobarbital, is highly effective in aborting SE. Unfortunately, adverse side effects are many and often severe. Hypotension is ubiquitous and requires vasopressors. Infections, especially pneumonia, ileus, and liver toxicity, occur in most patients treated with a barbiturate drip for more than 2 days. Consequently, we tend to reserve this option for those patients who fail to be controlled with other anesthetic medications.

We have tried other alternatives with variable success in our most challenging cases. We have found that isoflurane is the only effective rescue therapy in patients dependent on high doses of pentobarbital. However, the appearance of significant brain and brainstem abnormalities on magnetic resonance imaging (MRI) in two of our isoflurane-treated patients suggesting a neurotoxic effect has markedly tempered our enthusiasm for its prolonged use. Isoflurane is remarkably effective, but can be used only for a very brief period and therefore is much less useful.

What more can be considered? We have also tried electroconvulsive therapy as a last resort. How electroconvulsive therapy works is not known and may be simply through a "rebooting" phenomenon. Inducing ketosis in these critically ill patients is difficult, but when achieved, it can be helpful. Cooling was not effective in treating convulsive SE in the Hypothermia for Brain Enhancement Recovery by Neuroprotective and Anticonvulsivant Action after Convulsive Status Epilepticus (HYBERNATUS).

Finally, some seizures can only be controlled by treating the underlying cause that provoked them. Searching for treatable forms of encephalitis, brain lesions amenable to resection, and some specific systemic illnesses (e.g., thrombotic thrombocytopenic purpura) is important. Around half of patients presenting with new-onset refractory SE have no identifiable cause, and these patients tend to have poor prognosis. In the worst cases, one must accept at some point that the SE is untreatably refractory; in these rare instances, the status eventually "burns out" at the expense of rapid brain loss, which can be documented by the accelerated atrophy on serial neuroimaging. Yet, aggressive treatment of nonanoxic SE, even in cases lasting much longer than 1 week, can result in good functional outcome.

All these considerations can be summarized in treatment protocol, and ours is shown in Figure 21.1. It has been said that protocols are only as good as the data on which they are based, and they change all the time, but we think this approach would be on target when compared to other medical institutions. But previous judgments often become obsolete for no good reason.

Back to our patient. After another seizure in the emergency department, she received 0.1 mg/kg of intravenous lorazepam. The abnormal eye movements resolved for a few minutes but then recurred. Because valproate discontinuation likely triggered the seizures, we loaded her with valproic acid 40 mg/kg and then transferred her to our neurosciences intensive care unit. Emergency EEG showed continuous epileptiform activity. After delivering a bolus of 0.2 mg/kg, we initiated a midazolam infusion in the intensive care unit at a rate of 0.2 mg/kg/h and then

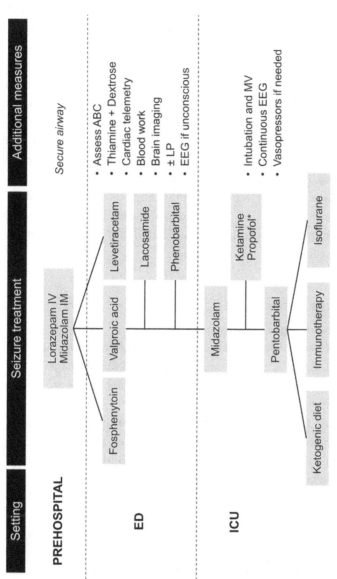

FIGURE 21.1 Algorithm for the management of status epilepticus. ABC, airway, breathing, circulation; ED, emergency department; EEG, electroencephalography; ICU, intensive care unit; LP, lumbar puncture; MV, mechanical ventilation.

*The risk of propofol infusion syndrome is substantial and this complication may be fatal. Use only briefly.

titrated until the electrographic seizures abated. (Infusion rate reached 0.5 mg/kg/h.) We then adjusted the dose of valproic acid according to the serum level. Within the following 24 hours, we were able to wean her off the infusion of midazolam. The patient became more alert and could be extubated without problems.

Treatment of refractory SE may be summarized as follows: treat aggressively, protect and support the patient, and try to find a treatable cause. Even when prolonged anesthetic treatment is needed, outcome can still be favorable in young patients, particularly if there is no MRI evidence of severe permanent brain damage. We, and others, have benefited from epilepsy consultants continuously watching the EEG during the initial treatment phase to full suppression of seizures.

The epileptologist and historian Simon Shorvon has identified the development of treatment protocols as one of the landmarks in treatment of SE and has speculated that it has reduced morbidity and even mortality. We think that is right.

KEY POINTS TO REMEMBER

- SE is a neurological emergency.
- Seizures become more resistant to antiepileptics over time, and prolonged SE can produce irreversible brain damage.
- It is best to use a treatment protocol and to decisively progress from step to step.
- Make sure the right drugs and the right doses are being used.
- If two anticonvulsants fail to abort generalized SE, consider intubating the patient, using continuous EEG monitoring, and starting a continuous infusion of an anesthetic agent.
- When treating focal SE, try additional anticonvulsants before moving to anesthetics.
- Among anesthetics, midazolam provides the best balance between safety and effectiveness. Ketamine can be a good addition. Propofol and pentobarbital are also highly effective, but their use is associated with a greater risk of severe—and even fatal—medical complications.

Further Reading

Cooper, A. D., J. W. Britton, and A. A. Rabinstein. "Functional and Cognitive Outcome in Prolonged Refractory Status Epilepticus." [In eng]. *Arch Neurol* 66, no. 12 (Dec 2009): 1505–9. https://doi.org/10.1001/archneurol.2009.273.

Cornwall, C. D., T. Krøigård, J. S. S. Kristensen, et al. "Outcomes and Treatment Approaches for Super-Refractory Status Epilepticus: A Systematic Review and Meta-Analysis." [In eng]. *JAMA Neurol* 80, no. 9 (Jul 31 2023): 959–68. https://doi.org/10.1001/jamaneurol.2023.2407.

Ferlisi, M., and S. Shorvon. "The Outcome of Therapies in Refractory and Super-Refractory Convulsive Status Epilepticus and Recommendations for Therapy." [In eng]. *Brain* 135, Pt 8 (Aug 2012): 2314–28. https://doi.org/10.1093/brain/aws091.

Gettings, J. V., Mohammad Alizadeh Chafjiri, F., Patel, A. A., Shorvon, S., Goodkin, H. P., Loddenkemper, T. "Diagnosis and management of status epilepticus: improving the status quo." *Lancet Neurol* 24. no. 1 (Jan 2025): 65–76. doi: 10.1016/S1474-4422(24)00430-7. Epub 2024 Dec 2. PMID: 39637874.

Hocker, S. E., J. W. Britton, J. N. Mandrekar, et al. "Predictors of Outcome in Refractory Status Epilepticus." [In eng]. *JAMA Neurol* 70, no. 1 (Jan 2013): 72–77. https://doi.org/10.1001/jamaneurol.2013.578.

Hocker, S., E. F. Wijdicks, and A. A. Rabinstein. "Refractory Status Epilepticus: New Insights in Presentation, Treatment, and Outcome." [In eng]. *Neurol Res* 35, no. 2 (Mar 2013): 163–68. https://doi.org/10.1179/1743132812y.0000000128.

Iyer, V. N., R. Hoel, and A. A. Rabinstein. "Propofol Infusion Syndrome in Patients With Refractory Status Epilepticus: An 11-Year Clinical Experience." [In eng]. *Crit Care Med* 37, no. 12 (Dec 2009): 3024–30. https://doi.org/10.1097/CCM.0b013e318 1b08ac7.

Kapur, J., J. Elm, J. M. Chamberlain, et al. "Randomized Trial of Three Anticonvulsant Medications for Status Epilepticus." [In eng]. *N Engl J Med* 381, no. 22 (Nov 28 2019): 2103–13. https://doi.org/10.1056/NEJMoa1905795.

Meierkord, H., P. Boon, B. Engelsen, et al. "EFNS Guideline on the Management of Status Epilepticus in Adults." [In eng]. *Eur J Neurol* 17, no. 3 (Mar 2010): 348–55. https://doi.org/10.1111/j.1468-1331.2009.02917.x.

Misirocchi F, Quintard H, Kleinschmidt A, Schaller K, Pugin J, Seeck M, De Stefano P. ICU-Electroencephalogram Unit Improves Outcome in Status Epilepticus Patients: A Retrospective Before-After Study. *Crit Care Med* 2024 Nov 1; 52(11):e545–e556. doi: 10.1097/CCM.0000000000006393. Epub 2024 Aug 9. PMID: 39120451.

Shorvon, S. "Twelve Landmarks in the Treatment of Status Epilepticus." [In eng]. *Epilepsy Behav* 159 (Jul 30 2024): 109954. doi:10.1016/j.yebeh.2024.109954.

Sutter, R., S. Marsch, P. Fuhr, et al. "Anesthetic Drugs in Status Epilepticus: Risk or Rescue? A 6-Year Cohort Study." [In eng]. *Neurology* 82, no. 8 (Feb 25 2014): 656–64. https://doi.org/10.1212/wnl.0000000000000009.

Tharmaraja, T., J. S. Y. Ho, A. Neligan, and S. Rajakulendran. "The Etiology and Mortality of New-Onset Refractory Status Epilepticus (NORSE) in Adults: A Systematic Review and Meta-Analysis." [In eng]. *Epilepsia* 64, no. 5 (May 2023): 1113–24. https://doi.org/10.1111/epi.17523.

Trinka, E., H. Cock, D. Hesdorffer, et al. "A Definition and Classification of Status Epilepticus—Report of the ILAE Task Force on Classification of Status Epilepticus." [In eng]. *Epilepsia* 56, no. 10 (Oct 2015): 1515–23. https://doi.org/10.1111/epi.13121.

22 When Brain Metastasis Becomes a Neurocritical Emergency

A 64-year-old man with history of smoking was admitted after recurrent episodes of loss of consciousness over the previous 2 days. For the previous 3 to 4 weeks, he had been having worsening problems with concentration, gait, and balance. He also noticed vision loss on the right side and had difficulties with left hand movements. Upon evaluation in our emergency department, he was fully awake, but his answers were slow. He had a right visual field deficit and left-sided ataxia. A computed tomography (CT) scan showed masses in the left cerebellar hemisphere and the left parietooccipital region surrounded by extensive edema. He was started on dexamethasone. Anticipating decline despite administration of corticosteroids and the possibility of an urgent neurosurgical debulking, we admitted him to our neuroscience intensive care unit (ICU) for close observation. Twelve hours after arrival, his condition declined. On examination, he is difficult to awaken and has developed left facial and abducens nerve palsies.

What do you do now?

Malignancies may present anywhere in the brain and cause rapid decline even before the pathology is known. Patients with a primary malignant brain tumor may worsen quickly from tumor growth, but the most common causes for decline are brain edema and hemorrhage (Box 22.1). More aggressive tumors increase the likelihood of these two complications. Highly malignant tumors secrete angiogenic factors, which promote the rapid formation of intratumoral vessels. The lack of efficient, tight junctions in these vessels produces a disruption of the blood-brain barrier, which results in the formation of vasogenic edema. These vessels are also fragile and prone to rupture.

Patients with malignant brain tumors may also deteriorate from exacerbating factors that disturb ongoing compensatory mechanisms. For instance, seizures can produce hypoventilation and hypercapnia from a reduced respiratory drive, which in turn can lead to increased cerebral blood volume and worsening tissue shift in patients with exhausted intracranial compliance. Incremental administration of opiates for excruciating headaches can have similar consequences. Severe hyponatremia, sometimes related to inappropriate secretion of antidiuretic hormone as a paraneoplastic disorder or due to hydrocephalus, can worsen cerebral edema. Radiation therapy, although useful for the reduction of mass effect in the longer term, characteristically correlates with worsening inflammatory edema in the early phase.

What options can we offer our patient? Corticosteroids are particularly useful for the treatment of peritumoral vasogenic edema, and often high

---

BOX 22.1 **Causes of Neurological Deterioration in Patients With Malignant Brain Tumors**

Worsening of vasogenic peritumoral edema[a]

Intratumoral hemorrhage[a]

Seizures[a]

Obstructive hydrocephalus

Venous infarction from extension of the tumor to the dural sinus

Arterial infarction from vessel invasion or compression by the tumor

[a] By far the most common.

doses are necessary. We adjust the dose depending on the severity of the edema. In patients with preserved alertness and no substantial brain tissue shift, the usual dose of 10 mg of dexamethasone may suffice. However, we administer intravenous bolus doses of 20 to 100 mg in severe and extreme cases. Maintenance doses then range from 4 to 10 mg every 4 to 6 hours. When using high-dose steroids, it is essential to minimize the risks and to initiate preventive measures (Table 22.1). Even if administered early, intravenous dexamethasone may take hours to reach its maximum effect, and patients may deteriorate before that time. Other antiedema medical treatments (mannitol or hypertonic saline) only have a role in emergency situations and are often used as a bridge to neurosurgical debulking.

Surgery is the most effective treatment. Even when complete resection is not possible, debulking can still help. Patients who present with rapid clinical worsening and signs of brainstem displacement, those

TABLE 22.1 **Side Effects and Preventive Measures Related to High-Dose Corticosteroids**

Side Effect	Preventive Measure
Hyperglycemia	Frequent glucose monitoring Insulin sliding scale or infusion
Increased susceptibility to infections (especially by *Pneumocystis jiroveci*)	Double-strength trimethoprim sulfamethoxazole 3 times per week
Psychosis	Antidopaminergics
Mood swings	Mood stabilizers (e.g., valproic acid)
Peptic ulcers[a]	H_2 blockers or proton pump inhibitors
High blood pressure	Monitoring and treatment as necessary
Myopathy	Minimize immobilization
Hypokalemia	Potassium monitoring and replacement

[a] Risk may only be increased with high doses, and after recent use of nonsteroidal anti-inflammatory agents.

with large intratumoral hemorrhages, and those failing increased doses of corticosteroids all require urgent surgery. Often, the decision to operate must be made without knowing the primary pathology and, thus, the prognosis. We generally discourage biopsies in patients with large masses and no space to expand. Even minor postoperative bleeding—a relatively frequent occurrence—can put patients at considerable further risk if the mass effect is not reduced during surgery. As illustrated by our case, cerebellar masses require surgery more often than supratentorial ones. Occasionally, a superimposed obstructive hydrocephalus causes the acute neurological decline, and in these cases, a ventriculostomy can be a acceptable invasive, temporary solution.

Whether patients with known malignant primary brain tumors need urgent or emergent surgery is a complex decision. The previous functional status of the patient, previously stated wishes, the possibility of effective future tumor treatment, and, most importantly, the potential for recovery of quality of life after surgery must be carefully considered. The major ethical question in some patients reaching this stage is whether a neurosurgical procedure is justified in a situation in which surgery only affords minimal gain in survival with poor quality of life. Some families are unable to decide, while others may turn to palliative care.

Our patient received 20 mg of dexamethasone and 4000 mg of levetiracetam (for suspected previous seizures) in the emergency department. When he worsened in the ICU, we administered an additional 20 mg of dexamethasone along with 1 g/kg of 20% mannitol. A repeat CT scan showed obstructive hydrocephalus from aqueduct compression. He underwent urgent surgery for excision of the cerebellar mass (Figure 22.1). His hydrocephalus resolved, and his neurological condition improved. He continued receiving dexamethasone, 6 mg every 6 hours, with subsequent taper. CT scan of the chest showed a nodular mass. Lung biopsy and brain pathology showed non–small cell carcinoma. He underwent further treatment and had a good functional status 6 months later.

Patients who undergo surgical resection of a brain metastasis from a highly malignant tumor are likely to succumb to progression of the cancer. Yet, aggressive treatment of the brain mass may afford quite acceptable quality of life for most of the remaining time. Other times, the

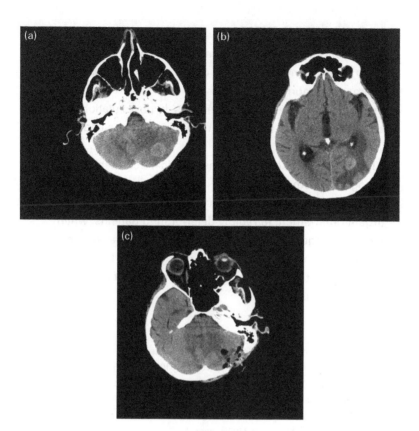

FIGURE 22.1 (A) Head CT scan showing a left cerebellar mass with associated edema producing effacement of the fourth ventricle. (B) At a higher level, a second mass is seen in the left parietooccipital area. Note the dilatation of the third ventricle. (C) After surgical excision of the cerebellar mass, the CT scan shows persistent edema with mass effect but less prominent than before and the appearance of a slit fourth ventricle.

primary tumor proves to be more treatable, and the emergent resection of a brain metastasis is followed by more prolonged survival with satisfactory function. A post craniotomy neurologic deficit still present months later or progression of the systemic cancer reduce overall survival.

For many years brain metastasis was considered an immediate death sentence but there are now useful medical treatment options for some patients (and certainly for metastatic melanoma).

KEY POINTS TO REMEMBER

- Acute neurological decline from brain metastasis or malignant brain tumor is most frequently due to worsening vasogenic edema or hemorrhage.
- Precipitating causes (such as seizures, hypoventilation, and hyponatremia) need to be recognized and treated without delay.
- Glucocorticosteroids are the best medical treatment for vasogenic edema.
- Surgical treatment (tumor removal or debulking) becomes urgent or emergent in rapidly deteriorating patients, when there is a large hemorrhage, and in patients refractory to medical treatments. When offering surgery as a life-saving intervention, the future prognosis and wishes of the patient must be discussed.

Further Reading

Achrol, A. S., R. C. Rennert, C. Anders, et al. "Brain Metastases." [In eng]. *Nat Rev Dis Primers* 5, no. 1 (Jan 17 2019): 5. https://doi.org/10.1038/s41572-018-0055-y.

Fiore, G., L. Tariciotti, G. A. Bertani, et al. "Surgery vs. Radiosurgery for Patients With Localized Metastatic Brain Disease: A Systematic Review With Meta-Analysis of Randomized Controlled Trials." [In eng]. *Cancers (Basel)* 15, no. 15 (Jul 26 2023): 3802. https://doi.org/10.3390/cancers15153802.

Lin, J., R. Jandial, A. Nesbit, et al. "Current and Emerging Treatments for Brain Metastases." [In eng]. *Oncology (Williston Park)* 29, no. 4 (Apr 2015): 250–57.

Linskey, M. E., D. W. Andrews, A. L. Asher, et al. "The Role of Stereotactic Radiosurgery in the Management of Patients With Newly Diagnosed Brain Metastases: A Systematic Review and Evidence-Based Clinical Practice Guideline." [In eng]. *J Neurooncol* 96, no. 1 (Jan 2010): 45–68. https://doi.org/10.1007/s11060-009-0073-4.

Nieblas-Bedolla, E., N. Nayyar, M. Singh, et al. "Emerging Immunotherapies in the Treatment of Brain Metastases." [In eng]. *Oncologist* 26, no. 3 (Mar 2021): 231–41. https://doi.org/10.1002/onco.13575.

Niedermeyer, S., M. Schmutzer-Sondergeld, J. Weller, et al. "Neurosurgical Resection of Multiple Brain Metastases: Outcomes, Complications, and Survival Rates in a Retrospective Analysis." [In eng]. *J Neurooncol* 169, no. 2 (Sep 2024): 349–58. doi:10.1007/s11060-024-04744-w.

Ryken, T. C., M. McDermott, P. D. Robinson, et al. "The Role of Steroids in the Management of Brain Metastases: A Systematic Review and Evidence-Based Clinical Practice Guideline." [In eng]. *J Neurooncol* 96, no. 1 (Jan 2010): 103–14. https://doi.org/10.1007/s11060-009-0057-4.

Suh, J. H., R. Kotecha, S. T. Chao, et al. "Current Approaches to the Management of Brain Metastases." [In eng]. *Nat Rev Clin Oncol* 17, no. 5 (May 2020): 279–99. https://doi.org/10.1038/s41571-019-0320-3.

23 The Surgical Urgency With Pituitary Apoplexy

A 73-year-old man awoke unable to open his right eye. He also noted a mild headache over the vertex that had begun the night before. He was on warfarin for a prior pulmonary embolus. On neurological examination, he had a right third-nerve palsy with complete ptosis, a nonreactive 6-mm pupil, and ophthalmoparesis. Bedside visual field testing revealed bitemporal hemianopia. Computed tomography (CT) scan of the brain demonstrated a heterogenous sellar and suprasellar mass (Figure 23.1). A CT angiogram of the head showed no evidence of intracranial aneurysm, but there was displacement of the internal carotid and anterior cerebral arteries. Laboratory studies showed an international normalized ratio of 3.5 and serum sodium of 133 mmol/L.

What do you do now?

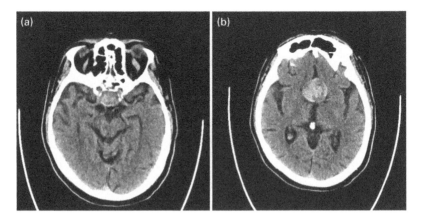

FIGURE 23.1 CT (noncontrast) shows a heterogenous hyperdense sellar (A) and suprasellar mass (B).

Pituitary apoplexy is sometimes the startling first announcement of a pituitary adenoma. Acute hemorrhage from necrosis of the pituitary adenoma is rare, clinically affecting less than 10% of patients with adenomas. Most pituitary adenomas with hemorrhage are only discovered on magnetic resonance imaging (MRI) studies. In fact, we now know that patients with hemorrhage into a pituitary adenoma may have mild symptoms. The classical Greek word apoplexia meaning "suddenly struck senseless and motionless," does not, in fact, characterize the usual presentation of hemorrhage within a pituitary adenoma. Most of the time, pituitary apoplexy occurs spontaneously, although some precipitating factors have been identified including anticoagulation or some intrinsic coagulopathy, pregnancy, bromocriptine, hypertension, pituitary irradiation, and estrogen therapy. A disproportionate number of cases present de novo after cardiac or general surgery. Unlike non-post-operative cases that most often present in young women, two-thirds of these patients are male, usually in the sixth or seventh decade of life.

Several theories attempt to explain the pathophysiology of pituitary apoplexy. Most surgeons accept that ischemic infarction of pituitary adenomas is frequently the product of intrinsic features of these tumors and that the main explanation is a tenuous balance between high metabolic demand and marginal tissue perfusion. The vascularity of pituitary tumors may contribute to hemorrhage when growth escalates. Ischemic necrosis in a tumor outgrowing its blood supply and compression by large tumors of the superior hypophysial artery against the sella are mechanisms that may contribute to the development of hemorrhage. Pituitary apoplexy occurring during cardiac surgery may be caused by acute pituitary edema from hemodilution induced by crystalloid priming of the cardiopulmonary bypass tubing, inadequate superior vena cava drainage, or release of vasoactive substances. Pituitary ischemia from a low-flow state (reduced mean arterial pressure) or pituitary hemorrhage from anticoagulation can occur with any type of surgical procedure.

Acute enlargement of the tumor may compress the neighboring optic chiasm and optic nerves. Compression of the oculomotor nerves in the cavernous sinus may cause ophthalmoplegia. Acute compression of the hypothalamus or acute Addison disease may explain stupor. Extravasation of hemorrhage into the subarachnoid space with obstructive hydrocephalus is another situation that requires attention.

Destruction of the pituitary gland causes hypopituitarism of varying severity and duration (partial, total, transient, or permanent). Because the posterior pituitary has its own blood supply, diabetes insipidus is not encountered as commonly as anterior pituitary failure.

Patients classically present with dramatic—and sometimes catastrophic— symptoms such as thunderclap headache, blurred vision, neck stiffness, vomiting, and altered consciousness. Headache is the most common presenting symptom, followed by visual abnormalities, which the patient commonly describes as blurred vision. A unilateral third cranial nerve palsy is the most common cranial nerve abnormality found on examination. CT scan is diagnostic in more severe cases, but MRI scans are much more sensitive than CT scans for this diagnosis (nearly 90% compared to 40%). MRI is valuable for making the diagnosis as well as delineating the extent of compression of the optic chiasm and cavernous sinus, which will be important for surgical planning. Thickening of the sphenoid sinus mucosa is suggestive of acute onset as the pressure exerted by a large pituitary tumor on the sphenoid sinus lining can lead to mucosal thickening.

Acute care of pituitary apoplexy focuses on stabilizing the patient's physiology, supplementing corticosteroids and other deficient hormones, and maintaining electrolyte balance. Box 23.1 depicts the serum pituitary-axis hormones that should be checked. Half of patients have decreased cortisol levels, and other hormonal deficiencies may be present. There is

> **BOX 23.1 Pituitary Hormones to Monitor in Pituitary Apoplexy**
>
> Cortisol (at 8 am)
>
> ACTH
>
> TSH and free T4
>
> Prolactin
>
> IGF-1
>
> Testosterone (total, free, bioavailable)
>
> ACTH, adrenocorticotropic hormone; IGF-1, insulin-like growth factor 1; T4, thyroxine; TSH, thyroid-stimulating hormone.

no consensus on whether to administer corticosteroids routinely or reserve them for patients with hypotension or low serum cortisol levels (typically measured in the early morning). Postural hypotension and tachycardia may be seen before frank hypotension.

The greatest concerns are cortisol and thyroid hormone deficiencies. If hypotension occurs or if a decreased morning cortisol level proves a deficiency, hydrocortisone is generally the preferred replacement steroid. Glucocorticoid replacement (e.g., intravenous hydrocortisone, 200 mg per 24 hours, either continuously or intermittently as 50 mg every 6 hours) is the first course of action, and thyroid hormone replacement, if needed, should be administered only after glucocorticoids have been given.

Hypopituitarism occurs in up to 80% of operated cases, with hypogonadism in 50%, hypothyroidism in 60%, and adrenocorticotropic hormone deficiency in 80%. In a series from Mayo Clinic, 70% of 87 patients had surgery within 10 days (as early as 3 days), and a minority had delayed (≥2 months) surgery. Intensive care admission was needed in 40% of patients.

Early transsphenoidal resection surgery is ultimately the definitive treatment, but timing remains in the hands of the neurosurgeon, who will not hesitate in patients with progressive neuroophthalmological symptoms. Some claim benefit from endoscopic endonasal resection of macroadenomas with apoplexy to spare part of the pituitary gland.

Preservation of the normal gland led to preservation of posterior pituitary function. Preoperative imaging can determine the location of the normal pituitary gland and stalk, but this may not be possible with large hemorrhagic tumors.

Often, those with stable or resolving neuro-ophthalmic symptoms receive conservative management. Currently, with increased recognition of mild or asymptomatic presentations of pituitary apoplexy by MRI, some neurosurgeons support more conservative management (delayed surgery or medical management) but only for medically stable patients with no neurological or progressive ophthalmological deficits.

Patients with pituitary apoplexy often have favorable outcomes. Survivors usually resume an independent lifestyle, with little or no symptoms. Limitations in eye movements tend to improve with time. One study of 15 cases with pituitary apoplexy with a mean follow-up of 30 months found that in surgically treated patients with pituitary apoplexy, all cranial nerve deficits normalized or improved. In this study, the cranial nerve deficits present at admission were visual deficit in a third, unilateral third-nerve palsy in approximately half, and a sixth-nerve palsy in one of four patients. No fourth-nerve palsies were observed. The improvement occurs rapidly; more than half of the patients with preoperative visual deficit had normal visual fields postoperatively. Similarly, most patients with preoperative third- and sixth-nerve palsies returned to normal function after surgery.

Establishing care with an endocrinologist is necessary because long-term hormonal replacement with hormones (e.g., hydrocortisone, levothyroxine, and testosterone for men) is often needed. Anterior pituitary hormone deficits are commonly seen in follow-up, but there is partial or complete recovery in up to 50% of cases. Completely normal pituitary function is reported in 5% to nearly 40% across reported series.

Our patient underwent urgent transsphenoidal, endoscopically assisted resection of the hemorrhagic pituitary mass. At 1-month follow-up, he had mild interval improvement in his ptosis and ophthalmoparesis and was taking hydrocortisone and levothyroxine replacement.

KEY POINTS TO REMEMBER

- Pituitary apoplexy should be suspected in a patient with sudden headache, oculomotor palsy, and a sellar mass.
- MRI is twice as sensitive as CT in detecting hemorrhage in pituitary tumors.
- Acute medical care consists of stabilizing physiology with corticosteroid replacement and management of electrolyte and fluid derangements.
- Most patients with pituitary apoplexy do not need emergency (i.e., same-day) surgery and do not have critical endocrine failure, yet some may worsen quickly.
- Transsphenoidal resection should be urgently performed in patients with a reduced level of consciousness or acute neuro-ophthalmic symptomatology, particularly when it threatens vision.

Further Reading

Alahmari, M., F. Alkherayf, A. Lasso, et al. "Recovery of Cranial Nerve Deficits in Patients Presenting With Pituitary Apoplexy: A Case Series." [In eng]. *J Neurol Surg B Skull Base* 83, no. Suppl 2 (Jun 2022): e1–6. https://doi.org/10.1055/s-0040-1722668.

Arnold, M. A., J. M. Revuelta Barbero, G. Pradilla, and S. K. Wise. "Pituitary Gland Surgical Emergencies: The Role of Endoscopic Intervention." [In eng]. *Otolaryngol Clin North Am* 55, no. 2 (Apr 2022): 397–410. https://doi.org/10.1016/j.otc.2021.12.016.

Bujawansa, S., S. K. Thondam, C. Steele, et al. "Presentation, Management and Outcomes in Acute Pituitary Apoplexy: A Large Single-Centre Experience From the United Kingdom." [In eng]. *Clin Endocrinol (Oxf)* 80, no. 3 (Mar 2014): 419–24. https://doi.org/10.1111/cen.12307.

Donegan, D., and D. Erickson. "Revisiting Pituitary Apoplexy." [In eng]. *J Endocr Soc* 6, no. 9 (Sep 1 2022): bvac113. https://doi.org/10.1210/jendso/bvac113.

Glezer, A., and M. D. Bronstein. "Pituitary Apoplexy: Pathophysiology, Diagnosis and Management." [In eng]. *Arch Endocrinol Metab* 59, no. 3 (Jun 2015): 259–64. https://doi.org/10.1590/2359-3997000000047.

Johnston, P. C., A. H. Hamrahian, R. J. Weil, and L. Kennedy. "Pituitary Tumor Apoplexy." [In eng]. *J Clin Neurosci* 22, no. 6 (Jun 2015): 939–44. https://doi.org/10.1016/j.jocn.2014.11.023.

Rajasekaran, S., M. Vanderpump, S. Baldeweg, et al. "UK Guidelines for the Management of Pituitary Apoplexy." [In eng]. *Clin Endocrinol (Oxf)* 74, no. 1 (Jan 2011): 9–20. https://doi.org/10.1111/j.1365-2265.2010.03913.x.

Rosso, M., S. Ramaswamy, H. Sucharew, et al. "Isolated Third Cranial Nerve Palsy in Pituitary Apoplexy: Case Report and Systematic Review." [In eng]. *J Stroke Cerebrovasc Dis* 30, no. 9 (Sep 2021): 105969. https://doi.org/10.1016/j.jstrokece rebrovasdis.2021.105969.

Salle, H., M. Cane, M. Rocher, et al. "Pituitary Apoplexy Score, Toward Standardized Decision-Making: A Descriptive Study." [In eng]. *Pituitary* 27, no. 1 (Feb 2024): 77–87. doi:10.1007/s11102-023-01372-x. Epub 2023 Dec 27.

Singh, T. D., N. Valizadeh, F. B. Meyer, et al. "Management and Outcomes of Pituitary Apoplexy." [In eng]. *J Neurosurg* 122, no. 6 (Jun 2015): 1450–57. https://doi.org/10.3171/2014.10.Jns141204.

Spiegel, S. J., and H. E. Moss. "Neuro-Ophthalmic Emergencies." [In eng]. *Neurol Clin* 39, no. 2 (May 2021): 631–47. https://doi.org/10.1016/j.ncl.2021.01.004.

24 Eclampsia and Its Neurologic Consequences

A 25-year-old female, 7 days postpartum from an uncomplicated vaginal delivery, was admitted to the neurosciences intensive care unit (ICU) for seizure management and subarachnoid hemorrhage. She had a normal postdelivery course, after which she had two seizures. She described bifrontal headache over 2 to 3 days earlier, which was severe and throbbing without nausea or emesis. On arrival, she was markedly hypertensive (up to 190s mmHg systolic). Head computed tomography (CT) demonstrated a small subarachnoid hemorrhage confined to the anterior right frontal sulci. We immediately proceeded with a magnetic resonance angiogram and magnetic resonance venogram of the brain, which were unremarkable. Magnetic resonance imaging (MRI) showed T2 fluid-attenuated inversion recovery hyperintensities in the bilateral occipital lobes (Figure 24.1) and confirmed the hemorrhage in the sulcus. She was drowsy but attentive when addressed, and there were no overt neurologic deficits, particularly no visual disturbances.

What do you do now?

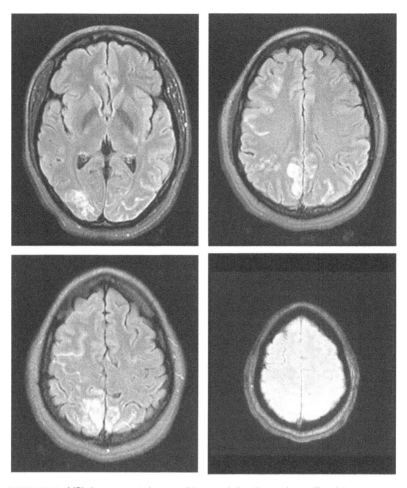

FIGURE 24.1 MRI shows a posterior reversible encephalopathy syndrome–like picture seen with eclampsia. Note hyperintensity in the sulcus on the right that corresponded with the (not shown) CT scan findings.

Given the distribution of magnetic resonance abnormality and clinical scenario, the findings were most consistent with acute postpartum eclampsia. We found no definite arterial luminal irregularity, which can be seen sometimes, and there was no evidence of cerebral venous thrombosis. We wanted to make certain that thrombosis was not present because pregnancy is a physiologically hypercoagulable state due to an increase in several prothrombotic factors, and the risk for venous thromboembolism is higher in the postpartum period. Postpartum eclampsia remains a formidable clinical management problem, and we can expect patients to be admitted to the neuro-ICU when the CT scan of the brain shows that hemorrhage or seizures are recurrent.

More than 75% of patients with eclampsia present before or during delivery, but eclampsia may occur up to 7 days after delivery. The reported incidence of eclampsia is 1.6 to 10 per 10,000 deliveries in developed countries and 50 to 151 per 10,000 deliveries in developing countries. Eclampsia is more common in patients with preexisting hypertension or renal disease, prior episodes of eclampsia, nulliparity or multiple gestation, triploidy, molar pregnancy, and hydrops fetalis. Working groups on high blood pressure in pregnancy have defined preeclampsia as the presence of hypertension, proteinuria, or pitting edema after 20 weeks of gestation. (Hypertension was defined as a blood pressure above 140/90 mmHg on two occasions several hours apart and proteinuria as urinary excretion of protein exceeding 300 mg daily.) Hypertensive disorders of pregnancy remain a leading cause of maternal morbidity and mortality but are potentially preventable. During pregnancy, prompt recognition, antihypertensive treatment, and speedy delivery reduce the risk of severe maternal morbidity or death, but patients remain at risk in the postpartum period, when hypertension may worsen. Most women who present with postpartum preeclampsia and stroke recall headaches or other symptoms in the days preceding admission. The American College of Obstetricians and Gynecologists therefore recommends that patients with hypertensive disorders of pregnancy have blood pressure evaluation no later than 7 to 10 days postpartum and that those with severe hypertension be seen within 72 hours. Aggressive management of hypertension is needed, but the optimal drugs are different than for other hypertensive patients.

Once in the ICU, the goal of blood pressure management is to keep it below 140/90 mmHg. Treatment should involve the immediate use of intravenous (IV) magnesium sulfate, Magnesium sulfate also acts centrally to inhibit N-methyl-D-aspartate receptors, providing anticonvulsant activity by raising the seizure threshold. In fact, several randomized trials have found that magnesium sulfate is more effective than phenytoin to reduce the incidence of seizures. Magnesium sulfate is well tolerated and beneficial in treating eclampsia for both mother and infant. Magnesium sulfate clears renally, with 90% of the dose excreted within 24 hours after infusion. The half-life of magnesium sulfate in patients with normal renal function is 4 hours; hence, a 24-hour treatment period is typically recommended, although some systematic reviews suggest shorter periods may be equally effective. Magnesium sulfate is started with an IV load of 4 to 6 g of magnesium sulfate (20 mL of a 20% solution), followed by an infusion of magnesium sulfate of 2 g/h. Magnesium levels are kept between 4 and 7 mEq/L. Because magnesium sulfate is excreted exclusively in the urine, serum magnesium levels will increase quickly with renal failure, which places patients with impaired kidney function at risk of significant adverse effects. The dose must be adjusted when the tendon reflexes disappear, and usually this clinical finding corresponds to a serum magnesium level of 8 to 12 mEq/L—one of the few instances when a reflex hammer helps an obstetrician. Magnesium sulfate can be highly toxic, leading to respiratory distress, loss of all motor function (becoming "locked in"), and need for intubation, but usually this degree of toxicity occurs if magnesium levels are allowed to exceed 12 mg/dL. This is not a trivial issue and a number of mishaps with severe toxicity have been reported even recently.

Lower infusion rates (1–2 g/h) may stop seizures more effectively than higher rates. Differences in volume of distribution (antepartum or postpartum) and higher body mass index also affect the dosage and duration needed to achieve the desired magnesium level.

Magnesium sulfate administration continues for 24 hours and then can be stopped. Very few other antihypertensives are effective or allowed. Specifically, nitroprusside should be strictly avoided because it can lead to cyanide toxicity of the fetus even if used only for several hours. Angiotensin-converting enzyme inhibitors are contraindicated. Adjunctive treatment is with labetalol, 10 to 20 mg IV, and in refractory cases, nicardipine 5 to 15 mg/h IV infusion. Nicardipine is also a better choice for puerperium eclampsia and breastfeeding. The consensus is first to reduce the blood pressure below 160/100 mmHg with an ultimate target of keeping the blood pressure below 140/90 mmHg. However, blood pressure should be lowered gradually because patients with cerebral vasoconstriction or substantial brain swelling may develop hypoperfusion if the systemic blood pressure is dropped too rapidly.

After discontinuation of magnesium sulfate, blood pressure may creep up again and require additional doses of IV labetalol. This actually happened to our patient. Labetalol improved her blood pressure levels, but not consistently. Therefore, we inserted an arterial line and treated her with nicardipine infusion, titrating up to 7.5 mg/h. We also started nifedipine XL, 60 mg orally. Long-term treatment was needed, and nifedipine was chosen because she was breastfeeding. The dose of nifedipine XL is 30 to 60 mg daily and titrated to a maximum of 120 mg/d. Alternatively, labetalol, 200 mg three times a day, can be titrated to a maximum of 800 mg three times a day as a reasonable option for maintenance therapy.

Most neurointensivists have little experience with eclampsia and major pregnancy complications. It is essential to collaborate closely and daily with the obstetrics department to coordinate care.

KEY POINTS TO REMEMBER

- Postpartum headache should be taken seriously and prompt consideration of brain MRI.
- The first priority is IV magnesium sulfate for 24 hours. Magnesium works to treat hypertension and prevent/treat seizures.
- The second priority is to prescribe long-acting antihypertensive therapy to prevent severe rebound hypertension.
- With persistent hypertension, initiate nifedipine XL or use labetalol.

Further Reading

Ali, M., E. S. van Etten, S. Akoudad, et al. "Hemorrhagic Stroke and Brain Vascular Malformations in Women: Risk Factors and Clinical Features." [In eng]. *Lancet Neurol* 23, no. 6 (Jun 2024): 625–35. doi:10.1016/S1474-4422(24)00122-4. PMID: 38760100.

Duley, L., A. M. Gülmezoglu, D. J. Henderson-Smart, and D. Chou. "Magnesium Sulphate and Other Anticonvulsants for Women With Pre-Eclampsia." [In eng]. *Cochrane Database Syst Rev* 2010, no. 11 (Nov 10 2010): CD000025. https://doi.org/10.1002/14651858.CD000025.pub2.

Euser, A. G., and M. J. Cipolla. "Magnesium Sulfate for the Treatment of Eclampsia: A Brief Review." [In eng]. *Stroke* 40, no. 4 (Apr 2009): 1169–75. https://doi.org/10.1161/strokeaha.108.527788.

Fishel Bartal, M., and B. M. Sibai. "Eclampsia in the 21st Century." [In eng]. *Am J Obstet Gynecol* 226, no. 2s (Feb 2022): S1237–53. https://doi.org/10.1016/j.ajog.2020.09.037.

Friedman-Korn, T., Y. Lerner, S. Haggiag, et al. "Pearls and Oysters: Reversible Postpartum Pseudo-Coma State Associated With Magnesium Therapy: A Report of 2 Cases." [In eng]. *Neurology* 99, no. 10 (Sep 6 2022): 433–6. https://doi.org/10.1212/wnl.0000000000200956.

Gibson, K. S., C. A. Combs, S. Bauer, et al. "Society for Maternal-Fetal Medicine Special Statement: Quality Metric for Timely Postpartum Follow-up After Severe Hypertension." [In eng]. *Am J Obstet Gynecol* 227, no. 3 (Sep 2022): B2–8. https://doi.org/10.1016/j.ajog.2022.05.045.

Lazard, E. M. "A Preliminary Report on the Intravenous Use of Magnesium Sulphate in Puerperal Eclampsia." *Am J Obstet Gynecol* 9, no. 2 (1925): 178–88. https://doi.org/https://doi.org/10.1016/S0002-9378(25)90068-3.

Lu, J. F., and C. H. Nightingale. "Magnesium Sulfate in Eclampsia and Pre-Eclampsia: Pharmacokinetic Principles." [In eng]. *Clin Pharmacokinet* 38, no. 4 (Apr 2000): 305–14. https://doi.org/10.2165/00003088-200038040-00002.

Mai, H., Z. Liang, Z. Chen, et al. "MRI Characteristics of Brain Edema in Preeclampsia/Eclampsia Patients With Posterior Reversible Encephalopathy Syndrome." [In eng]. *BMC Pregnancy Childbirth* 21, no. 1 (Oct 3 2021): 669. https://doi.org/10.1186/s12884-021-04145-1.

McDonnell, N. J., N. A. Muchatuta, and M. J. Paech. "Acute Magnesium Toxicity in an Obstetric Patient Undergoing General Anaesthesia for Caesarean Delivery." [In eng]. *Int J Obstet Anesth* 19, no. 2 (Apr 2010): 226–31. https://doi.org/10.1016/j.ijoa.2009.09.009.

Okonkwo, M., and C. M. Nash. "Duration of Postpartum Magnesium Sulphate for the Prevention of Eclampsia: A Systematic Review and Meta-Analysis." [In eng]. *Obstet Gynecol* 139, no. 4 (Apr 1 2022): 521–28. https://doi.org/10.1097/aog.0000000000004720.

Poon, L. C., A. Shennan, J. A. Hyett, et al. "The International Federation of Gynecology and Obstetrics (FIGO) Initiative on Pre-Eclampsia: A Pragmatic Guide for First-Trimester Screening and Prevention." [In eng]. *Int J Gynaecol Obstet* 145, no. Suppl 1 (May 2019): 1–33. https://doi.org/10.1002/ijgo.12802.

Sullivan, M., K. Cunningham, K. Angras, and A. D. Mackeen. "Duration of Postpartum Magnesium Sulfate for Seizure Prophylaxis in Women With Preeclampsia: A Systematic Review and Meta-Analysis." [In eng]. *J Matern Fetal Neonatal Med* 35, no. 25 (Dec 2022): 7188–93. https://doi.org/10.1080/14767058.2021.1946505.

25 Targeted Temperature Management After Cardiopulmonary Resuscitation

A 62-year-old man was playing tennis with a friend when he suddenly complained of chest pain and immediately collapsed. His friend called 911 and started chest compressions. When paramedics arrived, the patient was unresponsive and pulseless. The defibrillator indicated a shockable rhythm. He was shocked three times before achieving return of spontaneous circulation (ROSC). Total time to ROSC was 12 minutes. On arrival to the emergency department, we intubated him and sedated him with a low-dose propofol infusion. Neurological examination off sedation showed that he was comatose with preserved pupillary light reflexes and no motor responses to pain. Head computed tomography scan was unremarkable. Temperature was 35.5°C.

What do you do now?

After many failed clinical trials (barbiturates and calcium channel blockers) in comatose survivors of cardiac arrest, two clinical trials published back to back in the *New England Journal of Medicine* in 2002 purported to demonstrate that induced hypothermia to a core temperature of 32°C to 34°C for the first 12 to 24 hours after cardiac arrest improved the functional outcome of patients who did not regain consciousness after resuscitation. These trials were small and methodologically weak but generated a dramatic change in practice. "Therapeutic hypothermia" as it became known, was the standard of care for comatose survivors after cardiac arrest and spurred a new industry of cooling devices that became staples in any intensive care unit (ICU) treating these patients. These are sophisticated cooling systems with pads placed on the patients connected to a temperature-regulating console and endovascular systems (the invasive devices were mostly later abandoned in the United States due to catheter thrombosis). The general excitement of having an effective treatment to improve the prognosis of these comatose brain-injured patients drowned out the few dissenting voices.

As it is so often in critical care trials (think trials in sepsis, acute respiratory distress syndrome, and hyperglycemia), later trials debunk the results of earlier ones. More than a decade elapsed before solid evidence shattered the universal acceptance of therapeutic hypothermia after cardiac arrest. First, the Targeted Temperature Management (TTM) trial showed no differences in functional outcomes when comparing temperature targets of 33°C vs. 36°C. Eight years later—and nearly 20 years after the trials that led to the generalized adoption of therapeutic hypothermia—the TTM2 trial showed that a temperature target of 37.8°C (i.e., maintenance of normothermia or avoidance of fever) was as good as 33°C. Furthermore, the hypothermia group had higher risk of arrythmia with hemodynamic compromise.

In defense of those ardent proponents of hypothermia, there are physiolologic arguments to support the neuroprotective value of hypothermia in post-CPR coma and any other severe, acute cerebral disease. Experimental studies have indisputably indicated that hypothermia lessens early ischemic injury by attenuating cerebral metabolism, mitigate mitochondrial damage, limit the effect of extracellular calcium and excitotoxic neurotransmitters, and reduce intracellular edema. Hypothermia could also diminish the subsequent reperfusion injury by lowering free radical production, curtailing cortical spreading depolarization, lessening apoptosis, and moderating the inflammatory response. Despite these experiment results, the clinical reality was different and, hypothermia did not achieve the predicted therapeutic benefit particularly when thoroughly evaluated in prospective clinical studies. Neither patients in trials of post anoxic injury after CPR for cardiac arrest nor patients with severe traumatic brain injury, acute bacterial meningitis, or status epilepticus have benefited from hypothermia. Furthermore, a large randomized controlled trial showed that strict fever prevention did not improve outcomes in critically ill patients with acute ischemic or hemorrhagic strokes.

The fuss and bother attending therapeutic hypothermia after cardiac arrest is instructive. The medical community embraced the results of flawed trials without sufficient scrutiny. These early trials were insufficiently powered (i.e., cohorts were too small), had poorly standardized care in the control patients, and did not account for differences in rates of withdrawal of life support. A veritable hypothermia industry sprung up. Adequate trials debunking hypothermia were possible thanks to the sustained efforts of investigators motivated by a healthy dose of skepticism. It took years for their efforts to be rewarded.

A subgroup of patients might benefit from induction of hypothermia, but these patients remain unidentified. The Therapeutic Hypothermia After Cardiac Arrest in Non Shockable Rhythm (HYPERION) trial tested hypothermia in 581 patients with initial nonshockable rhythm and reported a benefit in functional recovery among survivors, but the results has a fragility index of 1 (i.e., in this cohort, a hypothetical shift of one patient from the good-recovery to the poor-recovery category would have made the difference in functional outcome nonsignificant). Also, subanalysis of the TTM and TTM2 trials did not show any benefit of 33°C in patients with nonshockable rhythm. Hypothermia did not improve outcomes in trials of patients with in-hospital arrest. Deeper or longer cooling was also not beneficial in other trials. Intranasal cooling was not superior to other cooling methods, and early cooling not only is not useful but also can even be harmful. Intra-arrest cooling decreased the rate of achieving ROSC in the Rapid Infusion of cold Normal Saline by paramedics during CPR (RINSE) trial. Prehospital cooling demonstrated greater risk of pulmonary edema and recurrent cardiac arrest in a large trial conducted in Washington state. Although both the intervention and control groups of the TTM trials included fever prevention for the first 72 hours after admission, the value of prolonged maintenance of strict normothermia after out-of-hospital cardiac arrest remains unproven. A recent study addressed this uncertainty by testing whether a shorter period of fever prevention after an out-of-hospital cardiac arrest would be beneficial or harmful, but it showed that active, device-based fever prevention for 36 or 72 hours after cardiac arrest did not significantly change the percentages of patients dying or having severe disability as compared with a shorter period of fever control. The Influence of Cooling duration on Efficacy in Cardiac Arrest Patients (ICECAP) trial, designed to evaluate different degrees of cooling duration (up to 72–96 hours) in multiple patient groups, is ongoing. With new trials sprung up it seems it is hard to let go, but perhaps there is benefit from other approaches.

Induction of hypothermia has disadvantages. It reduces the clearance of sedatives, which in turn confounds the neurological examination. It produces shivering, which requires pharmacological treatment because it can increase metabolic demands if left untreated. Hypokalemia is very prevalent during hypothermia, and hyperkalemia can ensue as temperature rises. More serious adverse effects are possible, such as pneumonia, bleeding (from coagulation abnormalities), and cardiac arrhythmias during rewarming.

However, while hypothermia may not be useful, we should at least avoid fever. Patients in the control arm of the early trials assessing hypothermia after cardiac arrest were often febrile because treatment of fever in these patients was not a priority. Yet, fever can exacerbate damage to the acutely injured brain, and therefore, the concept of targeted temperature management to maintain normothermia remains valid and worth implementing in practice. Preventing fever should be a goal throughout the ICU stay. Also, we discourage active rewarming in patients presenting with spontaneous hypothermia shortly after the cardiopulmonary arrest. Current international guidelines concur in recommending fever prevention after cardiac arrest.

We treated our patient with targeted temperature management to keep his body temperature less than 37.8°C. He required external cooling to maintain this target. He regained alertness on the third day after arrest and returned to his cognitive baseline 3 months later.

We have learned a lesson and can only conclude that hypothermia is not effective for most—if not all—patients who remain comatose after attaining resumption of circulation (Box 25.1). Back to the drawing board—perhaps—but what will we draw?

> **BOX 25.1 Recommendations for TTM**
>
> - OHCA (VF): The present data *do not support* the use of hypothermia.
> - OHCA (PEA, asystole): The present data *may support* the use of targeted hypothermia.
> - IHCA: The present data *do not support* the use of hypothermia.
> - OHCA/IHCA: The present data *support* temperature control to avoid fever.
>
> TTM, targeted temperature management; IHCA, in-hospital cardiac arrest; OHCA, out-of-hospital cardiac arrest; PEA, pulseless electrical activity; VF, ventricular fibrillation.

KEY POINTS TO REMEMBER

- Targeted temperature management to prevent fever (keep body temperature <37.8°C) is necessary for all patients who remain comatose after cardiopulmonary resuscitation.
- Active cooling of the patient has no or little proven value after cardiac arrest.
- Avoid prehospital cooling because it can be detrimental.
- Allow temperature to rise passively in spontaneously hypothermic patients shortly after cardiac arrest, avoiding both active rewarming and fever.

Further Reading

Bernard, S. A., T. W. Gray, M. D. Buist, et al. "Treatment of Comatose Survivors of Out-of-Hospital Cardiac Arrest With Induced Hypothermia." [In eng]. *N Engl J Med* 346, no. 8 (Feb 21 2002): 557–63. https://doi.org/10.1056/NEJMoa003289.

Bernard, S. A., K. Smith, J. Finn, et al. "Induction of Therapeutic Hypothermia During Out-of-Hospital Cardiac Arrest Using a Rapid Infusion of Cold Saline: The RINSE Trial (Rapid Infusion of Cold Normal Saline)." [In eng]. *Circulation* 134, no. 11 (Sep 13 2016): 797–805. https://doi.org/10.1161/circulationaha.116.021989.

Dankiewicz, J., T. Cronberg, G. Lilja, et al. "Hypothermia Versus Normothermia After Out-of-Hospital Cardiac Arrest." [In eng]. *N Engl J Med* 384, no. 24 (Jun 17 2021): 2283–94. https://doi.org/10.1056/NEJMoa2100591.

Greer, D. M., Helbok, R., Badjatia, N., et al; INTREPID Study Group. "Fever Prevention in Patients With Acute Vascular Brain Injury: The INTREPID Randomized Clinical Trial." *JAMA* 332, no.18 (Nov 2024) :1525–1534. doi: 10.1001/jama.2024.14745.

Hassager, C., H. Schmidt, J. E. Møller, et al. "Duration of Device-Based Fever Prevention After Cardiac Arrest." [In eng]. *N Engl J Med* 388, no. 10 (Mar 9 2023): 888–97. https://doi.org/10.1056/NEJMoa2212528.

Hypothermia After Cardiac Arrest Study. "Mild Therapeutic Hypothermia to Improve the Neurologic Outcome After Cardiac Arrest." [In eng]. *N Engl J Med* 346, no. 8 (Feb 21 2002): 549–56. https://doi.org/10.1056/NEJMoa012689.

Kim, F., G. Nichol, C. Maynard, et al. "Effect of Prehospital Induction of Mild Hypothermia on Survival and Neurological Status Among Adults With Cardiac Arrest: A Randomized Clinical Trial." [In eng]. *Jama* 311, no. 1 (Jan 1 2014): 45–52. https://doi.org/10.1001/jama.2013.282173.

Laffey, J. G., and B. P. Kavanagh. "Negative Trials in Critical Care: Why Most Research Is Probably Wrong." [In eng]. *Lancet Respir Med* 6, no. 9 (Sep 2018): 659–60. https://doi.org/10.1016/s2213-2600(18)30279-0.

Lascarrou, J. B., H. Merdji, A. Le Gouge, et al. "Targeted Temperature Management for Cardiac Arrest With Nonshockable Rhythm." [In eng]. *N Engl J Med* 381, no. 24 (Dec 12 2019): 2327–37. https://doi.org/10.1056/NEJMoa1906661.

Meurer, W. J., F. F. Schmitzberger, S. Yeatts, et al.; ICECAP trial investigators. "Influence of Cooling Duration on Efficacy in Cardiac Arrest Patients (ICECAP): Study Protocol for a Multicenter, Randomized, Adaptive Allocation Clinical Trial to Identify the Optimal Duration of Induced Hypothermia for Neuroprotection in Comatose, Adult Survivors of After Out-of-Hospital Cardiac Arrest." [In eng]. *Trials* 25, no. 1 (Jul 23 2024): 502. doi:10.1186/s13063-024-08280-w.

Nielsen, N., J. Wetterslev, T. Cronberg, et al. "Targeted Temperature Management at 33°C Versus 36°C After Cardiac Arrest." [In eng]. *N Engl J Med* 369, no. 23 (Dec 5 2013): 2197–206. https://doi.org/10.1056/NEJMoa1310519.

Sandroni, C., J. P. Nolan, L. W. Andersen, et al. "ERC-ESICM Guidelines on Temperature Control After Cardiac Arrest in Adults." [In eng]. *Intensive Care Med* 48, no. 3 (Mar 2022): 261–69. https://doi.org/10.1007/s00134-022-06620-5.

26 Surviving Cardiac Arrest but Disabling Twitches

A 62-year-old hospitalized man was resuscitated after a cardiac arrest. He was intubated and sedated but extubated a day later after fully awakening and being able to follow commands. Several days later, he noted that his arms and legs were "shaking" when he tried to move them. There was no twitch when lying flat in bed, and he could then relax fully. He could not control these movements or move a glass to his mouth without violent shaking. When he tried to stand, his balance lapsed quickly, and any voluntary movement initiated a burst of arrhythmic jerks in his extremities. His neurologic examination, including a brief cognitive test of recall and memory, was otherwise normal. No structural lesions were found on computed tomography or magnetic resonance imaging (MRI). We are asked to diagnose and treat this disabling movement disorder, which was impeding his overall functional recovery.

What do you do now?

We diagnosed his condition as action myoclonus (or Lance-Adams syndrome). This syndrome is rare (<0.5% in a large series of patients who had cardiac arrest). This has also been our experience.

Myoclonus can improve or persist long term; certainly, many will remain significantly hampered by myoclonus if not appropriately treated. In patients who improve, the legs often jerk less than the arms, and some can eventually stand and walk. Adams said, "We assume there must be cerebellar lesions disinhibiting the cerebral cortex, and that is one of the forms of cortical polymyoclonus." Indeed, a multimodality monitoring study has shown that the myoclonus in patients wtih Lance Adams syndrome originate in the cortex.

We do not expect Lance-Adams syndrome to be confused with myoclonus status in a comatose patient because the baseline characteristics and phenotype are so different (Table 26.1). But it is useful briefly to explore myoclonus in the intensive care setting. Existing literature focuses more on the presence or absence of myoclonus and less on types, underlying causes, or movements that can be mistaken for myoclonus.

Myoclonus is classically defined as very brief, shock-like, jerky, completely jolting, involuntary movement, mostly affecting a group of muscles. Myoclonus is further classified according to its distribution (focal, multifocal, segmental, or generalized) or its origin generator (cortical, subcortical, brainstem, spinal, or segmental). What do we see at the bedside? Basically, it is a very quick movement of a body part and a movement that is not rhythmic and does not flow. We can see it in any muscle group—for example, eyelids (looks like blinking), face (looks like mimicry), abdomen (looks like hiccups), legs (looks like sleep starts), and, in status myoclonus, all of the above, continuous, and powerful.

Further differentiation is possible. For example, cortical myoclonus is more prominent in the distal extremities. It may be focal and confined to the upper limbs or multifocal. Jerks may be elicited by touch, tap, or acoustic stimuli. On the other hand, spinal myoclonus affects the axial muscles, recruited via the polysynaptic propriospinal pathways. Segmental myoclonus is usually confined to one or two contiguous segments with rhythmic jerks occurring at the rate of one to two per minute, and this myoclonus persists during sleep. Brainstem myoclonus typically results in generalized myoclonic jerks and has an exaggerated motor response to unexpected, typically auditory, stimuli. After cardiac arrest and cardiopulmonary

TABLE 26.1 **Clinical and EEG Differences Between Postarrest Myoclonus and Posthypoxic Action Myoclonus**

Postarrest Myoclonic Status	Posthypoxic Action Myoclonus
After cardiac arrest	Usually after respiratory arrest
Gone within a few days	Persists
Severe brain damage on physical examination and ancillary tests	No evidence of severe brain damage on physical examination and ancillary tests
EEG often with burst suppression and CT abnormalities	EEG with normal or nearly normal background and vertex spike-wave discharges. CT is usually normal
Poor outcome	Good cognitive recovery but ataxia

resuscitation, we expect cortical myoclonus, but in more severe insults, neuropathology has shown that the spinal cord and (less commonly) the brainstem may be part of anoxic-ischemic onslaught.

Movements superficially resembling myoclonus are tremors (not jerk-like and rhythmic) and asterixis (lapses of postural tone, sometimes called negative myoclonus). However, for neurologists, the differences are easy to recognize. As clinicians, we must be able to separate myoclonus status (continuous) from myoclonus jerks (occasional) and action myoclonus (initiated by movement and does not occur at rest).

Electroencephalographic (EEG) recordings from patients with myoclonus status have been classified into four patterns. Pattern 1 consists of burst-suppression, high-amplitude polyspikes, and pattern 2 involves continuous background and narrow, vertex spike-wave discharges. Patterns 1 and 2 are closely time-locked with myoclonus jerks. Pattern 3 shows myoclonus but without the epileptiform discharges associated with myoclonic jerks, and pattern 4 includes the remaining, more variable epileptiform patterns. Outcome is poor, and only the second pattern is seen in survivors. The EEG pattern 2 are patients who presumably have Lance-Adams syndrome.

Taking all comers, a large study from Berlin concluded that basal ganglia injury was the most likely neuroanatomical correlate of movement disorders as indicated by T1 hyperintensities and hypometabolism of this region on MRI and positron emission tomography. However, in our series we noted no basal ganglia abnormalities. Levomepromazine and intrathecal baclofen offered the first promising, usually fast-acting responses to control posthypoxic movement disorders and even hyperkinetic storms. In contrast, posthypoxic myoclonus responded best to combination of clonazepam, levetiracetam, and primidone. Remission rates of posthypoxic movement disorders were around 50%. Affected patients seemed to present with good recovery of cognitive functions in contrast to the often more severe physical deficits. Our experience is similar.

We should recognize that status myoclonus correlates with poor outcomes as found in our large contemporary series of patients with postresuscitation encephalopathy. We also found that not all forms of myoclonus portend the same prognosis. Markers of severe neurologic injury were more prevalent in patients with status myoclonus and included absent pupillary reflexes, extensor posturing, absent motor response, and malignant EEG findings defined as burst suppression or marked uppression with no reactivity unrelated to sedation. In addition, postarrest cardiac dysfunction requiring an intra-aortic balloon pump, ischemia/ reperfusion injury signified by higher creatinine levels, hypotension requiring pressors, and persistent precipitating comorbidities, such as chronic kidney disease, correlated with status myoclonus. In other words, patients with myoclonus status represent the category of patients hit the hardest. No wonder they are worse off.

Although after cardiac arrest the enormous majority of myoclonus is due to anoxic-ischemic injury, we should not forget that renal failure and medications (fentanyl, midazolam, carbapenem, antibiotics, and amiodarone) can also cause myoclonus. Occasionally, toxic doses of phenytoin and valproic acid may also be implicated.

In our experience, postresuscitation status myoclonus may be refractory to levetiracetam, benzodiazepines, and valproic acid. Moderate to high doses of propofol or neuromuscular junction blockers suppress "violent" myoclonus most effectively. On the other hand, treatment of Lance-Adams syndrome can be successful even in patients who are initially nearly immobilized from these movements. Our first line of treatment has been levetiracetam or valproate sodium, but benzodiazepines such as clonazepam or diazepam can be most effective. Others have reported good response with zonisamide. Combination of these agents is often necessary to achieve adequate control of the action myoclonus. There is a concern that polytherapy can cause sedation (and falls) and careful titration is needed. In Europe, a placebo-controlled, randomized study found that piracetam, 4 g/d daily to a maximal dose of 24 g, when used in combination with other drugs, significantly improved disability in some patients. (Piracetam is only available in Europe or Asia and shares pharmacological similarities with levetiracetam.) The rationale for these treatments is far from established, but benzodiazepines control myoclonus by acting on gamma-aminobutyric acid receptors. Treatment-refractory myoclonus is likely due to reticular reflex myoclonus rather than cortical myoclonus, in which case 5-hydroxytryptophan can be considered. Lifelong continuation of anti-seizure medication is usually required. In patients with treatment-refractory myoclonus due to other conditions, globus pallidus deep brain stimulation has been performed to palliate the myoclonus, but similar attempts have not been reported in Lance-Adams syndrome.

We treated our patient successfully with levetiracetam, 1000 mg twice daily, in combination with valproate (maximum of 60 mg/kg/d). The disabling myoclonus was much improved and weeks later he was symptom-free. Tapering of the medication resulted in some relapse, albeit less severe, and required continuation of the medication. One lesson here is that long-term polypharmacy may be needed.

KEY POINTS TO REMEMBER

- Most myoclonus following cardiac resuscitation is myoclonus status, but exclusively in comatose patients.
- Myoclonus status typically correlates with severe brain and systemic injury and is thus indicative of a poor outcome.
- Action myoclonus (Lance-Adams syndrome) but can be disabling, and untreated patients may be wheelchair bound.
- Action myoclonus can be treated, often with a combination of anti-seizure medication.

Further Reading

Aicua Rapun, I., J. Novy, D. Solari, et al. "Early Lance-Adams Syndrome After Cardiac Arrest: Prevalence, Time to Return to Awareness, and Outcome in a Large Cohort." [In eng]. *Resuscitation* 115 (Jun 2017): 169–72. https://doi.org/10.1016/j.resuscitation.2017.03.020.

Brown, P., M. J. Steiger, P. D. Thompson, et al. "Effectiveness of Piracetam in Cortical Myoclonus." [In eng]. *Mov Disord* 8, no. 1 (1993): 63–68. https://doi.org/10.1002/mds.870080112.

Caviness, J. N. "Myoclonus." [In eng]. *Continuum (Minneap Minn)* 25, no. 4 (Aug 2019): 1055–80. https://doi.org/10.1212/con.0000000000000750.

Chakraborty, T., S. Braksick, A. Rabinstein, and E. Wijdicks. "Status Myoclonus With Post-Cardiac-Arrest Syndrome: Implications for Prognostication." [In eng]. *Neurocrit Care* 36, no. 2 (Apr 2022): 387–94. https://doi.org/10.1007/s12028-021-01344-8.

Elmer, J., J. C. Rittenberger, J. Faro, et al. "Clinically Distinct Electroencephalographic Phenotypes of Early Myoclonus After Cardiac Arrest." [In eng]. *Ann Neurol* 80, no. 2 (Aug 2016): 175–84. https://doi.org/10.1002/ana.24697.

Fahn, S. "Newer Drugs for Posthypoxic Action Myoclonus: Observations From a Well-Studied Case." [In eng]. *Adv Neurol* 43 (1986): 197–99.

Harper, S. J., and R. G. Wilkes. "Posthypoxic Myoclonus (the Lance-Adams Syndrome) in the Intensive Care Unit." [In eng]. *Anaesthesia* 46, no. 3 (Mar 1991): 199–201. https://doi.org/10.1111/j.1365-2044.1991.tb09409.x.

Lance, J. W., and R. D. Adams. "The Syndrome of Intention or Action Myoclonus as a Sequel to Hypoxic Encephalopathy." [In eng]. *Brain* 86 (Mar 1963): 111–36. https://doi.org/10.1093/brain/86.1.111.

Lee, H. L., and J. K. Lee. "Lance-Adams Syndrome." [In eng]. *Ann Rehabil Med* 35, no. 6 (Dec 2011): 939–43. https://doi.org/10.5535/arm.2011.35.6.939.

Marcellino, C., and E. F. M. Wijdicks. "Posthypoxic Action Myoclonus (the Lance-Adams Syndrome)." [In eng]. *BMJ Case Rep* 13, no. 4 (Apr 16 2020): e234332. doi:10.1136/bcr-2020-234332. PMID: 32303528; PMCID: PMC7199192.

Obeso, J. A., J. Artieda, J. C. Rothwell, et al. "The Treatment of Severe Action Myoclonus." [In eng]. *Brain* 112, Pt 3 (Jun 1989): 765–77. https://doi.org/10.1093/brain/112.3.765.

Polesin, A., and M. Stern. "Post-Anoxic Myoclonus: A Case Presentation and Review of Management in the Rehabilitation Setting." [In eng]. *Brain Inj* 20, no. 2 (Feb 2006): 213–17. https://doi.org/10.1080/02699050500442972.

Scheibe, F., W. J. Neumann, C. Lange, et al. "Movement Disorders After Hypoxic Brain Injury Following Cardiac Arrest in Adults." [In eng]. *Eur J Neurol* 27, no. 10 (Oct 2020): 1937–47. https://doi.org/10.1111/ene.14326.

Wijdicks, E. F. M. "Looking Back at the Lance-Adams Syndrome: Uncommon and Unalike." [In eng]. *Neurocrit Care* (2024 Oct);41(2):695–699.

Vellieux, G., Apartis, E., Baudin, P., et al; Lance-Adams coinvestigators. "Multimodal Assessment of the Origin of Myoclonus in Lance-Adams Syndrome." *Neurology* 103, no.11 (Dec 10 2024): e209994. doi: 10.1212/WNL.0000000000209994. Epub 2024 Nov 5.

27 Hypertensive Emergency and Brain Edema

A man brought his 48-year-old girlfriend to the emergency department because she had been unwell for 3 months. For 2 weeks prior to her presentation, she developed progressive symptoms including headache, episodic dizziness, and difficulty standing with recurrent falls. In the 2 days before her presentation, she became confused, missed work, and slept a lot. She had a history of hypertension and received a prescription for antihypertensive medications 3 years earlier but never filled it.

On arrival, her blood pressure was shockingly high and 290/170 mmHg, and she was afebrile. On examination, she was drowsy and disoriented but arousable to tactile stimulation. She did not blink to threat or track the examiner. During our examination, we witnessed an episode of head and eye deviation to the right with tonic posturing of all four extremities. Laboratory evaluation revealed kidney injury and anemia of unclear chronicity. A peripheral blood smear was normal. Head computed tomography (CT) scam showed diffuse cerebral and cerebellar edema and hydrocephalus (Figure 27.1, top row).

What do you do now?

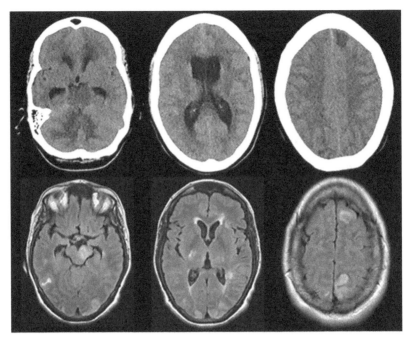

FIGURE 27.1 Top row: CT scan of the head on the day of presentation showing diffuse cerebral and cerebellar edema with a diffusely enlarged ventricular system. Bottom row: MRI of the brain 3 days after presentation shows a decrease in edema and resolution of hydrocephalus. Still present are patchy zones of fluid-attenuated inversion recovery (FLAIR) signal change in the frontal, parietal, and occipital lobes consistent with vasogenic edema.

The pattern to recognize here is the diffuse, symmetric, predominantly subcortical cerebral and cerebellar edema in connection with severe hypertension and clouding of consciousness. This condition was named reversible posterior leukoencephalopathy syndrome by Hinchey and colleagues in 1996. However, in 2000, cortical lesions were found on magnetic resonance imaging (MRI), and Casey and colleagues implied that the prefix "leuko" was incorrect. This led to renaming the diagnosis as posterior reversible encephalopathy syndrome and to the introduction of the acronym PRES—a catchy misnomer that seems to have settled permanently. Many subcortical areas other than the posterior regions are involved with frontal lobe edema being almost just as typical. Brainstem, basal ganglia, and in particular cerebellar involvement—as in our example—is seen in at least a third of the cases. Furthermore, we have repeatedly found the characteristic clinical syndrome without any vasogenic edema on brain MRI. We are convinced that MRI is useful to confirm the diagnosis when the edema is visible, but we cannot exclude the diagnosis when it is not. Reversibility of edema is the general rule, but not in areas with restricted diffusion on MRI—often indicating infarction and not edema. Intraparenchymal and sulcal subarachnoid hemorrhage and petechial hemorrhages are seen, but this was already noted by neuropathologists when the entity was still called hypertensive encephalopathy. Patients have died from increased intracranial pressure associated with severe brain edema and hemorrhages—so much for reversibility.

The insertion of encephalopathy in the moniker is also problematic. Some patients are confused because they cannot see (cortical blindness) or are postictal (generalized tonic-clonic seizures). Focal findings uncharacteristic of other forms of encephalopathy are also frequent (5%–15%). This clinical entity is therefore much more diverse in presentation and thus clinically more difficult to diagnose. We suspect PRES may have been present in many patients previously (and perhaps even now) diagnosed with "toxic-metabolic encephalopathy" in whom MRI was not available or not obtained. In fact, PRES may occur in patients with sepsis and renal failure.

Acute onset of neurologic symptoms in the setting of one of the following risk factors should alert the clinician to a potential diagnosis of PRES: severe hypertension, abrupt blood pressure fluctuations in the setting of sepsis or dysautonomia, calcineurin inhibitors, chemotherapy, acute kidney injury, dialysis and end-stage renal failure, autoimmune disease, or eclampsia (Box 27.1). Again, patients may present with any combination of encephalopathy, seizures, headache, visual disturbances, focal neurologic deficits such as aphasia or apraxia, and even hemiparesis. Visual disturbances may manifest as visual hallucinations, decreased visual acuity, a discrete visual field cut, or cortical blindness. Rarely, patients present with thunderclap headache or signs of a spinal cord lesion.

PRES may mimic other, less common conditions (Box 27.2). Cerebrospinal fluid (CSF) analysis is indicated in patients with fever, hypothermia, peripheral leukocytosis or leukopenia, recent viral prodrome, subacute onset of symptoms, or accompanying infectious or psychiatric symptoms. Neuroimaging showing any of the following should raise concern for an alternative diagnosis: unilateral abnormalities, isolated brainstem or

> **BOX 27.1 Risk Factors for Posterior Reversible Encephalopathy Syndrome**
>
> Severe hypertension or blood pressure fluctuations
>
> Renal failure (any chronicity)
>
> Eclampsia or preeclampsia
>
> Immunosuppressant therapy or chemotherapy
>
> Autoimmune disorder

cerebellar edema, or primarily confluent and periventricular signal abnormalities. Some noted that 4% of patients had imaging findings of a "central variant" PRES, revealing brainstem or deep gray nuclei lesions without involvement of the cerebral hemispheres. Extensive edema of central brain structures may result in brainstem compression and hydrocephalus. With a large number of atypical cases published, PRES is not easily excluded.

Rapid recognition of the syndrome, exclusion of alternative diagnoses, and removal or correction of the precipitant are paramount in the overall approach to these patients. Examples include treatment of hypertension, sepsis or acute kidney injury, or removal of a cytotoxic drug, such as tacrolimus or cyclosporine. These cytotoxic drugs should be withheld, when possible, even in the setting of normal drug concentrations as there is no association between PRES risk and drug serum levels. Switching from tacrolimus to sirolimus is a good option, as sirolimus carries minimal (if

> **BOX 27.2 Differential Diagnoses of PRES**
>
> Encephalitis
>   Infectious
>   Postinfectious (acute disseminated encephalomyelitis)
>   Antibody mediated (autoimmune or paraneoplastic)
>
> Progressive multifocal leukoencephalopathy
>
> Gliomatosis
>
> Severe subcortical leukoaraiosis
>
> Central nervous system necrotic vasculitis
>
> Osmotic demyelination syndrome
>
> Drug-induced leukoencephalopathy

any) risk of causing PRES. These decisions should be made in conjunction with the transplant team and not taken lightly.

Severe cerebral edema can result in coma, and prominent edema in the posterior fossa may cause obstructive hydrocephalus. Some patients may require acute CSF diversion but should not require ventriculoperitoneal shunting. Some patients with PRES show transient vasoconstriction on angiography and perfusion deficits during its hyperacute phase. Severe PRES can present with ischemic strokes, intracerebral hemorrhage, or subarachnoid hemorrhage (in sulci not basal cisterns). These complications are more common in patients with cerebral vasoconstriction.

Patients with a suspicion of clinical seizures should undergo at least a 30-minute electroencephalogram (EEG) to monitor for nonconvulsive status epilepticus and be treated appropriately with antiseizure medications. Dose adjustment for renal function may be necessary when using levetiracetam or lacosamide and a case can be made to use an alternate drug such as fosphenytoin or valproate. Recurrent seizures after PRES are uncommon and typically associated with recurrent bouts of PRES; prolonged antiseizure therapy is not necessary.

Approximately 75% to 90% of patients fully recover in several days, but severely affected patients rarely may take up to several weeks. However, we have seen the dramatic cortical blindness resolve within 24 hours of treating hypertension. Recurrent PRES has been reported in 5% to 10 % of patients and is even more likely when hypertension was the precipitant and blood pressure surges again. Recurrence is also more likely in patients with severe chronic kidney failure.

Our patient had severe end-organ sequelae of poorly controlled hypertension including PRES, microangiopathic hemolytic anemia, and renal failure. The goal was to reduce the mean arterial blood pressure by 20% to 25% within a few hours. This target value is cautious because cerebral blood flow autoregulatory limits are altered in patients with long-standing hypertension, and these patients easily reach a zone of "relative hypotension" and potential brain ischemia. The patient was loaded with antiseizure medication. Approximately 12 hours later, her blood pressure was decreased by another 10%, and then gradually normalized over several days. We additionally treated her with both hypertonic saline and mannitol for the first 12 to 24 hours, during which time she became progressively more alert. Hyperosmolar therapy was weaned over the next 2 days. On the third hospital day an MRI showed persistent vasogenic edema but resolution of hydrocephalus (Figure 27.1, bottom row). We always felt that a ventriculostomy could wait. Continuous EEG monitoring for the first 24 hours showed several electrographic seizures that responded to low doses of lorazepam. She continued antiseizure medication for 3 months, and she was seizure-free at last follow-up, 9 months after phenytoin discontinuation. She ultimately fully recovered without recurrence of PRES. This might be because she visits her nephrologist regularly and her blood pressure remains controlled on a four-drug regimen. Her microangiopathic hemolytic anemia and renal failure have persisted.

We see it all the time: PRES is underrecognized. Over the years, we have frequently diagnosed PRES in the emergency department and in medical and surgical intensive care units. PRES should be in the differential for patients with encephalopathy and delirium. In our own unit, we have seen it with severe dysautonomia and Guillain-Barré syndrome and as a complication of blood pressure augmentation to treat cerebral vasospasm in aneurysmal subarachnoid hemorrhage. Indeed, these unique circumstances in the neurosciences intensive care unit caught us off guard.

KEY POINTS TO REMEMBER

- Consider a diagnosis of PRES in patients presenting with acute onset of headache, encephalopathy, seizure, or focal neurologic deficits in the setting of blood pressure fluctuations, renal failure, cytotoxic drug use, autoimmune disorders, or eclampsia.
- If PRES is considered likely, removal of the precipitant is critical and can serve as a diagnostic test as it should result in clinical improvement over a period of days.
- Monitor for complications including seizures, hemorrhagic or ischemic strokes, and rarely hydrocephalus as their occurrence may require specific treatment.
- The syndrome is fully reversible in the majority of cases, but only if recognized rapidly and when the inciting factor is promptly removed or corrected.

Further Reading

Bartynski, W. S., and J. F. Boardman. "Distinct Imaging Patterns and Lesion Distribution in Posterior Reversible Encephalopathy Syndrome." [In eng]. *AJNR Am J Neuroradiol* 28, no. 7 (Aug 2007): 1320–27. https://doi.org/10.3174/ajnr. A0549.

Battal, B., and M. Castillo. "Imaging of Reversible Cerebral Vasoconstriction Syndrome and Posterior Reversible Encephalopathy Syndrome." [In eng]. *Neuroimaging Clin N Am* 34, no. 1 (Feb 2024): 129–47. doi:10.1016/ j.nic.2023.07.004. Epub 2023 Aug 7.

Casey, S. O., R. C. Sampaio, E. Michel, and C. L. Truwit. "Posterior Reversible Encephalopathy Syndrome: Utility of Fluid-Attenuated Inversion Recovery MR Imaging in the Detection of Cortical and Subcortical Lesions." [In eng]. *AJNR Am J Neuroradiol* 21, no. 7 (Aug 2000): 1199–206.

Datar, S., T. Singh, A. A. Rabinstein, et al. "Long-Term Risk of Seizures and Epilepsy in Patients With Posterior Reversible Encephalopathy Syndrome." [In eng]. *Epilepsia* 56, no. 4 (Apr 2015): 564–68. https://doi.org/10.1111/epi.12933.

Fugate, J. E., D. O. Claassen, H. J. Cloft, et al. "Posterior Reversible Encephalopathy Syndrome: Associated Clinical and Radiologic Findings." [In eng]. *Mayo Clin Proc* 85, no. 5 (May 2010): 427–32. https://doi.org/10.4065/mcp.2009.0590.

Geocadin, R. G. "Posterior Reversible Encephalopathy Syndrome." [In eng]. *N Engl J Med* 388, no. 23 (Jun 8 2023): 2171–78. https://doi.org/10.1056/NEJMra2114482.

Hawkes, M. A., M. Hajeb, and A. A. Rabinstein. "Perfusion Deficits in Patients With Posterior Reversible Encephalopathy Syndrome: A Retrospective, Two-Center Study." [In eng]. *Neurocrit Care* 38, no. 3 (Jun 2023): 726–32. https://doi.org/ 10.1007/s12028-022-01642-9.

Hinchey, J., C. Chaves, B. Appignani, et al. "A Reversible Posterior Leukoencephalopathy Syndrome." [In eng]. *N Engl J Med* 334, no. 8 (Feb 22 1996): 494–500. https://doi.org/10.1056/nejm199602223340803.

Kumar, A., S. G. Keyrouz, J. T. Willie, and R. Dhar. "Reversible Obstructive Hydrocephalus From Hypertensive Encephalopathy." [In eng]. *Neurocrit Care* 16, no. 3 (Jun 2012): 433–39. https://doi.org/10.1007/s12028-011-9663-z.

Lee, V. H., E. F. Wijdicks, E. M. Manno, and A. A. Rabinstein. "Clinical Spectrum of Reversible Posterior Leukoencephalopathy Syndrome." [In eng]. *Arch Neurol* 65, no. 2 (Feb 2008): 205–10. https://doi.org/10.1001/archneurol.2007.46.

Legriel, S., O. Schraub, E. Azoulay, et al. "Determinants of Recovery From Severe Posterior Reversible Encephalopathy Syndrome." [In eng]. *PLoS One* 7, no. 9 (2012): e44534. https://doi.org/10.1371/journal.pone.0044534.

28 The Elusive Rapidly Progressive Brain Disease

A 36-year-old woman complained of worsening headaches, fatigue, and malaise and then developed rapidly progressive behavioral changes and presumed seizures prompting hospitalization. Magnetic resonance imaging (MRI) of the brain showed nonspecific T2 hyperintense lesions in bilateral corona radiata and cerebrospinal fluid (CSF) with 13 total nucleated cells per mm^3, protein concentration of 57 mg/dL without oligoclonal bands, and normal glucose content. She was readmitted 3 days later for recurrent spells of posturing associated with hypoxemia, which required intubation and sedation with propofol. Repeat brain MRI (Figure 28.1) showed marked progression of white matter abnormality in both cerebral hemispheres with perivascular enhancement. MRI of the spine showed discontinuous T2 hyperintensity in the spinal cord at the cervical and thoracic segments without enhancement. A right frontal brain biopsy was complicated by focal hemorrhage. Pathology showed nonspecific excessive histiocytes. The family requested transfer to our institution for a definitive diagnosis.

What do you do now?

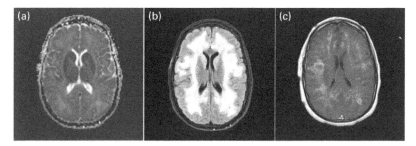

FIGURE 28.1 Examples of our patient's brain MRI upon presentation to our hospital. Apparent diffusion coefficient (A), fluid-attenuated inversion recovery (B), and postcontrast T1-weighted (C) sequences showing extensive white matter changes with perivascular contrast enhancement and restricted diffusion in basal ganglia.

Patients with rapidly progressive, diffuse, or multifocal brain disease requiring endotracheal intubation for coma represent a formidable diagnostic challenge and a state of uncertainty. Differential diagnoses are wide and seemingly endless, and the disorders typically have no pathognomonic features. When discussed in conferences, they could lead to wild, mostly wrong guesses and a game of one-upmanship. It may be impossible to arrive at a definitive diagnosis without pathological evaluation of diseased brain tissue. Our approach must therefore be systematic, and we must go through the common neuropathology such as vascular causes, infectious causes, parainfectious and autoimmune disorders, paraneoplastic variants, nutritional deficiencies, toxic encephalopathies from drugs, genetic metabolic disease, and brain hypoxia or ischemia. Often, the concept of a case discussion is not the expert's best guess but how the pathologic findings explain the clinical course and symptoms.

Clinical history remains especially important and certainly if it provides a good timeline. To acquire this history requires effort and discussions with family members. For example, progressive multifocal leukoencephalopathy presents in immunosuppressed patients or patients with AIDS. Even in those cases, definitive confirmation requires a specific test in the CSF (detection of polymerase chain reaction for JC virus) or brain biopsy. Certain brain structures may be preferentially involved and may provide further guidance (Table 28.1). The pattern of cerebral involvement on MRI can narrow the differential diagnosis, but MRI is rarely diagnostic.

TABLE 28.1 MRI in Rapid Progressive Brain Disease

Location	Causes
White matter	Acute disseminated encephalomyelitis Immunosuppression toxicity Posterior reversible encephalopathy syndrome Lymphomatosis cerebri Gliomatosis cerebri Solvents Chemotherapy Metabolic leukodystrophies Fulminant multiple sclerosis Autoimmune thyroiditis
Temporal lobes/hippocampi	Herpes simplex encephalitis Limbic encephalitis Fulminant multiple sclerosis Osmotic demyelination Wernicke-Korsakoff syndrome
Hemispheres	Astrocytoma Lymphoma Fungal and parasitic infections Neurosarcoidosis Fulminant multiple sclerosis Abscess Metastasis
Basal ganglia	Encephalitis (predominantly Eastern equine encephalitis) Methanol
Cortex/gray matter	Anoxic-ischemic injury Viral encephalitides such as West Nile or Powassan Carbon monoxide Creutzfeldt-Jakob disease Opioids
Cerebellum	Mitochondrial encephalomyopathy, lactic acidosis, and stroke-like episodes (MELAS) Primary and secondary vasculitis Mitochondrial encephalomyopathy (MELAS) Lymphoma Progressive multifocal leukoencephalopathy

Potentially treatment-responsive causes of rapid progressive dementia were diagnosed by brain biopsy in over 50% of patients in a multisite prospective cohort study. Autoimmune (34%), non-prion neurodegenerative (22%), and prion-related (16%) diseases were the most common causes of rapid progressive dementia.

Unusual types of disease mechanisms produce a clinical picture characterized by unrelenting neurological deterioration over days to weeks manifested by neurocognitive changes and bilateral long-track signs. If the cortex is involved, seizures may also occur. Abnormal movements, ataxia, and hypertonicity are common. Usually, none of these signs helps to discriminate among the various diagnostic possibilities.

Consider infectious and inflammatory processes first because of their eminently treatable nature. Subacute infections (e.g., fungal or mycobacterial) are typically associated with profound hypoglycorrhachia. Some forms of autoimmune encephalitis have distinctive MRI patterns (such as the radial periventricular enhancement observed in patients with antibodies against glial fibrillary acidic protein, initially considered a probable diagnosis in the case illustrated in this chapter). Yet, identification of the autoantibody is necessary to confirm the diagnosis. Brain biopsy is the only definitive method to diagnose malignancy (lymphoma should be an omnipresent consideration in these cases), neurosarcoidosis, histiocytosis, most cases of vasculitis, and occasional cases of Creutzfeldt-Jakob disease and cerebral amyloid angiopathy–related inflammation.

In fact, we encourage early consideration of brain biopsy in patients with rapidly progressive brain disease associated with extensive MRI abnormalities. While brain biopsy is certainly not risk-free, diagnostic delay, with successive MRIs only showing progression, may reduce the chance of a successful intervention if the chance exists. Yet, before proceeding with brain biopsy, we should explore safer biopsy targets in other parts of the body, which may be present even in patients without signs of systemic illness. Computed tomography (CT) scans with contrast of the chest, abdomen, pelvis and, particularly, whole-body positron emission tomography (PET) scans can identify areas of disease involvement, offering easier access for tissue diagnosis and reducing the need for brain biopsy. When the brain MRI shows no definite abnormalities, "blind" biopsy of meninges and cerebral tissue have an exceptionally low yield. It is worth having a second neuropathologist review the brain biopsy sample when the initial report fails to indicate a diagnosis. Moreover, samples might have skipped the lesion.

Empiric therapy is reasonable when there is a strong suspicion of a particular diagnosis (or at least a particular mechanism) but should not halt the search for the correct diagnosis. Particularly after administration of corticosteroids, a transient clinical response caused by attenuation of secondary inflammation and/or vasogenic edema can deceive the provider into a premature, incorrect diagnosis. As a rule, the clinician should never feel comfortable until reaching a definite diagnosis.

Our patient arrived in our hospital comatose with roving eye movements, bilateral extensor posturing, and sustained clonus in both ankle reflexes. She had frequent episodes of paroxysmal sympathetic hyperactivity but no seizures. We obtained a PET scan to look for underlying malignancy. It showed increased uptake in the right obturator muscle. CT-guided biopsy of that muscle tissue and review of the outside brain biopsy led to the diagnosis of ALK-positive histiocytosis. She was immediately started on alectinib, an ALK inhibitor. Unfortunately, she failed to respond. Subsequently, she received cladribine and high-dose methotrexate, also to no effect. After 3 months of chemotherapy, during which she developed systemic complications, the patient remained unresponsive. Follow-up brain MRI showed progressive parenchymal loss, and her family requested transition to comfort measures. Despite the intractable nature of the disease, the family was appreciative that we had achieved a definite diagnosis and gave her a chance for recovery.

Over the years, we have regularly seen cases of elusive, rapidly progressive brain disease leading to coma and intubation. We resort to (repeated) biopsies of the lesion when we are certain that there has been no toxin. The diagnosis often eludes us, and the disease progresses. If the family declines autopsy, we should carefully explain that it is our only chance to explain the disorder. Sometimes we are surprised later. (We have examples of later-discovered thallium poisoning and chlorobenzene inhalation.) Others have discussed clinicopathological conferences of cases with parainfectious encephalitides, Rocky Mountain spotted fever, schistosomiasis, and even neurosyphilis. Aaron Berkowitz summarized the challenges in complex, multielement cases, warned against anchoring, and suggested to: (1) seek the cause's cause by simply asking if something else could be causing the clinical findings, (2) to split the elements and not always lump them together, and (3) to take one element out or look for red herrings. For him, Hickham's dictum "a patient can have as many diseases as they want" may apply. However, transfers to tertiary centers often take place after a battery of negative test results. These patients are extraordinarily difficult to diagnose, and the reality is that we may not achieve a resolution—even if the referral physician or family thinks we may have a comparative advantage.

KEY POINTS TO REMEMBER

- Multiple disease mechanisms can cause rapid neurological decline, and MRI often demonstrates diffuse or multifocal abnormalities.
- Detailed history and evaluation of the radiological pattern can be helpful to guide diagnostic workup, but they are rarely sufficient in themselves to confirm the diagnosis.
- When serum and CSF investigations are nondiagnostic and there is no extracerebral biopsy target, perform brain biopsy on any accessible cerebral and/or meningeal target identified on MRI with contrast.
- Empiric treatment may be helpful, but apparent response should not preclude continuation of the diagnostic investigations.

Further Reading

Berkowitz, A. L. "Diagnostic Reasoning in Challenging Cases." [In eng]. *Pract Neurol* 24, no. 5 (Sep 13 2024): 376–81. doi:10.1136/pn-2023-003991.

Day, G. S. "Rapidly Progressive Dementia." [In eng]. *Continuum (Minneap Minn)* 28, no. 3 (Jun 1 2022): 901–36. https://doi.org/10.1212/con.0000000000001089.

Gelfand, J. M., G. Genrich, A. J. Green, et al. "Encephalitis of Unclear Origin Diagnosed by Brain Biopsy: A Diagnostic Challenge." [In eng]. *JAMA Neurol* 72, no. 1 (Jan 2015): 66–72. https://doi.org/10.1001/jamaneurol.2014.2376.

Josephson, S. A., A. M. Papanastassiou, M. S. Berger, et al. "The Diagnostic Utility of Brain Biopsy Procedures in Patients With Rapidly Deteriorating Neurological Conditions or Dementia." [In eng]. *J Neurosurg* 106, no. 1 (Jan 2007): 72–75. https://doi.org/10.3171/jns.2007.106.1.72.

Kuchenbecker, L. A., P. W. Tipton, Y. Martens, et al. "Diagnostic Utility of Cerebrospinal Fluid Biomarkers in Patients with Rapidly Progressive Dementia." [In eng]. *Ann Neurol* 95, no. 2 (Feb 2024): 299–313. doi:10.1002/ana.26822.

Lucas, C. G., A. Gilani, D. A. Solomon, et al. "ALK-Positive Histiocytosis With KIF5B-ALK Fusion in the Central Nervous System." [In eng]. *Acta Neuropathol* 138, no. 2 (Aug 2019): 335–37. https://doi.org/10.1007/s00401-019-02027-7.

Rossi, S., M. Gessi, S. Barresi, et al. "ALK-Rearranged Histiocytosis: Report of Two Cases With Involvement of the Central Nervous System." [In eng]. *Neuropathol Appl Neurobiol* 47, no. 6 (Oct 2021): 878–81. https://doi.org/10.1111/nan.12739.

Samuels, M. A., and A. E. Ropper. *Samuels and Ropper's Neurological CPCs From the New England Journal of Medicine*. 1st ed. New York: Oxford University Press; 2012.

Schuette, A. J., J. S. Taub, C. G. Hadjipanayis, and J. J. Olson. "Open Biopsy in Patients With Acute Progressive Neurologic Decline and Absence of Mass Lesion." [In eng]. *Neurology* 75, no. 5 (Aug 3 2010): 419–24. https://doi.org/10.1212/WNL.0b013e3181eb5889.

Satyadev, N., P. W. Tipton, Y. Martens, et al. "Improving Early Recognition of Treatment-Responsive Causes of Rapidly Progressive Dementia: The STAM$_3$P Score." [In eng]. *Ann Neurol* 95, no. 2 (Feb 2024): 237–48. doi:10.1002/ana.26812.

Vickrey, B. G., M. A. Samuels, and A. H. Ropper. "How Neurologists Think: A Cognitive Psychology Perspective on Missed Diagnoses." [In eng]. *Ann Neurol* 67, no. 4 (Apr 2010): 425–33. doi:10.1002/ana.21907.

29 Immune Checkpoint Inhibitors and Neuromuscular Disease

A 78-year-old man with previous treatment for metastatic melanoma presents to the hospital with diffuse muscle weakness 1 week after his second dose of pembrolizumab. He also noted that his voice was softer and his enunciation less clear. He had difficulty swallowing liquids and noted intermittent double vision. He found it hard to rise from a couch, but once he stood, he could walk unassisted. Neurologic examination showed bilateral ptosis, opthalmoparesis, and flaccid dysarthria (Figure 29.1). There was mild proximal muscle weakness of both the upper and lower extremities. Tendon reflexes were intact with no facilitation. Magnetic resonance imaging (MRI) of the brain and cervical spine was normal. Creatinine kinase was 1240 and aldolase was 42.9. Acetylcholine receptor antibodies were negative. Electromyography (EMG) showed brief, small, and polyphasic motor unit action potentials and fibrillation potentials. There was no evidence of a neuromuscular junction disorder on repetitive nerve stimulation.

What do you do now?

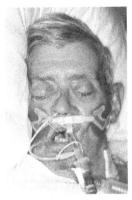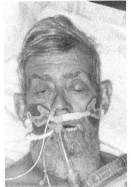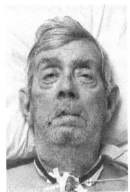

FIGURE 29.1 Severe ptosis, ophthalmoparesis, and bulbar weakness in a patient with lung cancer treated with pembrolizumab. Gradual improvement in 2 weeks (left to right) after corticosteroids, intravenous immunoglobulin, and plasma exchange administration.

The temporal association of weakness and pembrolizumab strongly suggested an immune-mediated myopathy, and the patient received prednisone, 80 mg daily. He underwent a muscle biopsy, which showed focal muscle fiber necrosis and inflammation. Antibody testing revealed an elevated, striated muscle antibody titer of 1:61,400. Paraneoplastic antibody panel was negative. Unfortunately, he worsened in a matter of days and developed severe respiratory weakness (profound respiratory paradox and use of accessory muscles) further complicated by mucous plugging, all leading to hypoxic respiratory failure and rapid endotracheal intubation. Given the severe deterioration and the underlying metastatic malignancy, the family opted for palliative care measures. An autopsy showed diffuse necrotic myositis of the diaphragm and lymphohistiocytic myocarditis. This presentation was one we had not previously seen in consultation. We have subsequently encountered equally severe cases (Figure 29.1).

This is a rare but increasingly recognized complication, and we now know that neurologic complications from anti-PD-1 therapy can involve both the central and peripheral nervous system (Figure 29.2). Often, these are case reports with variable neurologic details and granularity, and the overall incidence is highly variable, ranging from less than 1% to 15% in series of patients treated with pembrolizumab/nivolumab. It seems much

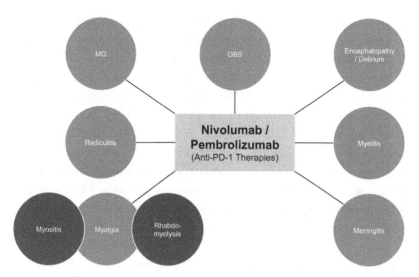

FIGURE 29.2 Neurologic complications with anti-PD-1 therapy. GBS, Guillain-Barré syndrome; MG, myasthenia gravis; PD, programmed death.

less common (<0.5%) in those receiving ipilimumab, with increased rates only in combinations of nivolumab plus ipilimumab.

Why are we seeing these complications? This warrants review of its putative mechanism. Pembrolizumab is an antibody that binds to PD-1 and blocks its interaction with the abnormal PD-L1 expressed by tumor cells. Programmed death 1 (PD-1) is a surface molecule expressed on antigen-stimulated T cells, monocytes, B cells, and dendritic cells. In normal cells, PD-1 acts as an immune checkpoint receptor. Immune checkpoints are a normal part of the immune system. Their role is to prevent an immune response from being so strong that it causes an autoimmune attack. PD-1 normally acts as a type of "off switch" that helps keep the T cells from attacking other cells in the body. It does this when it attaches to PD-L1, a protein on some normal (and cancer) cells. When PD-1 binds to PD-L1, it basically tells the T cell to leave the other cells alone. Tumor cells (such as melanoma) have substantial amounts of PD-L1. This allows them to suppress cytotoxic T-cell activity and enables the tumor cells to avoid a major attack by the immune system. Monoclonal antibodies that target either PD-1 or PD-L1 can block this binding and boost the immune response against cancer cells. But as an unintended but not surprising consequence, disruption of immune checkpoint receptors can lead to autoimmunity. The autoimmune response is cell-mediated (via T-cell and macrophage activation), causing damage to all components of the nervous system.

Neurologic complications tend to occur early, more often within 6 weeks of starting treatment. Published reports warn of aseptic meningitis and transverse myelitis within the first 6 weeks of treatment with ipilimumab (anti-CTLA-4), nivolumab, and pembrolizumab. Documented presentations that improve spontaneously after discontinuation of treatment include Tolosa-Hunt syndrome, granulomatous inflammation of the central nervous system, and encephalitis with seizures and MRI changes. An unusual complication is hypophysitis, which is frequently (10%) associated with anti-CTLA-4 therapy and usually occurs months later from initiation of therapy. Patients may develop headaches and hypopituitarism requiring hormonal replacement across the board. MRI may show an enlarged and enhancing pituitary gland.

The peripheral nerves and muscles are more frequently affected. Myositis is by far the most common, complication and it may be combined with myocarditis and signs suggestive of myasthenia gravis. Though not typically appreciated in other myopathies, immune checkpoint inhibitor (ICI) related myopathy can present with ocular findings, including ptosis and ophthalmoparesis which can suggest myasthenia gravis. However, in most patients, fluctuations or fatiguability are not part of the clinical presentation. Laboratory testing cannot distinguish between these diagnoses. For example, CK can be normal in oculobulbar ICI myopathy, and acetylcholine receptor antibodies can be detected in the absence of electrodiagnostic evidence of a neuromuscular junction disorder (abnormal jitter on single fiber testing) or vice versa. MRI of the orbits may show abnormal signal in the extraocular muscles suggestive of myopathy. Lack of response to acetylcholinesterase inhibitors also can argue against the diagnosis of myasthenia gravis. It is possible that cases of ICI toxicity initially attributed to myasthenia gravis were actually oculobulbar forms of ICI myopathy. If the diagnosis remains unclear, muscle biopsy should be pursued. Cases of ICI myopathy demonstrate multifocal necrotic fiber clusters. Positron emission tomography in myositis will show hot spots, often in the legs. However, myositis and myasthenia gravis may co-exist. In fact, the designation *Triple M syndrome* (combination of myocarditis, myositis, and myasthenia gravis) is commonly used, but we think it may not be as common as claimed and there may be anchoring relying on symptoms alone.

Specific types of peripheral neuropathy (e.g., mononeuritis multiplex, sensory neuronopathy, small-fiber autonomic neuropathy, and chronic inflammatory demyelinating polyneuropathy) have been reported. Guillain-Barré syndrome (GBS) showing the typical ascending progression has resulted from treatment with pembrolizumab and with nivolumab in combination with ipilimumab.

Our patient developed severe weakness of the bulbar musculature, with relative sparing of the limbs and, thus, a selection of certain muscle groups. Nivolumab, ipilimumab, pembrolizumab, and combination therapy, in that order, have induced reported cases of ICI–induced myasthenia gravis. In the largest case series of nivolumab-induced myasthenia gravis, patients received combinations of pyridostigmine, steroids, plasma exchange, and intravenous immunoglobulin. In an uncorroborated observation, patients with nivolumab-induced myasthenia gravis more often presented in myasthenic crisis than patients with idiopathic forms. Unfortunately, patients may not improve despite aggressive intervention of myasthenia gravis. Development of ptosis may predict concomitant myocarditis. At Mayo Clinic we identified 24 patients with immune checkpoint inhibitor–associated myopathy and 38 patients with immune-mediated necrotizing myopathy, and the study identified respiratory involvement in 20% to 30%.

Treatment of these complications naturally involves discontinuing pembrolizumab and giving high-dose corticosteroids (2 mg/kg body weight), but this is a difficult decision because it nullifies an expensive and often efficacious treatment of the malignancy. Plasma exchange (traditionally, 5 full exchanges) has occasionally attained success. The worst cases (defined as severe disability) receive intravenous high-dose methylprednisolone (1–2 mg/kg/d). If there is no benefit, the addition of tacrolimus, 0.15 mg/kg twice a day, or mycophenolate mofetil, 500 mg twice a day, could stabilize the symptoms. Another option is rituximab, a monoclonal antibody therapy targeting anti-CD20 on B cells administered as an infusion of 1 gram, usually every 4 weeks.

Neurological side effects could persist despite treatment with high-dose corticosteroids or other immunomodulating treatments.

If the patient survives and severe symptoms persist, methotrexate, azathioprine, and mycophenolate mofetil can be used, but they often take months to show full effect. Patients may experience undefined muscle pain and tingling for days, which subsequently worsens to severe neurologic manifestations. Arthralgia and myositis are very debilitating, but therapy with corticosteroids and anti-inflammatory drugs rapidly improves symptoms. Reintroduction of immune checkpoint inhibitors is inadvisable, although there is insufficient data.

Anderson and colleagues proposed performing a battery of studies: MRI of the spine with contrast (to rule out a concomitant lesion of the spinal cord and to look for enhancement of nerve roots), EMG, nerve conduction studies (NCSs) (to rule out a concurrent polyneuropathy), cerebrospinal fluid (CSF) analysis for flow cytometry, and cytology to rule out leptomeningeal carcinomatosis, in addition to measuring onconeural antibodies to assess for paraneoplastic disease. Investigation for a patient presenting with GBS is similar to that of a patient with meningoradiculitis, which must include MRI of the spine with contrast to rule out an acute myelopathy that can present with areflexia and flaccid paralysis. EMG and NCSs are critical to determine GBS types (i.e., axonal vs. demyelinating); the axonal variant of GBS portends a worse prognosis. CSF analysis should demonstrate albuminocytological dissociation to support the diagnosis of GBS, but lymphocytic pleocytosis in the CSF should raise suspicion of leptomeningeal carcinomatosis, infection, or paraneoplastic disease. In patients who present with fatigable ocular and proximal muscle weakness, look for myasthenia gravis (but remember the oculobulbar variant of myositis). NCSs should demonstrate an electro-decremental response with slow repetitive stimulation to support the diagnosis of myasthenia gravis. The increased jitter on single fiber EMG may clinch the diagnosis.

The increased frequency of these complications may eventually require a dedicated group with multidisciplinary expertise in managing these immunotherapy complications. We have added this neurocritical illness to our case collection because we expect to see these cases more often in consultation in the oncology ward, medical intensive care unit (ICU), or in our own neurosciences ICU.

KEY POINTS TO REMEMBER

- Neurologists must be aware of these immune-related complications. The use of these drugs in cancer treatment is expanding rapidly. Complications may too.
- The time between treatment and the development of complications can vary from weeks to months.
- Treatment of this complication naturally involves discontinuing pembrolizumab and high-dose corticosteroids (2 mg/kg).
- Treatment for steroid-refractory myocarditis can include mycophenolate mofetil, tacrolimus, antithymocyte globulin, IV immunoglobin (IVIG), abatacept, and plasmapheresis.

Further Reading

Barnhart, C. "Pembrolizumab: First in Class for Treatment of Metastatic Melanoma." [In eng]. *J Adv Pract Oncol* 6, no. 3 (May–Jun 2015): 234–38. https://doi.org/10.6004/jadpro.2015.6.3.5.

Beecher, G., Pinal-Fernandez, I., Mammen, A. L., Liewluck, T. "Immune checkpoint inhibitor myopathy: the double-edged sword of cancer immunotherapy." *Neurology* 103, n. 11 (Dec 10 2024): e210031. doi: 10.1212/WNL.0000000000210031.

Boutros, A., A. Bottini, G. Rossi, et al. "Neuromuscular and Cardiac Adverse Events Associated with Immune Checkpoint Inhibitors: Pooled Analysis of Individual Cases from Multiple Institutions and Literature." [In eng]. *ESMO Open* 8, no. 1 (Feb 2023): 100791. doi:10.1016/j.esmoop.2023.100791. Epub 2023 Feb 13.

Dubey, D., W. S. David, K. L. Reynolds, et al. "Severe Neurological Toxicity of Immune Checkpoint Inhibitors: Growing Spectrum." *Ann Neurol* 87, no. 5 (May 2020): 659–69. https://doi.org/10.1002/ana.25708. https://www.ncbi.nlm.nih.gov/pubmed/32086972.

Farina, A., C. Birzu, M. H. Elsensohn, et al. "Neurological Outcomes in Immune Checkpoint Inhibitor-Related Neurotoxicity." [In eng]. *Brain Commun* 5, no. 3 (2023): fcad169. https://doi.org/10.1093/braincomms/fcad169.

Farooq, M. Z., S. B. Aqeel, P. Lingamaneni, et al. "Association of Immune Checkpoint Inhibitors With Neurologic Adverse Events: A Systematic Review and Meta-Analysis." [In eng]. *JAMA Netw Open* 5, no. 4 (Apr 1 2022): e227722. https://doi.org/10.1001/jamanetworkopen.2022.7722.

Haanen, J., M. Obeid, L. Spain, et al. "Management of Toxicities from Immunotherapy: ESMO Clinical Practice Guideline for Diagnosis, Treatment and Follow-Up." [In eng]. *Ann Oncol* 33, no. 12 (Dec 2022): 1217–38. https://doi.org/10.1016/j.annonc.2022.10.001.

Hamada, N., A. Maeda, K. Takase-Minegishi, et al. "Incidence and Distinct Features of Immune Checkpoint Inhibitor-Related Myositis From Idiopathic Inflammatory Myositis: A Single-Center Experience With Systematic Literature Review and Meta-Analysis." [In eng]. *Front Immunol* 12 (2021): 803410. https://doi.org/10.3389/fimmu.2021.803410.

Lau, K. H., A. Kumar, I. H. Yang, and R. J. Nowak. "Exacerbation of Myasthenia Gravis in a Patient With Melanoma Treated With Pembrolizumab." [In eng]. *Muscle Nerve* 54, no. 1 (Jun 2016): 157–61. https://doi.org/10.1002/mus.25141.

Läubli, H., C. Balmelli, M. Bossard, et al. "Acute Heart Failure Due to Autoimmune Myocarditis Under Pembrolizumab Treatment for Metastatic Melanoma." [In eng]. *J Immunother Cancer* 3 (2015): 11. https://doi.org/10.1186/s40425-015-0057-1.

Okada, K., M. Seki, H. Yaguchi, et al. "Polyradiculoneuropathy Induced by Immune Checkpoint Inhibitors: A Case Series and Review of the Literature." [In eng]. *J Neurol* 268, no. 2 (Feb 2021): 680–88. https://doi.org/10.1007/s00415-020-10213-x.

Pepys, J., R. Stoff, R. Ramon-Gonen, et al. "Incidence and Outcome of Neurologic Immune-Related Adverse Events Associated With Immune Checkpoint Inhibitors in Patients With Melanoma." [In eng]. *Neurology* 101, no. 24 (Dec 12 2023): e2472–e2482. doi:10.1212/WNL.0000000000207632. Epub 2023 Aug 31.

Roth, P., S. Winklhofer, A. M. S. Müller, et al. "Neurological Complications of Cancer Immunotherapy." [In eng]. *Cancer Treat Rev* 97 (Jun 2021): 102189. https://doi.org/10.1016/j.ctrv.2021.102189.

Salam, S., T. Lavin, and A. Turan. "Limbic Encephalitis Following Immunotherapy Against Metastatic Malignant Melanoma." [In eng]. *BMJ Case Rep* 2016 (Mar 23 2016). https://doi.org/10.1136/bcr-2016-215012.

Vallet, H., A. Gaillet, N. Weiss, et al. "Pembrolizumab-Induced Necrotic Myositis in a Patient With Metastatic Melanoma." [In eng]. *Ann Oncol* 27, no. 7 (Jul 2016): 1352–53. https://doi.org/10.1093/annonc/mdw126.

Vicino, A., A. F. Hottinger, S. Latifyan, et al. "Immune Checkpoint Inhibitor-Related Myositis and Myocarditis: Diagnostic Pitfalls and Imaging Contribution in a Real-World, Institutional Case Series." [In eng]. *J Neurol* 271, no. 4 (Apr 2024): 1947–58. doi:10.1007/s00415-023-12134-x. Epub 2023 Dec 23.

Zhang, B., X. Li, T. Yin, et al. "Neurotoxicity of Tumor Immunotherapy: The Emergence of Clinical Attention." [In eng]. *J Oncol* 2022 (2022): 4259205. https://doi.org/10.1155/2022/4259205.

Zhu, J., and Y. Li. "Myasthenia Gravis Exacerbation Associated With Pembrolizumab." [In eng]. *Muscle Nerve* 54, no. 3 (Sep 2016): 506–7. https://doi.org/10.1002/mus.25055.

Zimmer, L., S. M. Goldinger, L. Hofmann, et al. "Neurological, Respiratory, Musculoskeletal, Cardiac and Ocular Side-Effects of Anti-PD-1 Therapy." [In eng]. *Eur J Cancer* 60 (Jun 2016): 210–25. https://doi.org/10.1016/j.ejca.2016.02.024.

30 Neurotoxicity of CAR T-Cell Therapy

A 58-year-old woman with large B-cell lymphoma proven refractory to conventional chemotherapy received infusion of CD19 chimeric antigen receptor (CAR) T-cell therapy. She had previously undergone chemotherapy and lymphodepleting conditioning with fludarabine and cyclophosphamide. She was neurologically asymptomatic before the CAR T-cell infusion. CAR T-cell infusion proceeded without complications. However, 4 days later she developed fever, tachycardia, hypotension, and hypoxemia. We obtained cultures and treated her with crystalloid fluids and empiric broad-spectrum antibiotic coverage for sepsis. Apart from persistent neutropenia, there was a markedly elevated C-reactive protein. Once admitted to the intensive care unit (ICU) because of worsening hypoxemia, she promptly received intravenous (IV) tocilizumab (8 mg/kg). Within the following hours, she became increasingly confused and then less responsive. On neurological examination, she would only awaken briefly to vigorous tactile stimulation.

What do you do now?

New oncologic approaches have dramatically changed outcome, but risks for major adverse effects can occur. We are increasingly involved in seeing these neurologic problems in medical ICUs. CAR T-cell therapy can induce remission in previously intractable cases of relapsed/refractory B-cell malignancies (acute lymphoblastic leukemia, large B-cell lymphoma, and mantle cell lymphoma) and multiple myeloma. However, the powerful immune activation it provokes can produce serious and potentially life-threatening complications, including severe neurotoxicity.

CAR T-cell therapy consists of harvesting T cells (the main orchestrators of the immune response) from the patient to modify their genetic code to express new receptors, called CARs, on their surface. Once they are reintroduced in the patient's circulation, these T cells can attach to a specific cancer cell antigen. Most current CAR T-cell products target the CD19 antigen. CAR T-cell activation leads to the release of effector cytokines, including interferon-gamma, tumor necrosis factor-alpha, and interleukin (IL)-2, which in turn trigger the release of proinflammatory cytokines (IL-1, IL-6, IL-10, monocyte chemoattractant protein-1). This resulting inflammatory response is the basis of the untoward effects.

Cytokine release syndrome (CRS) is the most common complication of CAR T-cell therapy, heralded by fever. Patients often complain of malaise and may have headache, myalgias, arthralgias, diarrhea, and skin rash. Tachycardia and tachypnea are common. More severe cases develop hypotension and hypoxemia, which may result in circulatory collapse, respiratory failure, and ICU admission. CRS presents in most patients within 1 to 2 weeks of CAR T-cell infusion; severe CRS manifestations can occur in 10% to 30% of cases. CRS is treated with supportive measures, prompt administration of tocilizumab (8 mg/kg IV up to 800 mg), and high-dose corticosteroids in the more severe cases (some patients have a variant of CRS that manifests as a hemophagocytic lymphohistiocytosis–like syndrome, which needs additional treatment with anakinra and basiliximab). Because these patients are ubiquitously neutropenic, and sepsis remains a real possibility broad-spectrum antibiotics are administered until sepsis is ruled out. Neurotoxicity is not part of CRS, although patients occasionally present nonspecific neurological symptoms.

Neurotoxicity from CAR T-cell therapy is best known in the literature as the *immune effector cell–associated neurotoxicity syndrome*, or *ICANS*.

It often coexists with CRS, but it can develop in its absence. An estimated 20% to 60% of patients treated with CAR T-cell therapy have signs of ICANS; severe ICANS occurs in 15% to 30%. Younger age, greater tumor disease burden, preexistent cerebral disease (although currently questioned), early severe CRS, and more profound cytopenias before CAR T-cell infusion have been risk factors for severe ICANS.

ICANS typically starts 3 to 10 days after CAR T-cell infusion. Grading of this condition has been variable, but a consensus seems to have been reached (with different monitoring tools for pediatric patients) by experts from all aspects of the field at a meeting supported by the American Society for Transplantation and Cellular Therapy (Table 30.1). Intracranial hemorrhage due to coagulopathy or other causes with or without associated edema is not part of this clinical syndrome and not graded.

The diagnosis of ICANS is clinical and demands exclusion of alternative diagnoses (most notably central nervous system infection). It manifests with confusion and reduced alertness that can range from mild drowsiness to coma. Headache, tremors, aphasia, and other, seldom assessed higher brain function abnormalities such as dysgraphia, dyscalculia, apraxia, and visual/proprioceptive skills can be prevalent. Patients may report visual and auditory hallucinations. Seizures and cerebral edema are the major potential complications. Although fortunately infrequent, status epilepticus and massive brain swelling are possible explanations in patients who become unresponsive and these conditions, obviously, must be immediately treated. In the RocKet trial, a study evaluating anti-CD19 CAR T-cell therapy in adult patients with B-cell acute lymphoblastic leukemia, five patients developed fatal cerebral edema, leading to early termination of the study. Other experiences with fatal diffuse cerebral edema have also been published. Some patients have more localized edema in the white matter, and in ICANS there may be some posterior predominance as in posterior reversible encephalopathy syndrome (Figure 30.1).

The trajectory of cerebral edema is unknown, and only extremes have been published. Experts in the field strongly feel that patients with any degree of cerebral edema should receive urgent treatment with osmotic agents and methylprednisolone. The pathophysiology of cerebral edema following CAR T-cell therapy has not been elucidated, Histological and neuroimaging

TABLE 30.1 **Consensus Grading for Cytokine Release Syndrome and Neurologic Toxicity Associated With Immune Effector Cells**

Neurotoxicity Domain	Grade 1	Grade 2	Grade 3	Grade 4
ICE score[a]	7–9	3–6	0–2	0 (patient is unarousable and unable to perform ICE)
Depressed level of consciousness[b]	Awakens spontaneously	Awakens to voice	Awakens only to tactile stimulus	Patient is unarousable or requires vigorous or repetitive tactile stimuli to arouse. Stupor or coma
Seizure	N/A	N/A	Any clinical seizure focal or generalized that resolves rapidly or nonconvulsive seizures on EEG that resolve with intervention	Life-threatening prolonged seizure (>5 minutes) or repetitive clinical or electrical seizures without return to baseline in between
Motor findings[c]	N/A	N/A	N/A	Deep focal motor weakness such as hemiparesis or paraparesis
Elevated ICP/cerebral edema	N/A	N/A	Focal/local edema on neuroimaging[d]	Diffuse cerebral edema on neuroimaging; decerebrate or decorticate posturing; cranial nerve VI palsy; papilledema; Cushing triad

ICANS grade is determined by the most severe event (ICE score, level of consciousness, seizure, motor findings, raised ICP/cerebral edema) not attributable to any other cause; for example, a patient with an ICE score of 3 who has a generalized seizure is classified as grade 3 ICANS.

ICANS, immune effector cell–associated neurotoxicity syndrome; IEC, immune effector cell; ICP, intracranial pressure; N/A, not applicable.

[a] A patient with an ICE score of 0 may be classified as grade 3 ICANS if awake with global aphasia, but a patient with an ICE score of 0 may be classified as grade 4 ICANS if unarousable according to CTCAE v5.0.

TABLE 30.1 **Continued**

[b] Depressed level of consciousness should be attributable to no other cause (e.g., no sedating medication).
[c] Tremors and myoclonus associated with immune effector cell therapies may be graded according to CTCAE v5.0, but they do not influence ICANS grading.
[d] Intracranial hemorrhage with or without associated edema is not considered a neurotoxicity feature and is excluded from ICANS grading. It may be graded according to CTCAE v5.0.
From D. W. Lee et al. *Biol. Blood Marrow Transplant* 25 (2019): 625–638, used with permission.

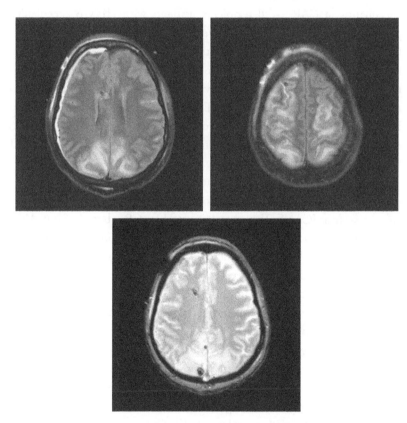

FIGURE 30.1 Profound white matter (vasogenic edema) in another patient treated with CAR T-cell therapy (CT and MRI). The edema was noted in the occipital, parietal, and cerebellar lobe but clinical examination only showed a mild encephalopathy. The gradient echo showed a few additional microhemorrhages in the areas with vasogenic edema in the white matter. (The patient's platelets were kept more than 20,000 after CAR T-cell therapy.) This patient suffered a devastating cerebellar hemorrhage 3 days into ICANS.

evidence supports vasogenic edema triggered by cytokine-mediated blood-brain barrier breakdown.

We also tailor neurological testing to the specific case and do not hesitate to obtain brain imaging and electroencephalography (EEG) in patients with diminished alertness and to perform lumbar puncture in those who are febrile. Severe (grade 3 and particularly grade 4) ICANS requires continuous EEG monitoring and serial brain imaging.

There is one infectious disease that warrants special consideration in the differential diagnosis. There are cases of human herpesvirus type 6 (HHV-6) encephalitis in CAR T-cell recipients. Patients with HHV-6 encephalitis present differently with cognitive changes and seizures and no fever. Cerebrospinal fluid (CSF) lymphocytic pleocytosis, temporal abnormalities shown on EEG, and hyperintense lesions in the limbic system shown on magnetic resonance imaging (MRI) are typical findings. CSF polymerase chain reaction is positive but should be differentiated from genome-integrated HHV-6 from prior exposure. There is no specific therapy for HHV-6 encephalitis, but consultants often prescribe ganciclovir or foscarnet. MRI findings may predict a poor outcome.

High-dose corticosteroids (dexamethasone IV 10 mg every 6 hours or, in high-grade cases, methylprednisolone 1g IV daily for at least 3 days) are effective to treat ICANS. Tocilizumab is useful for CRS, but not for ICANS; there is, in fact, evidence that tocilizumab might even contribute to ICANS by increasing circulating IL-6. Therefore, tocilizumab is only administered when the patient has substantial concomitant signs of CRS. We reserve anti-seizure medication and osmotic agents for patients with evidence of seizures or brain swelling. Anakinra (an IL-1-type receptor antagonist) and siltuximab (an anti-IL-6 drug) may help in cases of steroid-refractory ICANS, but this remains unproven. Most patients respond well to prompt administration of cortico steroids. Recovering patients usually tolerate rapid tapering of the cortico steroid dose, though they remain under careful clinical monitoring to exclude signs of recrudescence.

Because of her rapid neurological deterioration, our patient started methylprednisolone, 1g IV daily. She did not have papilledema and the head computed tomography scan was not suspicious for focal or diffuse brain edema. EEG showed generalized slowing without epileptiform activity. CSF revealed no signs of infection, and blood cultures remained negative.

The patient's neurological condition started improving gradually after the second day of high-dose methylprednisolone, and after the third day, we rapidly tapered the dose of steroid as she continued to improve.

CAR T-cell therapy is a potent accelerant of immune responses, and they may involve the brain. Varying degrees of neurotoxicity exist, and it is hard to predict which patients might be vulnerable. Once involved, we need to stay engaged until the clinical course has defined itself and we do not anticipate recurrent seizures and progressive brain swelling.

KEY POINTS TO REMEMBER

- CAR T-cell therapy is a valuable therapeutic option for patients with previously untreatable relapsing/recurrent hematological malignancies, but neurotoxicity is a frequent complication.
- Despite the absence of pathognomonic features, neurotoxicity from CAR T-cell therapy (ICANS) usually follows a predictable course.
- ICANS is a clinical diagnosis. Order neurological tests to diagnose complications (cerebral edema, seizures) and exclude alternative diagnoses (e.g., infection).
- Treat ICANS with high-dose steroids. Tocilizumab only if severe concurrent CRS. Osmotherapy only to patients who develop cerebral edema and antiseizure medication only to patient who had seizures.
- Fulminant fatal cerebral edema has been reported with ICANS.

Further Reading

Alsalem, A. N., L. A. Scarffe, H. R. Briemberg, et al. "Neurologic Complications of Cancer Immunotherapy." [In eng]. *Curr Oncol* 30, no. 6 (Jun 19 2023): 5876–97. https://doi.org/10.3390/curroncol30060440.

Freyer, C. W., and D. L. Porter. "Cytokine Release Syndrome and Neurotoxicity Following CAR T-Cell Therapy for Hematologic Malignancies." [In eng]. *J Allergy Clin Immunol* 146, no. 5 (Nov 2020): 940–48. https://doi.org/10.1016/j.jaci.2020.07.025.

Gea-Banacloche, J. C. "Infectious Complications of Chimeric Antigen Receptor (Car) T-Cell Therapies." [In eng]. *Semin Hematol* 60, no. 1 (Jan 2023): 52–58. https://doi.org/10.1053/j.seminhematol.2023.02.003.

Hayden, P. J., C. Roddie, P. Bader, et al. "Management of Adults and Children Receiving CAR T-Cell Therapy: 2021 Best Practice Recommendations of the European Society for Blood and Marrow Transplantation (EBMT) and the Joint Accreditation Committee of ISCT and EBMT (JACIE) and the European Haematology Association (EHA)." [In eng]. *Ann Oncol* 33, no. 3 (Mar 2022): 259–75. https://doi.org/10.1016/j.annonc.2021.12.003.

Karschnia, P., J. T. Jordan, D. A. Forst, et al. "Clinical Presentation, Management, and Biomarkers of Neurotoxicity After Adoptive Immunotherapy With CAR T Cells." [In eng]. *Blood* 133, no. 20 (May 16 2019): 2212–21. https://doi.org/10.1182/blood-2018-12-893396.

Lee, D. W., B. D. Santomasso, F. L. Locke, et al. "ASTCT Consensus Grading for Cytokine Release Syndrome and Neurologic Toxicity Associated With Immune Effector Cells." [In eng]. *Biol Blood Marrow Transplant* 25, no. 4 (Apr 2019): 625–38. https://doi.org/10.1016/j.bbmt.2018.12.758.

Lin, Y., L. Qiu, S. Usmani, et al.; International Myeloma Working Group. "Consensus Guidelines and Recommendations for the Management and Response Assessment of Chimeric Antigen Receptor T-Cell Therapy in Clinical Practice for Relapsed and Refractory Multiple Myeloma: A Report from the International Myeloma Working Group Immunotherapy Committee." [In eng]. *Lancet Oncol* 25, no. 8 (Aug 2024): e374–e387. doi:10.1016/S1470-2045(24)00094-9. Epub 2024 May 28. Erratum in: *Lancet Oncol* 25, no. 8 (Aug 2024): e336. doi:10.1016/S1470-2045(24)00337-1.

Neelapu, S. S., S. Tummala, P. Kebriaei, et al. "Chimeric Antigen Receptor T-Cell Therapy—Assessment and Management of Toxicities." [In eng]. *Nat Rev Clin Oncol* 15, no. 1 (Jan 2018): 47–62. https://doi.org/10.1038/nrclinonc.2017.148.

Pensato, U., L. Muccioli, P. Zinzani, et al. "Fulminant Cerebral Edema Following CAR T-Cell Therapy: Case Report and Pathophysiological Insights From Literature Review." [In eng]. *J Neurol* 269, no. 8 (Aug 2022): 4560–63. https://doi.org/10.1007/s00415-022-11117-8.

Rebechi, M. T., J. T. Bork, and D. J. Riedel. "HHV-6 Encephalitis After Chimeric Antigen Receptor T-Cell Therapy (CAR-T): 2 Case Reports and a Brief Review of the Literature." [In eng]. *Open Forum Infect Dis* 8, no. 11 (Nov 2021): ofab470. https://doi.org/10.1093/ofid/ofab470.

Rubin, D. B., H. H. Danish, A. B. Ali, et al. "Neurological Toxicities Associated With Chimeric Antigen Receptor T-Cell Therapy." [In eng]. *Brain* 142, no. 5 (May 1 2019): 1334–48. https://doi.org/10.1093/brain/awz053.

Wijdicks EFM, Rabinstein AA, Lin Y. CAR-T Cell Therapy and the Neurointensivist. *Neurocrit Care.* 2024 Oct;41(2):691-694. doi: 10.1007/s12028-024-01995-3. Epub 2024 May 28.

31 Failure to Awaken After Surgery

A 56-year-old woman underwent emergent repair of a perforated duodenal ulcer. Surgery was uncomplicated with no major blood loss or marked hypotension. There was no documented perioperative atrial fibrillation. Following surgery, the patient seemed agitated, which was viewed as emergence delirium or withdrawal from known substance abuse. She received lorazepam. This calmed her down, but she continued to "wake up slowly." The surgical intensive care service noted that she did not speak and barely responded to voice. Later, her speech was "unintelligible."

On neurologic examination, the patient had a markedly dysarthric speech, limited upgaze, and vertical nystagmus. There was a severe appendicular dysmetria. Computed tomography (CT) scan showed acute bilateral cerebellar hypodensities and acute hydrocephalus (Figure 31.1).

What do you do now?

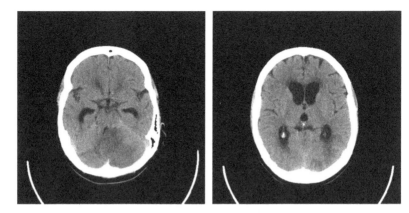

FIGURE 31.1 CT scan shows bilateral cerebellar strokes with acute obstructive hydrocephalus.

Abnormal responsiveness and awakening after a surgical procedure is a common reason for neurological consultation in surgical intensive care units (ICUs). The term "altered mental status" typically applies to patients who do not fully awaken following a major surgical repair and who do not respond well to the surgeon's questions during rounds. The total incidence of postoperative coma (≥24 hours) in one exceptionally large study of 858,606 patients was small (0.06%), but the investigators offered no precise causes or mechanisms. There are a few well-defined causes for failure to awaken after surgery, and the main ones are listed in Box 31.1.

The risk of perioperative stroke is higher within the first 72 hours after surgery. The first 24 hours carry the highest risk and offer the greatest challenge in identifying stroke symptoms because of lingering effects of anesthetic medications. Rapid recognition of strokes (quickly ordering CT and CT angiography [CTA] of the brain) could lead to clot retrieval through endovascular means in appropriate patients and, rarely, in patients with short procedures, use of intravenous thrombolysis if the estimated window is still within 4.5 hours. Obviously, it is all about recognition and calling the neurologist. But there are also several covert (silent) strokes, and recognition depends on the frequency and type of neuroimaging. It begs the question: covert to whom? Most studies have looked at so-called "overt" strokes. In those patients there is an unmistakable, unmissable acute onset of a major neurological deficit. But we have repeatedly received calls more than 24 hours from presumed presentation, which often leaves us with little to do. Delays to

> **BOX 31.1 Causes to Consider in Patients Who Fail to Awaken After Surgery**
>
> Excessive opioid use
>
> Prolonged clearance of benzodiazepines with multiorgan failure
>
> Postoperative hemispheric or brainstem strokes
>
> Postoperative cerebellar stroke with mass effect or hydrocephalus
>
> Postoperative posterior reversible encephalopathy syndrome[a]
>
> Acute hyponatremia
>
> Acute hypoglycemia or hyperglycemia
>
> Acute hypercapnia with hypoxemia
>
> Acute uremia
>
> Acute hyperammonemia
>
> Nonconvulsive status epilepticus
>
> [a] Aortic dissection repair.

consult us may occur due to other more pressing medical issues or from attributing clinical signs to sedation. Moreover, perioperative stroke in non-cardiac surgery is quite uncommon. In the most recent VISION (Vascular Events in Noncardiac Surgery Patients Cohort Evaluation) study with 40,004 patients older than 45 years of age who underwent noncardiac surgery, stroke occurred in 132 patients (0.3%). The incidence was not specifically higher in certain types of surgery. However, the risk of stroke after emergency noncardiac surgery was manifold higher in patients with a prior stroke within the preceding 3 months. Complex cardiac or vascular procedures are more often associated with ischemic stroke. Most surgeons anticipate "trouble ahead" when they find mobile atherosclerotic plaques or if prolonged hypotension occurs during major vascular surgery; both strongly predicting insults to the brain.

Once we have determined a patient has had a perioperative stroke, we should search for a possible underlying mechanism (changes in intraoperative and postoperative hemodynamics) and investigate for cardioembolism, including a screen for atrial fibrillation sometimes with extended continuous monitoring. (Perioperative atrial fibrillation is often transient but, once observed, may recur in up to 50% of patients.) Still in our experience we are often unsuccessful in pinpointing a definitive mechanism.

Ischemic stroke involving major arterial territories is a well-known complication of any type of vascular surgery (e.g., aortic arch replacement, surgery for aortic dissection) or any type of open-heart surgery. Vertebral occlusions (e.g., dissecting aorta occluding the vertebral artery origins) are responsible for strokes in the cerebellum, but the posterior circulation is often involved in cardiogenic stroke. The diagnostic yield of magnetic resonance imaging (MRI) in a patient remaining stuporous can be substantial and can show multiple hemispheric and often cortical lesions accounting for failure to awaken after anesthesia.

In cases of postoperative, bithalamic infarct-associated stupor (explained by an embolus in the artery of Percheron—an anatomical variant where one artery feeds both paramedian thalami and rostral midbrain), MRI remains a highly informative test in postoperative patients whose decreased level of consciousness is due to something other than sedation. In patients undergoing a general (nonvascular-noncardiac) surgical procedure—as in our case example—we do not expect neurological complications. Multiple ischemic strokes after a general surgical procedure (e.g., urogenital, gastrointestinal, orthopedic, or chest surgery) that do not develop from manipulation of the vasculature are rare and hard to explain. They occur most often in patients with other risk factors for stroke (e.g., peripheral vascular disease or ischemic cardiomyopathy). Hypotension does not play a key role except when there is a large, unexpected blood loss or there is underlying advanced cervicocranial arterial stenosis.

When ischemic stroke involving the posterior circulation results in cerebellar infarcts with obstructive hydrocephalus (explaining stupor), the diagnosis is difficult and often goes unrecognized. In our patient, the sudden occurrence of a bilateral cerebellar infarct compressing the fourth ventricle led to an obstructive hydrocephalus. After placement of a ventriculostomy, the patient improved and eventually was weaned from the ventriculostomy. Worsening and outcome are related to the size of the infarct—larger volume cerebellar strokes cause more clinical worsening and these patients are candidates for suboccipital decompression. Medical management is a realistic option for patients with swelling without clinical worsening, although strategies are poorly defined and including use of osmotic diuretics which we often use until we see the swelling subside.

Finally, it is noteworthy that postoperative stupor in general surgical ICUs usually is due to prolonged clearance of sedative drugs or excessive opioid use. Intravenous naloxone in repeated doses of 0.4 mg may be needed and up to 2 mg at 3-minute intervals. Quick train-of-four testing is also needed to exclude persistent neuromuscular blockage. Additionally, multiorgan failure in critically ill patients may reduce clearance of most of these drugs, and a careful look at the medication dose, infusion rate, and expected clearance is necessary. Reduced renal clearance of sedatives and analgesics is a major determinant of prolonged awakening after cardiac surgery. (A focused 16-gene pharmacogenomics panel will look for genetic differences that could warn a patient about slow metabolism with future surgeries.)

Also rare, but often considered a diagnostic possibility, is the presence of nonconvulsive status epilepticus. This is a highly unusual occurrence after any type of surgical procedure and general anesthesia. It is more likely in patients with a history of seizures or a known seizure disorder but who did not have their antiseizure medications administered. We have encountered cases of status epilepticus particularly after cardiac surgery.

Always consider an acute metabolic derangement such as acute hyponatremia or acute hypoglycemia; occasionally, these derangements explain the clinical picture. In susceptible patients, a surgical procedure can lead to an acute increase in serum ammonia. (These are mostly teenaged females with an ornithine transcarbamylase deficiency or patients who have had a lung transplant.)

In any patient with postoperative coma, we need to go back to the basics of a coma examination and determine if the lesion started in one hemisphere, in both hemispheres, or in the brainstem. Then we would need an urgent CT scan and CTA that could show a new structural lesion on CT (hemorrhage, hydrocephalus, brain edema) or large cerebral vessel occlusion of the anterior or posterior circulation (CTA). MRI of the brain is more determinative and could show a new stroke or fat or air emboli. With no apparent structural injury, we need to exclude a new metabolic derangement (hypoglycemia, hyponatremia, hyperammonemia) or nonconvulsive status epilepticus.

What happened to our patient? We think it must have been an embolus to the vertebral artery, but also a dominant single PICA that perfused both cerebellar hemispheres. This situation is uncommon but we have seen more than a few similar cases over the years. In some there were additional infarctions in thalami and occipital lobes.

The next time you are asked to see a patient with postoperative stupor in the surgical ICU with "altered mental status," think of 5 causes starting with an S: sedatives, stroke, seizures, sudden metabolic derangement, and slow drug clearance due to altered pharmacokinetics and pharmacodynamics—not specifically in that order. We have seen a number of cases of functional postoperative coma that often declares itself with unusual neurologic findings (sudden fixation with eye opening, inability to do an oculocephalic test again due to eye fixation, changing eye deviation). But we also acknowledge that potent anesthetics (ketamine, opioids, propofol) may cause bizarre clinical pictures (read: inexplicable neurologic findings). But if we look at the grand scheme of things, the three major causes of failure to awaken postoperatively (or excessively slow recovery of consciousness) are drugs, drugs, and drugs and their poor clearance due to age and organ failure. It is Occam's razor—the simplest explanation is the correct one.

KEY POINTS TO REMEMBER

- Postoperative stupor is usually associated with excessive sedation. As a rule, the expected clearance of an opioid or benzodiazepine is usually five times its half-life.
- In stuporous patients, consider an ischemic stroke in the posterior circulation involving the thalamus or cerebellar infarction(s) causing acute hydrocephalus from compression.
- Hyponatremia and hypoglycemia are potential causes of postoperative stupor. Hypoglycemia requires immediate correction, while hyponatremia should be corrected more slowly.

Further Reading

Baki, E., L. Baumgart, V. Kehl, et al. "Predictors of Malignant Swelling in Space-Occupying Cerebellar Infarction." [In eng]. *Stroke Vasc Neurol* (Aug 29 2024): svn-2024-003360. doi:10.1136/svn-2024-003360. Epub ahead of print.

Benesch, C., L. G. Glance, C. P. Derdeyn, et al. "Perioperative Neurological Evaluation and Management to Lower the Risk of Acute Stroke in Patients Undergoing Noncardiac, Nonneurological Surgery: A Scientific Statement From the American Heart Association/American Stroke Association." [In eng]. *Circulation* 143, no. 19 (May 11 2021): e923–46. https://doi.org/10.1161/cir.0000000000000968.

Christiansen, M. N., C. Andersson, G. H. Gislason, et al. "Risks of Cardiovascular Adverse Events and Death in Patients With Previous Stroke Undergoing Emergency Noncardiac, Nonintracranial Surgery: The Importance of Operative Timing." [In eng]. *Anesthesiology* 127, no. 1 (Jul 2017): 9–19. https://doi.org/10.1097/aln.0000000000001685.

Limburg, M., E. F. Wijdicks, and H. Li. "Ischemic Stroke After Surgical Procedures: Clinical Features, Neuroimaging, and Risk Factors." [In eng]. *Neurology* 50, no. 4 (Apr 1998): 895–901. https://doi.org/10.1212/wnl.50.4.895.

Newman, J., K. Blake, J. Fennema, et al. "Incidence, Predictors and Outcomes of Postoperative Coma: An Observational Study of 858,606 Patients." [In eng]. *Eur J Anaesthesiol* 30, no. 8 (Aug 2013): 476–82. https://doi.org/10.1097/EJA.0b013e328 35dcc62.

Rodriguez, R. A., M. Bussière, M. Bourke, et al. "Predictors of Duration of Unconsciousness in Patients With Coma After Cardiac Surgery." [In eng]. *J Cardiothorac Vasc Anesth* 25, no. 6 (Dec 2011): 961–67. https://doi.org/10.1053/j.jvca.2010.10.001.

Spence, J., Y. LeManach, M. T. V. Chan, et al. "Association Between Complications and Death Within 30 Days After Noncardiac Surgery." [In eng]. *CMAJ* 191, no. 30 (Jul 29 2019): e830–37. https://doi.org/10.1503/cmaj.190221.

Vasivej, T., P. Sathirapanya, and C. Kongkamol. "Incidence and Risk Factors of Perioperative Stroke in Noncardiac, and Nonaortic and Its Major Branches Surgery." [In eng]. *J Stroke Cerebrovasc Dis* 25, no. 5 (May 2016): 1172–76. https://doi.org/10.1016/j.jstrokecerebrovasdis.2016.01.051.

Wang, Y., M. M. Binkley, M. Qiao, et al. "Rate of Infarct-Edema Growth on CT Predicts Need for Surgical Intervention and Clinical Outcome in Patients With Cerebellar Infarction." [In eng]. *Neurocrit Care* 36, no. 3 (Jun 2022): 1011–21. https://doi.org/10.1007/s12028-021-01414-x.

Wijdicks, E. F. M. *Solving Critical Consults.* Core Principles of Acute Neurology. New York: Oxford University Press; 2015.

Won, S. Y., S. Hernández-Durán, B. Behmanesh, et al. "Functional Outcomes in Conservatively vs Surgically Treated Cerebellar Infarcts." [In eng]. *JAMA Neurol* 81, no. 4 (Feb 26 2024): 384–93. doi:10.1001/jamaneurol.2023.5773. Epub ahead of print.

32 Stupor After Brain Surgery

A 23-year-old man underwent surgical resection of a tumor filling the fourth ventricle extending into the cerebellopontine angle and upper cervical spinal canal (Figure 32.1A). Pathology showed World Health Organization grade II ependymoma. Following surgery, he demonstrated dysarthria, dysphagia, and left hemiataxia and underwent a surgical reexploration with removal of an extradural hematoma in the posterior fossa. He recovered well; a week later, he unexpectedly became gradually more stuporous and developed a new hemiparesis. We decided to transfer him back to the neurosciences intensive care unit. On examination, he did not follow commands, was mute, and was grinding his teeth. He had increased bilateral grasp reflexes and snout reflexes. His brainstem reflexes were intact. He had significant right arm weakness, barely overcoming gravity. Computed tomography (CT) scan showed new multiple hemispheric hypodensities, mostly in the posterior frontal lobes (Figure 32.1B). Cerebral angiogram showed diffuse cerebral vasospasm in both anterior and posterior circulation (Figure 32.1C).

What do you do now?

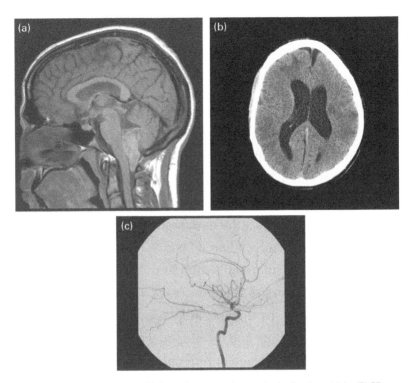

FIGURE 32.1 (A) Preoperative MRI shows large ependymoma in the fourth ventricle. (B) CT scan about 10 days after surgery shows multiple hypodensities. (C) The cerebral angiogram (sample of multiple series) shows cerebral vasospasm in the anterior circulation.

To detect deterioration, after brain tumor surgery, we often observe patients overnight in an intensive or intermediate care unit. Most leave the intensive care unit the next day. Neurosurgeons ask neurointensivists to become involved in postoperative care when the clinical condition is unexplained and unusual, because seizures have occurred, or because a major systemic complication needs close attention. Complications after craniotomy are uncommon but may be more frequent after extensive and complex neurosurgery. To know what to consider, Box 32.1 lists the causes of deterioration after a craniotomy.

A patient with early deterioration may be having seizures, but most patients who are stuporous or comatose from seizures will have already shown focal twitches that become more generalized and evolve into nonconvulsive

> **BOX 32.1 Causes of Deterioration After Craniotomy**
>
> Seizures (partial or generalized) and status epilepticus
>
> Postoperative hemorrhage (operative bed or remote)
>
> Cerebral infarction (sacrifice of an arterial branch or cerebral vein)
>
> Postoperative cerebral edema
>
> Diffuse cerebral vasospasm
>
> Medical complications (e.g., hyponatremia or hypernatremia after pituitary surgery)

status epilepticus. The cause may not be clear or may simply be related to removal of brain tumor tissue or postoperative swelling. The best treatment options in these patients include intravenous levetiracetam loading with 60 mg/kg or intravenous fosphenytoin loading with 20 mg/kg.

Postoperative hemorrhage in the surgical bed may or may not be symptomatic. When mass effect occurs, patients are more likely to decline. A more recently identified cause of neurologic deterioration is the appearance of a hematoma remote from the surgical site. Most hemorrhages are venous and may be in the opposite hemisphere or, most commonly, in the cerebellum in patients with surgery of the cerebral hemispheres. They may also occur after drainage of an acute subdural hematoma. The likely mechanism is mechanical shift of the brain ("sagging") after intracranial pressure reduction, either intraoperatively or by excessive postoperative suction drainage. These remote hemorrhages can become clinically relevant, and lobar hemorrhage may present with new seizures. Hemorrhages in the cerebellar peduncles produce new-onset slurred speech, cerebellar ataxia, and nystagmus. Often, the hemorrhages resolve without affecting functional recovery.

Cerebral infarction can occur after craniotomy when there is sacrifice of an arterial or venous branch. The typical example is a sizable meningioma extirpation with necessary sacrifice of large venous tributaries.

Certain neurosurgical procedures correlate with more specific complications in the postoperative days. These include patients with epilepsy surgery who have hemorrhagic complications associated with depth-electrode placement (rare) and patients after pituitary surgery with major adrenal or thyroid deficiencies (more common). A week after pituitary surgery, hyponatremia may occur and become acutely severe. Hypernatremia with major polyuria may follow hyponatremia and require treatment with desmopressin (Chapter 50).

Our patient had a well-described postoperative complication that may be more common than appreciated but is rarely considered. A cerebral angiogram may be necessary to identify a cerebral vasospasm. Early on, even a magnetic resonance angiogram may not be sufficiently sensitive to demonstrate vasospasm in smaller arterial branches. The onset of new neurologic signs, particularly when they do not easily fit a single syndrome, and the appearance of new-onset multifocal ischemia on CT scan should point toward this complication. Diffuse cerebral vasospasm can occur up to a week after surgery, and its development is associated with clear clinical deterioration. Patients may have fluctuating neurologic deficits that could point toward the diagnosis. Cerebral vasospasm may be more prevalent after certain types of neurosurgical procedures and, in particular, after skull base surgery. A commonly implicated surgery is pituitary adenoma resection via a transcranial or transsphenoidal approach.

Proposed causes for postsurgical cerebral vasospasm include significant blood loss during surgery and the release of vasoactive substances after resection of tumors encasing vasculature. However, the pathophysiology of cerebral vasospasm after tumor surgery is not known. Removal of tumor adjacent to the basal cisterns could release vasoactive substances, but this remains speculative. Intraoperative hemorrhage and postoperative blood in the subarachnoid cisterns were not prominent in reported cases and have not been factors in the cases we have seen. Mechanical manipulation with extensive mobilization of medium-sized arteries during surgery might be another cause. Yet, this does not explain the diffuse distribution of the vasospasm or its development after a prolonged interval. Therefore, neither what we know about delayed vasospasm following aneurysmal subarachnoid hemorrhage nor what we know about reversible cerebral vasoconstriction syndrome explains these cases of vasospasm after brain tumor surgery.

After establishing the diagnosis, there is some uncertainty about how to treat this condition. If the situation allows, the treatment should be (1) to increase cerebral perfusion by opening the larger arteries through angioplasty and smaller ones through intra-arterial infusion of vasodilators and (2) to increase cerebral perfusion pressure with traditional methods of hemodynamic augmentation (vasopressors and milrinone).

Our patient's significant diffuse cerebral vasospasm warranted immediate balloon angioplasty and intra-arterial infusion of verapamil in multiple arterial segments. He additionally received hemodynamic augmentation using vasopressors. He recovered gradually and eventually achieved an acceptable functional outcome.

Even though it is unusual, consider cerebral vasospasm after brain surgery in any patient with unexplained deterioration. Cerebral vasospasm, when severe, may require endovascular intervention, which is successful if done early.

KEY POINTS TO REMEMBER

- Cerebral vasospasm can explain neurological worsening after craniotomy for tumor surgery. It can be diffuse and extend beyond the surgical field. Often, only catheter cerebral angiogram can document the presence of vasospasm.
- Worsening can also occur because of hemorrhage in the surgical bed, remote hemorrhage, cerebral edema, or ischemic stroke from sacrifice of a large vein or artery.
- Postoperative seizures may present as focal seizures, which may evolve into generalized status epilepticus.

Further Reading

Alotaibi, N. M., and G. Lanzino. "Cerebral Vasospasm Following Tumor Resection." [In eng]. *J Neurointerv Surg* 5, no. 5 (Sep 1 2013): 413–18. https://doi.org/10.1136/neurintsurg-2012-010477.

Amini, A., A. G. Osborn, T. D. McCall, and W. T. Couldwell. "Remote Cerebellar Hemorrhage." [In eng]. *AJNR Am J Neuroradiol* 27, no. 2 (Feb 2006): 387–90.

Bejjani, G. K., L. N. Sekhar, A. M. Yost, et al. "Vasospasm After Cranial Base Tumor Resection: Pathogenesis, Diagnosis, and Therapy." [In eng]. *Surg Neurol* 52, no. 6 (Dec 1999): 577–83; discussion 83–84. https://doi.org/10.1016/s0090-3019(99)00108-1.

Budnick, H. C., S. Tomlinson, J. Savage, and A. Cohen-Gadol. "Symptomatic Cerebral Vasospasm After Transsphenoidal Tumor Resection: Two Case Reports and

Systematic Literature Review." [In eng]. *Cureus* 12, no. 5 (May 17 2020): e8171. https://doi.org/10.7759/cureus.8171.

Honegger, J., J. Zentner, J. Spreer, et al. "Cerebellar Hemorrhage Arising Postoperatively as a Complication of Supratentorial Surgery: A Retrospective Study." [In eng]. *J Neurosurg* 96, no. 2 (Feb 2002): 248–54. https://doi.org/10.3171/jns.2002.96.2.0248.

Krayenbuehl, H. "[A Contribution to the Problem of Cerebral Angiospastic Insult]." [In ger]. *Schweiz Med Wochenschr* 90 (Aug 27 1960): 961–65.

Sturiale, C. L., M. Rossetto, M. Ermani, et al. "Remote Cerebellar Hemorrhage After Supratentorial Procedures (Part 1): A Systematic Review." [In eng]. *Neurosurg Rev* 39, no. 4 (Oct 2016): 565–73. https://doi.org/10.1007/s10143-015-0691-6.

Williams JD, Lucas S, Breton J,et al. Cerebral vasospasm following tumor resection: Illustrative cases and review of the literature. *Clin Neurol Neurosurg.* 2024 Oct 10;246:108590. doi: 10.1016/j.clineuro.2024.108590. Epub ahead of print.

33 When Antiseizure Medication Causes Harm

A 72-year-old man with paroxysmal atrial fibrillation and a right middle cerebral artery stroke 1 year prior presented to the emergency department with focal seizures and secondary generalization. He received intravenous lorazepam and a loading dose of levetiracetam but then had another focal seizure. We administered lacosamide in a loading dose (400 mg). Shortly after his arrival at the intensive care unit, we noted a second-degree atrioventricular (AV) block (Mobitz type II) on the telemetry monitor. He was still asymptomatic with no bradycardia or hypotension. His electrocardiogram previously showed atrial fibrillation with normal ventricular response.

What do you do now?

Even antiseizure medications with a favorable side effect profile can cause major adverse events. The drugs we used in the not-so-distant past were known to be toxic and, therefore, we used them with more caution. But now there are more antiseizure medications perceived as benign and all too often prescribed without a second thought about potential complications. We cannot prescribe lacosamide without first reviewing an electrocardiogram for a prolonged PR interval. In this case, those prescribing lacosamide did attempt to check the PR interval on an electrocardiogram, but they could not complete the assessment because the patient was in atrial fibrillation. They did not think that the risk was high enough to withhold lacosamide. In fact, looking back, this patient had a prior electrocardiogram with a sinus rhythm and prolonged PR. Although the risk of cardiac complications from intravenous loading with lacosamide is low, we have seen serious AV blocks in more than one occasion and acknowledge this uncommon but serious risk.

It is imperative to know the side effect—and drug interaction—profile of antiseizure medications that one uses. And we must not underestimate these risks. It is a responsibility of the prescribing clinician, and not just the pharmacist, to think of potential adverse events and interactions. When approached conscientiously, this task may appear insurmountable given the number of possible adverse effects and interactions. Yet nowadays there are point-of-care tools that can facilitate the task and ensure the safe use of these medications. In the emergency setting, we may not always weigh the options.

Table 33.1 summarizes the main side effects and interactions of the most used medications in neurocritical care including some so frequent or dangerous that they deserve special attention.

Levetiracetam has become the most prescribed medication for acute treatment of seizures in the hospital. The main reason is its safety profile and absence of major interactions with other drugs. However, we have occasionally seen it cause severe agitation in young patients and persistent reduction of alertness (even stupor) in older ones. Excreted directly by the kidneys, levetiracetam can accumulate in patients with reduced renal filtration. Failure to adjust the dose for current renal function is a common error. Brivaracetam, which works similarly to levetiracetam, has fewer behavioral side effects, and requires no renal adjustment but is restricted

TABLE 33.1 **Clinically Meaningful Adverse Effects and Drug Interactions From Antiseizure Medications Used in the Emergency Setting**

Antiseizure Drug	Main Side Effects	Main Interactions With Other Drugs
Levetiracetam	Irritability, agitation (young patients) Sedation, drowsiness (older patients)	None
Brivaracetam	Less behavioral side effects than levetiracetam	None
Lacosamide	Prolongs PR interval Sedation, fatigue, dizziness at higher doses	Avoid using with AV node blockers (calcium channel blockers and beta-blockers)
Valproic acid	Liver toxicity Bleeding diathesis (thrombocytopenia, platelet dysfunction) Hyperammonemia Pancreatitis Acute encephalopathy	Increases phenytoin exposure Increases rufinamide exposure Its free fraction may increase when used with phenytoin Carbapenems reduce the effect Risk of severe skin rash when used with lamotrigine Increases effect of warfarin May decrease effect of direct oral anticoagulants

(continued)

TABLE 33.1 **Continued**

Antiseizure Drug	Main Side Effects	Main Interactions With Other Drugs
(Fos)phenytoin	Hypotension Sedation Hepatotoxicity Thrombocytopenia Serious skin reactions Cardiac arrhythmia Cognitive impairment Local reactions (phlebitis, cellulitis) in site of infusion	Reduces exposure to medications metabolized by cytochrome P450: Antiseizure drugs (such as carbamazepine, lamotrigine, felbamate) Anticoagulants (warfarin and direct anticoagulants) Protease inhibitors (used to treat HIV infection) Digoxin Nimodipine Chemotherapeutic agents (such as cyclosporine, paclitaxel, methotrexate) Fluconazole, ketoconazole, and voriconazole reduce (fos)phenytoin exposure Valproic acid increases (fos)phenytoin exposure Oxcarbazepine can increase risk of phenytoin toxicity Ethosuximide can increase risk of phenytoin toxicity

for use in patients with end-stage renal disease (and still prohibitively expensive in the out-of-hospital setting).

Valproic acid is a highly effective antiseizure drug, but its side effect profile is less favorable. In addition to the myriad, untoward effects seen with chronic use (weight gain, fatigue, dizziness, drowsiness, tremor, hair loss, nausea, and even parkinsonism in the elderly), its acute administration can cause hepatotoxicity, pancreatitis, thrombocytopenia, and platelet dysfunction, and hyperammonemia. Reported cases of acute encephalopathy have occurred in the absence of hyperammonemia. Also, its drug interactions are multiple and prominent. It competes for protein binding and reduces the metabolism of phenytoin; thus, concomitant use of these two medications often results in high free-serum concentrations of phenytoin. Carbapenems increase the metabolism of valproic acid and may render it ineffective; we have seen status epilepticus result from overlooking this major interaction. In patients taking lamotrigine, it is prudent to avoid the acute use of valproic acid because of the increased risk of Stevens-Johnson syndrome when these two drugs interact.

Phenytoin (and its prodrug fosphenytoin) also has major potential adverse effects. Its acute administration can produce hypotension, sedation, hepatotoxicity, thrombocytopenia, and serious skin reactions including toxic epidermal necrolysis and drug rash with eosinophilia and systemic symptoms (DRESS syndrome). It can manifest with diffuse lymphadenopathy, liver failure, and renal failure, in addition to rash and eosinophilia. Fosphenytoin has a lower risk of local infusion reactions (phlebitis and cellulitis) and has a faster infusion rate than phenytoin but still demands telemetry monitoring. We can reduce the risk of hypotension by infusing the drug more slowly (i.e., reserving the maximal rate of fosphenytoin infusion of 150 mg/min only for patients with convulsive status epilepticus), but other side effects are more difficult to predict and prevent. Rarely, phenytoin (and fosphenytoin) can induce cardiac arrhythmias—even ventricular tachycardia and fibrillation—and therefore it is best to avoid using this medication in patients with severe cardiomyopathies. Because phenytoin induces the cytochrome P450 enzymatic system, it can increase the hepatic metabolism of multiple medications including other antiseizure drugs (such as carbamazepine), anticoagulants (warfarin and direct anticoagulants including dabigatran, and anti-Xa inhibitors), protease inhibitors used to treat HIV infection, digoxin, and various chemotherapeutic agents (such as cyclosporine). When discharging a patient on phenytoin, consider other side effects including ataxia, dizziness, nystagmus, lethargy, drowsiness, cognitive impairment, osteoporosis, gingival hyperplasia, hirsutism, folate deficiency, and various other immunological reactions.

Phenobarbital remains a effective antiseizure drug, but its adverse effects are even more extensive. Sedation, respiratory depression, liver toxicity, hypotension, myocardial depression, ileus, and increased risk of pneumonia are the main ones. Barbiturates are also potent inducers of the cytochrome P450 system. When you start a patient on a barbiturate, try to discontinue it as soon as possible. Discontinuation after chronic use becomes a formidable task.

Lacosamide stabilizes excitable neuronal membranes by activating slow Na channels and is a commonly used drug. Avoid lacosamide in patients with liver failure, and adjust the dose as needed with renal dysfunction. Prolongation of the PR interval is the most common adverse effect and can result in AV block as illustrated by our patient. Severe toxicity of lacosamide can paradoxically cause both seizures and terminal cardiac arrhythmias. We have encountered refractory ventricular tachycardia that only responded to stellate ganglion blocks with lidocaine.

Our patient remained hemodynamically stable, and therefore we did not need to treat with beta-adrenergic agonists. We used transcutaneous cardiac pacing and kept atropine at the bedside. We emergently consulted cardiology, but transvenous pacing was not necessary because the AV block resolved spontaneously. We were lucky and we knew that the complication could have been much worse. We took advantage of the case to reinforce the policy of avoiding lacosamide in any patient with an abnormal PR interval.

With all these side effects, it seems that starting any antiseizure medication is scary business and in all seriousness it is not. But we should be prepared to encounter major adverse events from the use of antiseizure drugs. We cannot underestimate drug-drug interactions and the effect of liver and renal failure, which may not be initially present and may emerge later. We must protect patients from iatrogenic complications that can be serious.

KEY POINTS TO REMEMBER

- Do not underestimate the risk of serious adverse events from antiseizure drugs, even when prescribing medications with a safer profile.
- Do not forget to check what other drugs the patient is receiving because drug interactions are common with most antiseizure medications.
- Except when treating convulsive status epilepticus, always consider the potential for harm before prescribing any antiseizure drug.

Further Reading

Abou-Khalil, B. W. "Update on Antiseizure Medications 2022." [In eng]. *Continuum (Minneap Minn)* 28, no. 2 (2022): 500–535. https://doi.org/10.1212/con.000000000 0001104.

Goldstein, R., A. R. Jacobs, L. Zighan, et al. "Interactions Between Direct Oral Anticoagulants (DOACs) and Antiseizure Medications: Potential Implications on DOAC Treatment." [In eng]. *CNS Drugs* 37, no. 3 (2023): 203–14. https://doi.org/ 10.1007/s40263-023-00990-0.

Kim, H. K., H. Lee, E. K. Bae, et al. "Cardiac Effects of Rapid Intravenous Loading of Lacosamide in Patients With Epilepsy." [In eng]. *Epilepsy Res* 176 (2021): 106710. https://doi.org/10.1016/j.eplepsyres.2021.106710.

Loser, V., J. Novy, I. Beuchat, et al. "Acute Valproate-Induced Encephalopathy in Status Epilepticus: A Registry-Based Assessment." [In eng]. *CNS Drugs* 37, no. 8 (2023): 725–31. https://doi.org/10.1007/s40263-023-01024-5.

Marcellino, C., C. C. Ransom, and E. F. Wijdicks. "Refractory Ventricular Tachycardia and Seizures With Lacosamide Overdose." [In eng]. *Cureus* 14, no. 9 (2022): e29547. https://doi.org/10.7759/cureus.29547.

Perucca, P., and F. G. Gilliam. "Adverse Effects of Antiepileptic Drugs." [In eng]. *Lancet Neurol* 11, no. 9 (2012): 792–802. https://doi.org/10.1016/s1474-4422(12)70153-9.

34 LVAD and Intracranial Hemorrhage

A 72-year-old man with a HeartMate II left ventricular assist device (LVAD) as destination therapy and chronic anticoagulation with warfarin presented to the emergency department after having a generalized seizure. He had no previous history of seizures or previous strokes. On examination, he was drowsy and had mild right hemiparesis. Head computed tomography showed an acute left frontal intracerebral hematoma (Figure 34.1). The international normalized ratio (INR) was 3.1. While still in the emergency department, his postictal state resolved but then he had another brief seizure.

What do you do now?

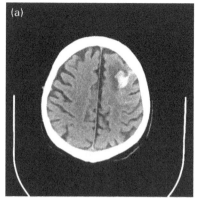 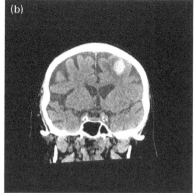

FIGURE 34.1 Head CT, axial (A) and coronal (B) views, showing a left frontal intracerebral hemorrhage with some surrounding edema but without tissue shift.

A rare situation until not long ago, this case illustrates a problem now relatively common in daily practice, at least in large-volume centers with sophisticated cardiothoracic surgery programs. Approaching end-stage heart failure encompasses several medical and surgical innovative therapies. End-stage heart failure is notable for persistent symptoms that interfere with daily life activities and lead to recurrent hospitalizations despite maximal medical therapy. Implantation of LVADs functions as a bridge to transplantation, a bridge to candidacy, or (palliative) destination therapy. Increasingly, LVADs are used as destination therapy with considerable success. As the survival of patients with end-stage heart failure and palliative LVADs lengthens, the chances of anticoagulation-related intracerebral hematoma (ICH) grow. Contemporary LVAD recipients are more severely ill than recipients in the past, but outcomes are better (survival times ranging from 1 month to more than 10 years with an estimated median of 5 years). Cardiovascular surgeons optimistically feel that with improving technology and miniaturization, the furthest goal could be to offer device therapy comparable to (or even surpassing) heart transplantations in the long term.

Patients with LVADs present a series of unique challenges compared to other patients with anticoagulation-associated ICH. The first decision is whether to reverse anticoagulation. Anticoagulation reversal is necessary when ICH is life-threatening and most certainly in patients presenting within the first few hours from symptom onset when the risk of hematoma expansion is greatest. However, given the particularly considerable risk of thrombotic complications (device malfunction, cerebral and systemic embolism), we may avoid reversal agents when the chances of expansion are relatively low, such as in patients with a small ICH or subdural hematoma and patients with delayed presentation. Four-factor prothrombin complex concentrate along with intravenous vitamin K are also typically used here (see Chapter 2). Fresh frozen plasma is generally not a viable alternative because of the heightened risk of inducing volume overload in these patients with underlying severe heart failure.

Intracranial hemorrhage in patients with LVADs is most commonly intracerebral and spontaneous, but it can be posttraumatic (most often subdural or multicompartmental) or related to device-associated infection (sulcal subarachnoid or intracerebral). Hemorrhagic conversion of an embolic ischemic infarction should also be considered. Close attention to the radiological pattern of the hemorrhage and concurrent signs of infection helps clarify the cause of the bleeding.

In cases of subdural hemorrhage or intraparenchymal hematoma with major tissue shift, the best possible functional prognosis and cardiac risks of a major neurosurgery should be considered, sometimes with minimal time to make the decision. Yet, a combined discussion among the neurologist, the neurosurgeon, and the cardiologist should occur before committing to evacuation, assuming informed consent from the patient's surrogate.

These patients either await transplantation or receive mechanical circulatory support for palliation of their end-stage heart failure. In their situation, a disabling ICH may be a terminal disease, even when the bleeding is not fatal per se. For younger patients on a transplant list, prognosis is crucial because disabling neurological injury may potentially remove them from the list. Neurologists estimating prognosis must therefore be cognizant of the implications of their pronouncements. It is not out of the question that patients with non-incapacitating strokes could still receive a heart transplant.

In patients who survive the ICH, the need to resume anticoagulation is even more pressing than for patients with mechanical valves. While withholding anticoagulation is generally safe for at least 1 week in patients with metallic valves, LVADs are less forgiving. The risk of embolism may be higher, but the risk of LVAD malfunction makes cardiologists and cardiac surgeons extremely uncomfortable when these patients are not being fully anticoagulated. The optimal timing of anticoagulation resumption in patients with LVADs and ICH is unclear. In practice, we feel the pressure to restart anticoagulation as soon as possible and often resume it—with no small degree of discomfort—within 3 to 5 days of the hemorrhage. When the hemorrhage is subdural, we now pursue embolization of the middle meningeal cerebral artery before restarting the anticoagulant. Middle meningeal artery embolization has been best studied for the prevention of recurrent chronic subdural hemorrhage, but it may similarly reduce the risk of recurrent acute subdural hemorrhage in patients who require re-initiation of anticoagulation. It is tempting (but possibly unsafe) to start by "testing the waters" with a lower intensity of intravenous heparin infusion (i.e., targeting a slightly lower anti-Xa level than the therapeutic anticoagulation range). In patients with mechanical valves, we have noticed a higher risk of hemorrhagic expansion with heparin bridging. Yet, the stakes are so high in patients with LVADs that waiting for the INR to become therapeutic may take too long and the risk of heparin bridging may be justified. We do not know if bivalirudin is a good temporary option when resuming anticoagulation after ICH in patients with LVADs. We need better data to answer the many questions that come at us.

We promptly reversed our patient with four-factor prothrombin complex concentrate and vitamin K after the second seizure. Repeat head computed tomography revealed that the size of the hematoma was stable. His seizures were controlled on levetiracetam. Four days later, he was restarted on warfarin without heparin bridging. The INR became therapeutic 4 days later. Upon 1-year follow-up, the patient was doing well with no recurrent seizures (on levetiracetam) and had not suffered any thrombotic or recurrent hemorrhagic complications.

Unfortunately, the story of neurologic complications with LVADs does not end here, and we have seen more serious and fatal scenarios. With longer duration of LVAD placement, device-related complications are increasingly more common, and the most significant is pump thrombosis (approximately a year after implantation). Pump thrombosis is usually suspected with (1) lactate dehydrogenase elevation several-fold higher than baseline and often above 1000 IU/L, (2) power spikes or consistent new high pump powers noted upon device interrogation, (3) worsening heart failure not explained by other reasons, (4) tea-colored urine, or (5) believe it or not, grinding noises from the device. This may lead to device exchange or, more commonly, treatment with intravenous tirofiban. Tirofiban is a potent, reversible antagonist of the glycoprotein IIb/IIIa receptor, rendering the receptor ineffective in binding von Willebrand factor and fibrinogen, which play major roles in platelet adhesion and aggregation and, as a result, thrombus generation. Cardiologists or cardiovascular surgeons administer tirofiban while the patient is fully anticoagulated and on antiplatelet agents. When successful, they add prasugrel. Major hemorrhages may occur, and we and others have encountered fatal intracerebral hemorrhages (Figure 34.2). Reversal of tirofiban requires desmopressin 0.3 mcg/kg, platelet transfusion, plus infusion of 10 units of cryoprecipitate. Cangrelor, a reversible P2Y(12) platelet receptor inhibitor, may be a valuable alternative to IIb/IIIa receptor inhibitors because its very short half-life results in lower risk of bleeding complications.

LVADs "save lives," but with serious risks and consuming tremendous resources. When intracranial bleeding occurs in patients with LVADs, they may be transferred to the neurosciences intensive care unit for closer monitoring and neurosurgical involvement but accompanied by an LVAD

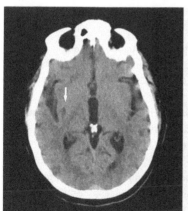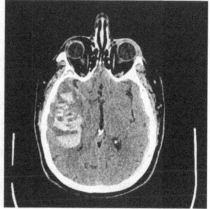

FIGURE 34.2 Cerebral hemorrhage into the putamen during tirofiban therapy in a patient on an LVAD for over 10 years. Note several fluid levels ("footsteps") due to anticoagulation inhibition to form a dense clot. This patient also had a minor stroke a week before device thrombosis was detected and on CT a small new hypodensity in the insula. (see left image and arrow) This was the patient's second treatment for device thrombosis in a year.

team. These patients require expertise found only in cardiovascular surgical intensive care units, and neurointensivists may become actively involved in a consulting role in these increasingly more common situations.

KEY POINTS TO REMEMBER

- When deciding whether to prescribe emergency anticoagulation reversal, clinicians should weigh the risk of hematoma expansion versus the particularly substantial risk of subsequent thromboembolic complications, including potentially life-threatening LVAD malfunction.
- When making emergency treatment decisions, such as neurosurgery for ICH evacuation or tracheal intubation and initiation of mechanical ventilation, we need to consider whether the LVAD is being used as a bridge to cardiac transplantation or as destination therapy.
- Resumption of anticoagulation the optimal timing to restart anticoagulation is unknown, but in patients with LVADs we must resume it (much) earlier than we would in other cases of anticoagulation-related ICH.

Further Reading

Boulet, J., M. R. B. Wanderley, Jr., and M. R. Mehra. "Contemporary Left Ventricular Assist Device Therapy as a Bridge or Alternative to Transplantation." [In eng]. *Transplantation* 108, no. 6 (Jun 1 2024): 1333–41. doi:10.1097/TP.0000000000004834.

Cho, S. M., N. Moazami, and J. A. Frontera. "Stroke and Intracranial Hemorrhage in HeartMate II and HeartWare Left Ventricular Assist Devices: A Systematic Review." [In eng]. *Neurocrit Care* 27, no. 1 (2017): 17–25. https://doi.org/10.1007/s12028-017-0386-7.

Cho, S. M., N. Moazami, S. Katz, et al. "Reversal and Resumption of Antithrombotic Therapy in LVAD-Associated Intracranial Hemorrhage." [In eng]. *Ann Thorac Surg* 108, no. 1 (2019): 52–58. https://doi.org/10.1016/j.athoracsur.2019.01.016.

Ibeh, C., D. L. Tirschwell, C. Mahr, et al. "Medical and Surgical Management of Left Ventricular Assist Device-Associated Intracranial Hemorrhage." [In eng]. *J Stroke Cerebrovasc Dis* 30, no. 10 (2021): 106053. https://doi.org/10.1016/j.jstrokecerebrovasdis.2021.106053.

Santos, C. D., N. L. Matos, R. Asleh, et al. "The Dilemma of Resuming Antithrombotic Therapy After Intracranial Hemorrhage in Patients With Left Ventricular Assist Devices." [In eng]. *Neurocrit Care* 32, no. 3 (2020): 822–27. https://doi.org/10.1007/s12028-019-00836-y.

Shoskes, A., C. Hassett, A. Gedansky, et al. "Implications of Causes of Intracranial Hemorrhage During Left Ventricular Assist Device Support." [In eng]. *Neurocrit Care* 37, no. 1 (2022): 267–72. https://doi.org/10.1007/s12028-022-01494-3.

Tellor, B. R., J. R. Smith, S. M. Prasad, et al. "The Use of Eptifibatide for Suspected Pump Thrombus or Thrombosis in Patients With Left Ventricular Assist Devices." [In eng]. *J Heart Lung Transplant* 33, no. 1 (2014): 94–101. https://doi.org/10.1016/j.healun.2013.11.002.

Varshney, A. S., E. M. DeFilippis, J. A. Cowger, et al. "Trends and Outcomes of Left Ventricular Assist Device Therapy: JACC Focus Seminar." [In eng]. *J Am Coll Cardiol* 79, no. 11 (2022): 1092–107. https://doi.org/10.1016/j.jacc.2022.01.017.

SECTION 2

THE BASICS OF BRAIN MONITORING

35 The Choice Between Spot and Continuous Electroencephalography

A 64-year-old man treated for acute pneumococcal meningitis suddenly had a left gaze preference with rhythmic movements of the left hemibody while he was still following simple commands. The gaze preference and movements resolved with intravenous (IV) fosphenytoin loading. A 20-minute electroencephalogram (EEG) showed no epileptiform abnormalities. Several hours later, he became stuporous, and we placed an external ventricular drain for treatment of hydrocephalus. By hospital day 6, he had improved substantially.

In the ensuing days, he appeared less responsive, although his eyes were open. He no longer followed commands and had infrequent arrhythmic twitching of both upper and lower extremities, of the eyelids, and around the mouth, which appeared consistent with multifocal myoclonus. His breathing also appeared more labored, but his oxygen saturation and respiratory rate did not change significantly. An EEG showed generalized, anterior-predominant, sharply contoured theta-to-delta-range rhythmic activity (Figure 35.1).

What do you do now?

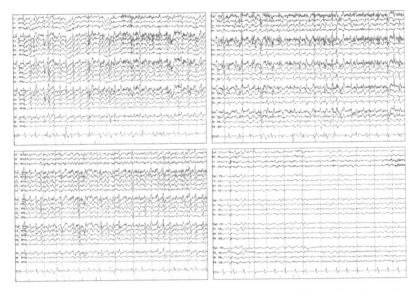

FIGURE 35.1 Top left, top right, and bottom left panels show generalized, anterior-predominant sharply contoured theta-to-delta range rhythmic activity. Bottom right panel after treatment with IV fosphenytoin shows a theta background without epileptiform abnormalities.

An unexpected sudden deterioration after successful management of a structural brain injury should always make us look for nonconvulsive seizures (NCS) or nonconvulsive status epilepticus (NCSE). NCSE is likely when there are diffuse spike or polyspike and wave complexes at frequencies of greater than 2.5 Hz. Frontal-central polyspike waves may occur in bursts of rapid generalized spikes mixed with slow activity. NCS may be more common than we realize, and between 20% and 30% of patients affected by various neurocritical care disorders undergo continuous EEG monitoring.

Nearly half of the patients who undergo EEG after a flurry of witnessed convulsive seizures have electrographic proof of NCS, and others will have NCSE after apparent control of convulsive status epilepticus. The incidence of NCS varies with several types of acute brain injury but seems more common with severe traumatic brain injury, subdural hematoma after craniotomy, central nervous system infection, recurrent brain tumors, and less common after acute ischemic stroke and aneurysmal subarachnoid hemorrhage. Surprisingly, studies have claimed that NCS occurred in 10% of "encephalopathic" patients with sepsis. We question these findings because studies examining the yield of continuous EEG monitoring often fail to discriminate between epileptiform discharges and NCS.

Clinical recognition of NCSE is difficult and sometimes impossible. We often incorrectly suspect NCSE. We are sometimes doubtful when it truly is NCSE. In fact, while awaiting the EEG result for our patient, we asked the bedside nurse, neurology resident, neurocritical care fellow, critical care medicine fellow, and senior attending neurologist whether the EEG would show NCSE, and there was no consensus.

Another snare is the increasing evidence that NCS correlate with worse neurologic outcome, and no prospective study to date has demonstrated that treatment of NCS or NCSE can improve functional outcomes or mortality. NCSE is associated with intracranial pressure elevations, increased cerebral metabolic distress, and, if prolonged, long-term hippocampal trophy. NCS have been associated with increased perihematomal edema in the setting of intraparenchymal hemorrhage and with mortality in acute bacterial meningitis. Yet, in the TELSTAR trial, which tested the value of treating epileptiform discharges and NCS after cardiac arrest, aggressive use of antiseizure medications did not improve outcome in patients with epileptiform discharges; results in a small number of patients with NCS were inconclusive, with a theoretical possibility of benefit.

Indications for EEG monitoring in the intensive care unit (ICU) are listed in Table 35.1, and many are straightforward. For some, EEG may hold promise for detecting changes in cortical perfusion before irreversible infarcts occur in patients with hemodynamic lesions and borderline flow or in the setting of cerebral vasospasm after aneurysmal subarachnoid hemorrhage, but no studies show superiority of EEG monitoring over current monitoring methods. Moreover, ischemia is difficult to identify in practice because it requires continuous real-time analysis of the raw and quantitative EEG.

After deciding to initiate EEG monitoring, the next question is how long to continue. Certainly, if the clinical question is whether a patient's unexplained alteration in consciousness is due to NCS, a 30-minute EEG recording showing no epileptiform abnormalities is sufficient to exclude seizures as the cause. However, if the initial 30 minutes of EEG recording

TABLE 35.1 Indications and Rationale for EEG Monitoring in the ICU

Indication	Rationale
Unexplained coma or altered consciousness in the setting of acute brain injury (i.e., patient looks worse than the scan)	Exclude nonconvulsive status epilepticus
Fluctuating mental status or unexplained alteration of consciousness without acute brain injury	Exclude nonconvulsive seizures or status epilepticus
Otherwise unexplained focal neurologic deficits (i.e., aphasia or unilateral weakness)	Exclude nonconvulsive status epilepticus
Recent clinical seizure activity without obvious signs of improvement within 10 minutes or with any depressed consciousness after 30 minutes	Exclude transition into nonconvulsive status epilepticus or ongoing frequent nonconvulsive seizures
Periodic discharges (generalized, lateralized, or bilateral independent) on routine EEG	May evolve to nonconvulsive seizures and status epilepticus
Stereotyped paroxysmal clinical events	Exclude nonconvulsive seizures
Persistent change in consciousness following brain surgery	Exclude nonconvulsive status epilepticus
Patients with acute brain injury at considerable risk for seizures who require neuromuscular blockade	Monitor for seizures as paralysis prevents clinical manifestations of seizures
Initiation of anesthetic coma for treatment of refractory status epilepticus	Monitor degree of suppression and recurrence of seizures and guide weaning of the anesthetic agent

show generalized periodic discharges, monitoring must be extended. Some data exist to guide the decision of how long to monitor in these patients. In a study of 625 consecutive patients undergoing at least 48 hours of EEG monitoring, 27% of patients had seizures, and the first seizure occurred within 30 minutes in 58% of patients. In most others with later seizures, epileptiform discharges were seen early. Thus, in patients with epileptiform discharges, it is reasonable to monitor for 24 to 48 hours or until patients have recovered to their neurologic baseline.

Epileptologists and intensivists experienced in interpreting EEG in critical illness should take the lead. Triphasic waves or frontal, intermittent, rhythmic delta activity often appears in patients with multiorgan failure, and both are nonspecific (and definitively nonepileptogenic). The most common misinterpretation is to confuse triphasic waves with NCSE. Other patients have spikes or sharp waves that come and go without reaching a frequency greater than 2.5 Hz. (as said earlier, epileptiform discharges >2.5 Hz constitute a seizure.) Thus, it is often unclear which EEG abnormalities require treatment and which are epiphenomena of an injury (i.e., electrical changes that will resolve over time even if left untreated). Epileptologists debate which periodic lateralized discharges and other manifestations of the "ictal-interictal continuum" are suspicious for seizures, but that is outside the scope of this book. However, neurointensivists should be familiar with the preferred terminology for EEG reporting in ICU patients. (The document created by the American Clinical Neurophysiology Society is a good starting point.)

Management of EEG findings involves consideration of the clinical scenario (i.e., underlying cause and temporal association with a decline in the level or content of consciousness), patient comorbidities, and the patient's goals of care. Treatment of NCS and particularly NCSE is reasonable, but aggressively treating other EEG paroxysms that are not definitive seizures is unjustified. When making these decisions, it is also useful to distinguish between a patient who is (or may be) comatose because of seizures and a comatose patient with epileptiform changes on EEG. The former should always get at least a trial of antiseizure medications; the latter may not benefit (and may even be harmed) from them.

Our patient was in NCSE based on both clinical and electrographic criteria. There was no concomitant change in organ function, evidence of new systemic infection, or worsening meningitis. Additional neuro-imaging with brain magnetic resonance imaging and magnetic resonance venography did not show any abscess formation, thrombophlebitis, or cerebral infarctions. He had not received medications known to lower the seizure threshold. A free phenytoin level obtained the previous day was 1.4 mcg/mL. Resolution of the epileptiform discharges transiently occurred after a partial load of 10 mg/kg PE IV fosphenytoin, but our patient did not improve clinically, and the original ictal pattern recurred within several hours. The same electrographic response occurred after administration of 400 mg IV lacosamide, again with recurrence several hours later. Ultimately, we achieved persistent electrographic control approximately 12 hours after oral phenobarbital loading (Figure 35.1). Within 24 hours after we achieved electrographic seizure control, our patient was again interactive with family and staff. We discontinued EEG monitoring at that time. There had been no seizures for 36 hours, and we could reliably monitor the patient's neurological condition with serial bedside examinations. While he made significant gains over several weeks, he ultimately succumbed to complications related to prior cancer 2 months after discharge from the ICU.

Continuous EEG is available in major medical centers but not elsewhere. EEG monitoring is an important diagnostic tool for specific indications including diagnosis of NCS and NCSE, characterization of other paroxysmal events, and assessment of the efficacy of therapy for status epilepticus. Deciding when to transfer patients to centers with this capability depends on clinical urgency, but we do not know how to avoid a transfer. Deciding when to escalate treatment requires skill and experience, but how to proceed may still remain ambiguous. We may be doing serious harm if we are too aggressively pursuing EEG findings and most certainly if we intubate patients and treat with a number of potent anesthetics.

KEY POINTS TO REMEMBER

- Continuous EEG monitoring will increase the yield of detection of seizures but also nonspecific transient abnormalities.
- Interpretation of continuous EEG requires expertise, but even then, some ambiguity remains.
- NCS are common after control of convulsive seizures.

- NCS may occur in up to 20% to 30% of critically ill neurologic patients, and half are detected within the first 30 minutes of monitoring.
- Continue EEG monitoring until the clinical question is answered and either (1) the patient has recovered to their neurologic baseline or (2) no seizures have occurred for 2 hours in patients without epileptiform abnormalities or for 24 hours in patients with epileptiform abnormalities.

Further Reading

Alkhachroum, A., B. Appavu, S. Egawa, et al. "Electroencephalogram in the Intensive Care Unit: A Focused Look at Acute Brain Injury." [In eng]. *Intensive Care Med* 48, no. 10 (2022): 1443–62.

Brophy, G. M., R. Bell, J. Claassen, et al. "Guidelines for the Evaluation and Management of Status Epilepticus." [In eng]. *Neurocrit Care* 17, no. 1 (2012): 3–23.

Claassen, J., F. S. Taccone, P. Horn, et al. "Recommendations on the Use of EEG Monitoring in Critically Ill Patients: Consensus Statement From the Neurointensive Care Section of the ESICM." [In eng]. *Intensive Care Med* 39, no. 8 (2013): 1337–51.

Herman, S. T., N. S. Abend, T. P. Bleck, et al. "Consensus Statement on Continuous EEG in Critically Ill Adults and Children, Part I: Indications." [In eng]. *J Clin Neurophysiol* 32, no. 2 (2015): 87–95.

Hirsch, L. J., M. W. K. Fong, M. Leitinger, et al. "American Clinical Neurophysiology Society's Standardized Critical Care EEG Terminology: 2021 Version." [In eng]. *J Clin Neurophysiol* 38, no. 1 (2021): 1–29.

Long, B., and A. Koyfman. "Nonconvulsive Status Epilepticus: A Review for Emergency Clinicians." [In eng]. *J Emerg Med* 65, no. 4 (2023): e259–71.

Ruijter, B. J., H. M. Keijzer, M. C. Tjepkema-Cloostermans, et al. "Treating Rhythmic and Periodic EEG Patterns in Comatose Survivors of Cardiac Arrest." [In eng]. *N Engl J Med* 386, no. 8 (2022): 724–34.

Shafi, M. M., M. B. Westover, A. J. Cole, et al. "Absence of Early Epileptiform Abnormalities Predicts Lack of Seizures on Continuous EEG." [In eng]. *Neurology* 79, no. 17 (2012): 1796–801.

Westover, M. B., M. M. Shafi, M. T. Bianchi, et al. "The Probability of Seizures During EEG Monitoring in Critically Ill Adults." [In eng]. *Clin Neurophysiol* 126, no. 3 (2015): 463–71.

36 When to Place an Intracranial Pressure Monitor

A 53-year-old man fell 15 feet from a rooftop onto a cement surface. He remained unresponsive and motionless after he fell and developed irregular, shallow respirations. Paramedics found him comatose with no eyelid opening to pain and dilated pupils with preserved light reactivity. They brought him to our emergency department, and we intubated him for airway protection. Vital signs were stable; blood pressure was 127/75 mmHg, heart rate was 109 beats per minute, and oxygen saturation was 96%. His pupils were similar in size and reactive to light and he had extensor posturing with noxious stimulation to the nailbeds of his hands. A noncontrast head computed tomography (CT) scan showed acute traumatic right subdural hematoma with 1 cm of midline shift at the level of the septum pellucidum, effacement of the basilar cisterns, global edema, and a nondisplaced skull fracture (Figure 36.1).

What do you do now?

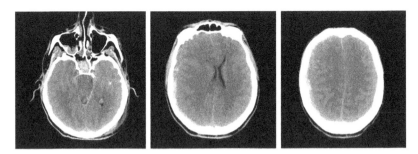

FIGURE 36.1 Noncontrast head CT in TBI shows acute right subdural hematoma with midline shift, effacement of basal cisterns, and global early edema and scattered shear lesions in the white matter.

Decisions on whether to place an intracranial pressure (ICP) monitor are never straightforward and all too often based on personal preference. One of the main reasons to monitor ICP is that sustained intracranial hypertension (defined in most studies as either >20 mmHg or 25 mmHg is strongly associated with mortality, particularly in patients with traumatic brain injury (TBI). In theory, high ICP compromises cerebral perfusion pressure and may put the patient at risk for global cerebral ischemia. Increased ICP compresses vital brain structures. These two neurophysiological attributes govern our approach. But there is more to the story than that. Monitors may also help us detect deterioration from increased ICP in patients who are difficult to assess clinically, evaluate response to treatment, and avoid iatrogenically induced elevations in ICP.

Recommendations are most clearly set for patients with TBI because this has been the disorder best studied. The neurosurgical and neurointensivist mantra in severe TBI is to place an ICP monitor if the patient is comatose and the CT scan is abnormal (contusions, edema, hemorrhage, compressed cisterns). Who can argue with that? But even if the CT scan is initially normal, ICP monitoring is advisable in comatose patients with TBI who meet two of the following three conditions: (1) age older than 40 years, (2) decerebrate or decorticate posturing, and (3) systolic blood pressure (SBP) less than 90 mmHg.

CT findings cannot reliably predict ICP, but obliteration of sulci, effacement of basal cisterns, and amount of midline shift may be suggestive of elevated ICP. When the ventricles are small, the monitoring method of choice is most often an intraparenchymal fiberoptic catheter through a bolt.

What about conditions not as well studied as TBI? In general, consider ICP monitoring in any patient with suspicion of elevated ICP or at-risk patients who are difficult to assess clinically because of sedation or neuromuscular blockade. Clinical scenarios where ICP monitors are fundamentally necessary for more appropriate care or could be potentially helpful are shown in Box 36.1.

Do ICP monitors improve outcomes? That is not the right question. Monitoring devices per se cannot improve outcomes. What matters is what to do with the information provided by the device. So, then, is management guided by ICP monitoring better than when ICP monitoring is not used? A randomized trial showed that a strict protocol of ICP treatment guided by clinical examination and serial brain imaging might be just as good as treatment guided directly by ICP monitors and raised doubt as to their added benefit. However, other investigators have raised questions

---

BOX 36.1 **Clinical Scenarios Indicating Need for ICP Monitors**

Traumatic brain injury
    Comatose patient and abnormal head CT
    Comatose patient and normal head CT and motor posturing
    (decorticate or decerebrate)
Aneurysmal Subarachnoid hemorrhage
    Acute obstructive hydrocephalus
    Global brain edema
Intracerebral hemorrhage
    Intraventricular extension and hydrocephalus
Acute bacterial meningitis
    Global brain edema and hydrocephalus
Fulminant hepatic failure
    Rapidly progressing grade III hepatic encephalopathy (incoherent
    speech, mostly sleeping)
    Grade IV hepatic encephalopathy (comatose, unresponsive to
    pain, motor posturing)

regarding the generalizability of this trial, and ICP monitoring continues to be routine in most academic medical centers because most experts recognize its value in the care of acutely brain-injured patients. Observational studies may be difficult to interpret because of selection bias (i.e. patients who undergo ICP monitoring are often more affected or considered to be at higher risk of neurological complications). In a review of 1448 patients from 43 intensive care units in Italy and Hungary, ICP monitoring correlated with worse outcome, more medical interventions, and more associated side effects. The investigators correctly surmised that such a finding requires further study and elaboration, which may include (1) patient selection for monitoring, (2) appropriateness of ICP thresholds, (3) comparison of algorithm-specific versus pathophysiology-specific interventions for intracranial hypertension, and (4) comparisons of urgent management of ICP elevations versus attempts to maintain ICP within an acceptable range. A recent international e-Delphi survey reached some consensus on how to define a best practice in the reporting of intracranial pressure monitoring data.

ICP monitor placement is standard in other acute neurological conditions such as aneurysmal subarachnoid hemorrhage (SAH), intracerebral hemorrhage (ICH), fulminant hepatic failure, and acute bacterial meningitis. Yet, there is substantial variation in the use of ICP monitoring in these conditions. Because obstructive hydrocephalus is common in SAH and ICH, an external ventricular drain (EVD) is usually the preferred method in these cases. In patients with intraventricular hemorrhage, the lateral ventricle that contains the least volume of blood seems the optimal target to minimize the risk of a clogged and nonfunctional catheter.

Patients with fulminant hepatic failure are at risk for rapidly progressive cerebral edema. ICP monitoring is common in this situation, but the high rate of monitor-related intracranial hemorrhage (10% or even higher) and lack of proven benefit in survival rates make neurosurgeons reluctant. Half of transplant programs in the United States routinely place ICP monitors in patients with fulminant hepatic failure, and a bolt is the preferred monitor. Noninvasive ways to estimate ICP have gained attention and would be advantageous in cases of marked coagulopathy but remain without validation for use in current clinical practice. Measurements of optic nerve sheath diameter by ultrasound and pulsatility index measured on transcranial Doppler are the most evaluated noninvasive modalities. A commonly used threshold for placing an ICP monitor in patients with fulminant hepatic failure is grade III, rapidly progressing hepatic encephalopathy (mostly sleeping, marked confusion, incoherent speech) or grade IV hepatic encephalopathy (comatose, unresponsive to pain, includes decorticate or decerebrate posturing). To minimize the risk of ICH, which is always increased with severe liver failure, continuous monitoring and reversal of coagulopathy with prothrombin complex concentrate and platelet transfusions are imperative in these patients.

Once intracranial hypertension becomes apparent, regardless of the cause, we follow a tiered approach to medical therapy. Basic measures include elevating the head of the bed to 30 degrees, maintaining excellent oxygenation (SpO_2 ≥95%), strict avoidance of hypercapnia ($PaCO_2$ of 35–40 mmHg), maintaining normothermia, and avoiding either hypoglycemia or marked hyperglycemia. Sedation with fentanyl, propofol, or midazolam infusions may be necessary.

In a very acute situation, the most rapidly effective measure to reduce ICP is hyperventilation to a goal $PaCO_2$ of approximately 30 mmHg. However, this should only be transient, intended to be a bridge to other treatments, as persistent hypocapnia can cause cerebral vasoconstriction and brain ischemia.

Hyperosmolar therapy with either mannitol (1–2 g/kg) or hypertonic saline (30 ml of 23.4%) is next in line. An advantage of mannitol in the hyperacute setting is the opportunity to administer it through a peripheral intravenous line, while hypertonic saline (if ≥3%) typically requires placement of a central venous catheter, though there are reports of safe peripheral administration of 23% saline with a rapid 2-5 minute push. Potentially adverse effects of mannitol include hypovolemia (and hypotension) from its diuretic effect in addition to acute kidney injury. Kidney injury is more common in patients with preexistent kidney disease and with accumulating and higher doses of mannitol. The kidney injury is usually reversible, and if needed, mannitol can be dialyzed out of the system. The most reliable way to assess whether a significant concentration of mannitol is still circulating is to calculate the osmolar gap (measured serum osmolality - calculated serum osmolality). Sources differ, but if the gap exceeds 20, the risk of kidney injury increases, so when such gap is present, we avoid administering mannitol until it clears further. Urine output will increase due to (sometimes potent) diuretic effect and will require fluid replacement. Mannitol given consistently over consecutive days may induce a systemic hyperosmolar state, causing brain cells to adapt to a new balance because of increased intracellular formation of "idiogenic osmoles." Once this occurs, any reduction in systemic osmolality theoretically might cause water to move into brain cells and could cause a "rebound edema" if mannitol infusion is stopped or decreased abruptly. Also, if the patient deteriorates while in a new steady state of hyperosmolarity, hyperosmolar therapy will "max out," and there will be no room to give additional mannitol or hypertonic saline. Yet, in practice, the efficacy of mannitol continues even after prolonged use.

The alternative hyperosmolar agent is hypertonic saline in various concentrations and, preferably, in boluses (from 250 ml of 3% saline to 30 or 60 ml of 23.4% saline). Hypertonic saline at 23.4% may be effective even after mannitol or lower concentrations of hypertonic saline have failed to reduce ICP, and the renal complications are much less frequent than with mannitol. Careful monitoring is still essential because hypotension may occur with a large bolus, or a metabolic acidosis may occur because of the high concentrations of chloride (mitigated by replacing sodium chloride with equimolar amounts of sodium acetate).

Hypertonic saline and mannitol have been compared in multiple small trials of patients with elevated ICP from various causes (TBI, stroke, SAH, ICH). Overall, available studies possibly favor hypertonic saline for TBI but show no difference between the two options for other diagnoses.

For patients with refractory intracranial hypertension, rescue craniectomy is the best solution. Once osmotic therapy, cerebrospinal fluid drainage (when possible), and deep sedation have failed, decompressive craniectomy can be life-saving. Needless to say, neurosurgeons proceed with prompt surgery to release mass effect from extra-axial hematomas or even in situations where hemorrhagic contusions cause major midline shift.

We sent our patient to the operating room for emergent right frontotemporoparietal craniectomy and evacuation of the right subdural hematoma with intraoperative placement of an ICP monitor. Postoperatively, he remained comatose. His ICP readings hovered in the high teens, occasionally requiring hyperosmolar therapy for readings greater than 20 mmHg. His neurological examination was unchanged with no eyelid opening to pain, pupils of equal diameter, intact brainstem reflexes, and persistent extensor posturing to stimulation. Due to failure to improve, his family requested withdrawal of life-sustaining treatments 2 weeks after the injury and he died shortly after extubation. Although we respected the right to autonomy, we would have preferred to wait longer before deciding to concede.

Our case illustrates that neurologic examination (along with head CT) provides the most valuable information to decide which patients may need emergency surgery and to determine the initial level of care after a severe brain injury. It also illustrates that ICP control is just one part of the larger picture of traumatic injury to the brain. In some, the severe primary impact damage (which may have included an ICP surge and brainstem displacement from compression) cannot be reversed with our current measures. Granted, at the time of the decision to place an ICP monitor we do not know whether reduction of ICP (and compressive effects from increased ICP) may help the patient. Aggressive treatment may not always improve outcome in TBI, which mainly is determined by the extent of primary neuronal injury (see Chapter 52).

KEY POINTS TO REMEMBER

- Place an ICP monitor in comatose TBI patients with an abnormal head CT scan or with a normal CT scan and motor posturing (decerebrate or decorticate).
- ICP monitors may be necessary in patients with SAH, ICH, fulminant hepatic failure, and acute bacterial meningitis.
- CT scan findings cannot reliably predict ICP.
- Persistent intracranial hypertension (ICP >25 mmHg) is associated with marked increase in morbidity and mortality.

Further Reading

Badri, S., J. Chen, J. Barber, et al. "Mortality and Long-Term Functional Outcome Associated With Intracranial Pressure After Traumatic Brain Injury." [In eng]. *Intensive Care Med* 38, no. 11 (2012): 1800–1809. https://doi.org/10.1007/s00 134-012-2655-4.

Carney, N., A. M. Totten, C. O'Reilly, et al. "Guidelines for the Management of Severe Traumatic Brain Injury, Fourth Edition." [In eng]. *Neurosurgery* 80, no. 1 (2017): 6–15. https://doi.org/10.1227/neu.0000000000001432.

Chesnut, R. M., N. Temkin, N. Carney, et al. "A Trial of Intracranial-Pressure Monitoring in Traumatic Brain Injury." [In eng]. *N Engl J Med* 367, no. 26 (2012): 2471–81. https://doi.org/10.1056/NEJMoa1207363.

Cook, A. M., G. Morgan Jones, G. W. J. Hawryluk, et al. "Guidelines for the Acute Treatment of Cerebral Edema in Neurocritical Care Patients." [In eng]. *Neurocrit Care* 32, no. 3 (2020): 647–66. https://doi.org/10.1007/s12028-020-00959-7.

Dawes, A. J., G. D. Sacks, H. G. Cryer, et al. "Intracranial Pressure Monitoring and Inpatient Mortality in Severe Traumatic Brain Injury: A Propensity Score-Matched Analysis." [In eng]. *J Trauma Acute Care Surg* 78, no. 3 (2015): 492–501; https://doi.org/10.1097/ta.0000000000000559.

Hawryluk, G. W. J., G. Citerio, P. Hutchinson, et al. "Intracranial Pressure: Current Perspectives on Physiology and Monitoring." [In eng]. *Intensive Care Med* 48, no. 10 (2022): 1471–81. https://doi.org/10.1007/s00134-022-06786-y.

Hawryluk, G. W. J., J. L. Nielson, J. R. Huie, et al. "Analysis of Normal High-Frequency Intracranial Pressure Values and Treatment Threshold in Neurocritical Care Patients: Insights Into Normal Values and a Potential Treatment Threshold." [In eng]. *JAMA Neurol* 77, no. 9 (2020): 1150–58. https://doi.org/10.1001/jamaneurol.2020.1310.

Helbok, R., D. M. Olson, P. D. Le Roux, et al. "Intracranial Pressure and Cerebral Perfusion Pressure Monitoring in Non-TBI Patients: Special Considerations." [In eng]. *Neurocrit Care* 21, no. Suppl 2 (2014): S85–94. https://doi.org/10.1007/s12028-014-0040-6.

Kommer, M., C. Hawthorne, L. Moss, et al. "International e-Delphi Survey to Define Best Practice in the Reporting of Intracranial Pressure Monitoring Recording Data." [In eng]. *Brain Spine* 4 (Jul 4 2024): 102860. doi:10.1016/j.bas.2024.102860.

Nattino, G., L. Gamberini, O. Brissy, et al. "Comparative Effectiveness of Intracranial Pressure Monitoring on 6-Month Outcomes of Critically Ill Patients With Traumatic Brain Injury." [In eng]. *JAMA Netw Open* 6, no. 9 (2023): e2334214. https://doi.org/10.1001/jamanetworkopen.2023.34214.

O'Brien SK, Koehl JL, Demers LB, Hayes BD, Barra ME. Safety and Tolerability of 23.4% Hypertonic Saline Administered Over 2 to 5 Minutes for the Treatment of Cerebral Herniation and Intracranial Pressure Elevation. [In eng]. *Neurocrit Care.* 2023 Apr;38(2):312-319. doi: 10.1007/s12028-022-01604-1

Perez-Barcena, J., J. A. Llompart-Pou, and K. H. O'Phelan. "Intracranial Pressure Monitoring and Management of Intracranial Hypertension." [In eng]. *Crit Care Clin* 30, no. 4 (2014): 735–50. https://doi.org/10.1016/j.ccc.2014.06.005.

Ropper, A. H. "Brain in a Box." [In eng]. *N Engl J Med* 367, no. 26 (2012): 2539–41. https://doi.org/10.1056/NEJMe1212289.

Shi, J., L. Tan, J. Ye, et al. "Hypertonic Saline and Mannitol in Patients With Traumatic Brain Injury: A Systematic and Meta-Analysis." [In eng]. *Medicine (Baltimore)* 99, no. 35 (2020): e21655. https://doi.org/10.1097/md.0000000000021655.

Vaquero, J., R. J. Fontana, A. M. Larson, et al. "Complications and Use of Intracranial Pressure Monitoring in Patients With Acute Liver Failure and Severe Encephalopathy." [In eng]. *Liver Transpl* 11, no. 12 (2005): 1581–89. https://doi.org/10.1002/lt.20625.

SECTION 3

CALLS, PAGES, TEXTS, AND OTHER ALARMS

37 Alert With a Fixed and Dilated Pupil

A 40-year-old woman awoke with a sudden severe headache with nausea, vomiting, photophobia, and retro-orbital pain. Looking into the mirror, she noted a drooping right eye and a wider pupil. There was no eye redness or swelling. Neurologic examination showed the right eye down and out and with an incomplete ptosis and consistent with an oculomotor palsy. Computed tomography (CT) suggested a posterior communicating artery aneurysm on the right. A cerebral angiogram demonstrated a 2.3 × 2 × 1.8 (neck) posterior communicating artery aneurysm (Figure 37.1). A lumbar puncture in the emergency department was normal, and there was no xanthochromia. She was anxious and hypertensive with blood pressures in the 190s. We admitted her for observation and further management to the neurosciences intensive care unit (ICU).

What do you do now?

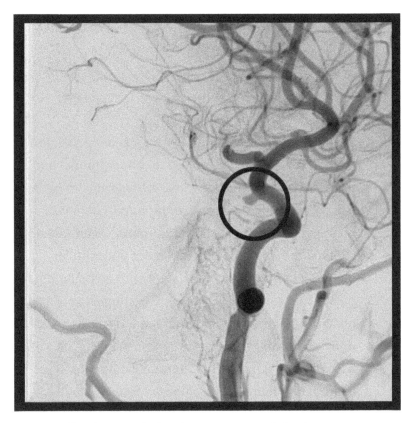

FIGURE 37.1 Posterior communicating artery aneurysm on cerebral angiogram.

The answer must be "fix the aneurysm," and do it as soon as feasible. A "blown" pupil—whether in a comatose or alert patient—often causes panic. The acutely fixed and dilated pupil is a dreaded neurologic sign, whatever the circumstances. Even neurology-naïve health care workers recognize these large pupils as emergent situations, and this sign has a much higher priority for alerts than the ubiquitously found insignificant mild to moderate anisocoria (<2 mm). We expect calls about a wide pupil, and of course, we see it in our own patients with expanding masses. The examination and interpretation (and, particularly, when we find an additional oculomotor palsy) must lead to urgent tests and, often, neuro-ICU admission. A fixed and dilated pupil may present de novo in the emergency department and requires a good understanding of the testing priorities. Finding an alert patient should not lessen our concern. Acute oculomotor palsy with preceding retro-orbital pain may warn us that rapid aneurysm formation (or growth) is happening or may be around the corner.

Our patient underwent balloon-assisted coiling. In addition. the left internal carotid artery angiogram demonstrated early filling of the ipsilateral cavernous sinus, and the right external carotid artery demonstrated early filling of the clival plexus suggestive of diffuse, bilateral, indirect cavernous-carotid fistulae. However, her symptoms fully resolved after endovascular coil placement, and several months later, the carotid-cavernous fistulae were also successfully endovascularly treated.

Certainly, painful oculomotor palsy may occur in a carotid-cavernous fistula, and the classic accompanying clinical signs, such as proptosis, bruit, or conjunctival injection, may not (yet) be present. In addition, there are no specific distinguishing features of third-nerve involvement in the cavernous sinus. Nonetheless, in this case, we consider it far more plausible that the aneurysm was the culprit. Moreover, we measured the (often forgotten) intraocular pressure, which was normal. Additional history revealed that she was in a car rollover several years previously and was told that she had some "vascular abnormalities" because of it. Again, in a carotid-cavernous fistula, the trauma to the orbit may occur belatedly (as in our patient) or early, such as after transsphenoidal pituitary surgery, carotid endarterectomy, or ethmoidal surgery. Lid swelling and orbital pain with characteristic pulsating exophthalmos and tortuous conjunctival vessels point to its diagnosis. Funduscopy may demonstrate pulsating venous dilation and, in more extreme forms, disc edema and ophthalmoplegia. Ophthalmoplegia may be due to restricted excursions or cranial nerve injury in the segments traversing the cavernous or petrosal sinus. Visual loss is a consequence of increased intraocular pressure and reversal of flow or thrombus in the superior ophthalmic vein. There is a need for full angiographic documentation. Immediate opacification of the cavernous sinus appears after carotid injection.

Oculomotor palsy is not difficult to diagnose (Figure 37.2), and the abnormal movement involves adduction of the affected eye with horizontal and vertical lagging. In extreme situations, ptosis is complete, and the affected eye is "down and out."

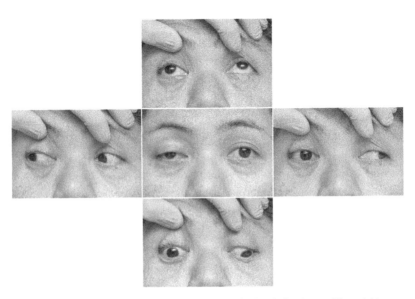

FIGURE 37.2 Complete right third-nerve palsy with key findings in four key positions: right ptosis, limitation of elevation, depression, and adduction in the right eye with a dilated pupil nonreactive to light.

Issues become more complex if other cranial nerves (i.e., IV and V) are involved, and the movement will be much more restricted. It may help to ask about one eye versus both eye involvement (i.e., no diplopia if one eye closes), how the images are separated (horizontal or vertical), and which direction of gaze has the greatest separation, change with near-versus-distant viewing, and diurnal variation.

We can localize the lesion based on other findings (Table 37.1). Aneurysms do compress the peripherally located pupillary fibers—but not always. Microvascular ischemia comprises most isolated pupil-sparing third-nerve palsies and frequently correlates with diabetes mellitus or systemic hypertension. (The peripherally located pupillary fibers may receive more collateral blood supply than the main central nerve trunk.)

Oculomotor nerve palsy is a well-recognized presentation of posterior communicating artery aneurysms that compress the nerve. Other

TABLE 37.1 Localization of the Lesion in Third Nerve Palsy

Where	Symptoms/Signs	Causes
Nucleus	Complete ipsilateral third plus contralateral ptosis and contralateral superior rectus weakness	Ischemic stroke Hemorrhage Tumor
Fascicles	Contralateral hemiparesis (Weber syndrome) Contralateral tremor (Benedikt syndrome) Ipsilateral ataxia (Nothnagel syndrome)	Ischemic stroke Hemorrhage Tumor Demyelination
Subarachnoid space	Thunderclap or orbital pain	ICA/Pcom/BA aneurysm Uncal herniation Tumor Meningitis Trauma
Cavernous sinus	CN IV and VI, V1, V2 Oculosympathetic dysfunction Facial pain may be extreme	Tumor Inflammation ICA aneurysm Microvascular thrombosis
Orbit	Proptosis Visual loss	Trauma Tumor Inflammation Arteriovenous fistula

BA, basilar artery; CN, cranial nerve; ICA, internal carotid artery; Pcom, posterior communicating.
Adapted From Biousse V, Newman NJ. Third Nerve Palsies. *Semin Neurol* 2000;20(1):55-75. Used with permission.

mechanisms may include pulsatile flow in the aneurysmal sac and irritation or inflammation of the nerve by the jet of blood released during aneurysmal rupture.

With the introduction of detachable coils for treatment of endovascular aneurysms, some worry that recovery from oculomotor palsy could be suboptimal because coiling does not relieve mass effect or that the coiled sac could even exacerbate nerve compression. But no studies have corroborated these concerns, and there is no effect in the size or direction of posterior communicating artery aneurysms once they are coiled. For patients with a partial recovery, the most frequent residual symptom is diplopia followed by ptosis. In one study, the overall rate of complete recovery of oculomotor palsy following clipping was 55% compared with 32% after coiling. In other studies including patients with complete oculomotor palsy, half of patients made a complete recovery after endovascular coiling, but only a handful made a partial recovery. Generally, we can expect that more than 25% of patients undergoing procedures for brain aneurysms have lingering disability from third nerve palsy-associated diplopia or ptosis, and despite later ophthalmic interventions.

This case also underlines that neurocritical ill patients do not always look "sick" in the traditional critical care sense, but they rapidly can become terminally ill when the aneurysm ruptures. We have actually seen rupture happen during a cerebral angiogram, which we were performing to further characterize the morphology of the aneurysm. Defining readily identifiable factors that predict aneurysmal rupture seems impossible, but some findings may play a role. These are, of course, the larger (>10 mm) aneurysms, but the critical threshold of risk has varied from 5 to 10 mm. Other factors are the presence of a daughter sac as opposed to a smooth wall or a morphologic structure that changes over time and a ratio greater than 1.6, calculated using the aneurysm height measurement divided by the aneurysm neck measurement. Honestly, we can never tell if a new oculomotor nerve palsy correlates with an unstable aneurysm unless we have documented recent growth. It is also well known that rupture can still occur in the absence of growth and in small aneurysms. Aneurysmal wall enhancement is a marker of wall inflammation, and cerebral aneurysms with wall enhancement are significantly more likely to be unstable. Yet, interpretation of these studies, which are often normal, is not easy. We may have to live with these uncertainties and offer repair to the patient if the intervention is deemed technically feasible and reasonably safe. Once we encounter a patient in this situation, we must remind ourselves that admission to a regular ward (rather than a neuro-ICU with close monitoring and rapid resuscitation opportunities) is asking for trouble.

> **KEY POINTS TO REMEMBER**
>
> - A wide, dilated pupil requires immediate testing.
> - If an oculomotor palsy appears, consider all localizations in the trajectory of the nerve.
> - Painful ophthalmoplegia has a broad spectrum of causes and needs urgent evaluation.
> - In oculomotor palsy caused by a compressing aneurysm, coiling or clipping results in (not always full) recovery within a month.

Further Reading

Güresir, E., P. Schuss, M. Setzer, et al. "Posterior Communicating Artery Aneurysm-Related Oculomotor Nerve Palsy: Influence of Surgical and Endovascular Treatment on Recovery: Single-Center Series and Systematic Review." [In eng]. *Neurosurgery* 68, no. 6 (Jun 2011): 1527–33; discussion 33–34. https://doi.org/10.1227/NEU.0b013e31820edd82.

Hoz SS, Ma L, Muthana A, Al-Zaidy MF, et al. Cranial nerve palsies and intracranial aneurysms: A narrative review of patterns and outcomes. *Surg Neurol Int.* 2024 Aug 9;15:277. doi: 10.25259/SNI_531_2024.

Leigh, R. J., and D. S. Zee. *The Neurology of Eye Movements.* 4th ed. NewYork: Oxford University Press; 2006.

Mocco, J., R. D. Brown, Jr., J. C.Torner, et al. "Aneurysm Morphology and Prediction of Rupture: An International Study of Unruptured Intracranial Aneurysms Analysis." [In eng]. *Neurosurgery* 82, no. 4 (Apr 1 2018): 491–96. https://doi.org/10.1093/neuros/nyx226.

Mulderink,T. A., B. R. Bendok,W.Y.Yapor, and H. H. Batjer. "Third Nerve Paresis Caused by Vascular Compression by the Posterior Communicating Artery." [In eng]. *J Stroke Cerebrovasc Dis* 10, no. 3 (May–Jun 2001): 139–41. https://doi.org/10.1053/jscd.2001.25469.

Phan, K., J. Xu, V. Leung, et al. "Orbital Approaches forTreatment of Carotid Cavernous Fistulas: A Systematic Review." [In eng]. *World Neurosurg* 96 (Dec 2016): 243–51. https://doi.org/10.1016/j.wneu.2016.08.087.

Shapiro, J. N., L. B. Delott, and J. D.Trobe. "Impact of Diplopia and Ptosis From LingeringThird Nerve Palsy AfterTreatment of Cerebral Aneurysms." [In eng]. *J Neuroophthalmol* 44, no. 3 (Sep 1 2024): 400–5. doi:10.1097/WNO.0000000000002052.

Sheehan, M. J., R. Dunne, J.Thornton, et al. "Endovascular Repair of Posterior Communicating Artery Aneurysms, AssociatedWith Oculomotor Nerve Palsy: A Review of Nerve Recovery." [In eng]. *Interv Neuroradiol* 21, no. 3 (Jun 2015): 312–16. https://doi.org/10.1177/1591019915583222.

Texakalidis, P., A. Sweid, N. Mouchtouris, et al. "Aneurysm Formation, Growth, and Rupture: The Biology and Physics of Cerebral Aneurysms." [In eng]. *World Neurosurg* 130 (Oct 2019): 277–84. https://doi.org/10.1016/j.wneu.2019.07.093.

Yanaka, K., Y. Matsumaru, R. Mashiko, et al. "Small Unruptured Cerebral Aneurysms Presenting With Oculomotor Nerve Palsy." [In eng]. *Neurosurgery* 52, no. 3 (Mar 2003): 553–57; discussion 56–57. https://doi.org/10.1227/01.neu.0000047 816.02757.39.

Zu, Q. Q., X. L. Liu, B. Wang, et al. "Recovery of Oculomotor Nerve Palsy After Endovascular Treatment of Ruptured Posterior Communicating Artery Aneurysm." [In eng]. *Neuroradiology* 59, no. 11 (Nov 2017): 1165–70. https://doi.org/10.1007/s00234-017-1909-9.

38 Sorting Through Delirium

A 72-year-old man with a history of hypertension, diabetes mellitus, and a right subcortical ischemic stroke 3 years before was admitted with acute abdominal pain. Exploratory laparotomy revealed perforated diverticulitis. He underwent partial colectomy and colostomy without complications. In the surgical intensive care unit (ICU), he received fluids, vasopressors, and antibiotics for sepsis. Complications included acute kidney injury and mild elevation of liver transaminases. He was kept on mechanical ventilation and sedated with a midazolam infusion. Three days after the surgery, his service called us because the patient became agitated every time the nurses tried to diminish the sedation. On examination, he fluctuated between drowsiness and agitation and had multifocal adventitious movements.

What do you do now?

Delirium is a common complication in the ICU—in any ICU. It can follow critical medical, surgical, or neurologic illness and presents in 15% to 80% of critically ill patients, depending on the severity of the underlying illness, age, and previous cognitive status. Another factor that explains the wide variation of reported rates of ICU delirium is that it is often underrecognized. Clinicians may accept a certain degree of drowsiness, agitation, or confusion in elderly critically ill patients. However, delirium is a form of brain dysfunction (there is undoubtedly pathology of the brain or encephalopathy) associated with poor clinical outcomes and has the potential for persistent cognitive decline or to worsen preexisting cognitive decline. Preliminary studies with functional magnetic resonance imaging found indications of a defective working memory and executive functioning.

The raving and raging patient is obvious, but patients with ICU delirium may not have pure or even predominant hyperactivity. The word "delirium" derives from the Latin *deliro-delirare*, or to be crazy, deranged, or out of one's wits or to rave, and so the term "hypoactive delirium," to stick with Latin, seems a *contradictio in terminis*. When patients are hallucinating, delusional, and totally disorientated, they may still be hypoactive, but to call every confused, quiet patient delirious is a stretch, and we have seen different neurologic illnesses with patients in a "hypoactive delirium" and some that were serious and needed immediate intervention. Leading experts have called delirium "a depersonalized state often driven by overuse of sedation and immobilization." But there are more causes.

First, we need to have our nursing staff recognize it so we can recognize it. Screening tools sensitive to manifestations of delirium help prevent cases from going unnoticed (Figure 38.1). Sedation holidays (stopping all sedatives at regular intervals) can decrease the duration of mechanical ventilation and the length of ICU stay. They also decrease the incidence of delirium. Still, the need for sedation holidays is underappreciated. In fact, it has been our experience that precisely the sickest patient is the one at highest risk for delirium and in whom sedation holidays are less frequently used.

We still know little about the causes and mechanisms of delirium in critically ill patients, but there is emerging research. Studies have definitively demonstrated that prolonged exposure to psychoactive drugs in general and sedative drugs in particular increase the risk and severity of delirium. Benzodiazepines are particularly prone to exacerbate delirium; we reserve them

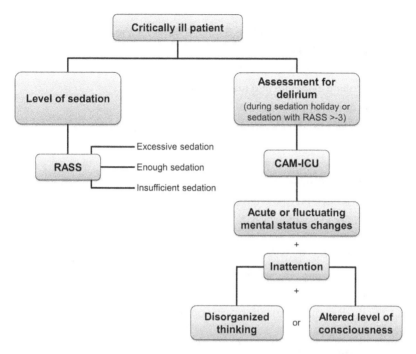

FIGURE 38.1 Assessment of level of sedation and delirium in the ICU. RASS, Richmond Agitation Sedation Scale (see Table 38.3); CAM-ICU, Confusion Assessment Method for the ICU: the presence of three of the four diagnostic features confirms the diagnosis of delirium.

for treatment of alcohol withdrawal–related delirium. Dexmedetomidine may be a safer option. Antidopaminergic agents are the best medications for agitation; the relative value of haloperidol versus atypical antipsychotics (such as quetiapine or olanzapine) in the ICU population requires more study. However, haloperidol is not beneficial in preventing delirium and should be limited to patients where agitation requires control. The risk of delirium with opiates has been less studied, but we often find them to be a major contributing factor. We have regularly seen patients withdraw abruptly after days of fentanyl infusion. The general principle is that we should be using all sedatives very judiciously, prescribing the lowest possible doses, and stopping them as soon as they are no longer necessary. In fact, a good first step would be to ensure that we avoid sedating critically ill patients who are already drowsy (when not stuporous or comatose); an everyday error in ICUs today. To that end, using a validated scale for monitoring the level of sedation,

> **BOX 38.1 Richmond Agitation Sedation Scale for the Assessment of Depth of Sedation**
>
> +4 Very combative, violent, dangerous to staff
>
> +3 Pulling catheters and tubes, aggressive
>
> +2 Frequent nonpurposeful movements, fights ventilator
>
> +1 Anxious but movements not aggressive or vigorous
>
> 0 Alert and calm
>
> −1 Awakens (eye contact) for >10 seconds in response to voice
>
> −2 Awakens (eye contact) for <10 seconds in response to voice
>
> −3 Eye opening or movement to voice without eye contact
>
> −4 No response to voice, but eye opening or movement to physical stimulation
>
> −5 No response to voice or physical stimulation

such as the Richmond Agitation Sedation Scale (RASS) (Box 38.1), is useful for the nursing staff.

We neurologists frequently receive calls to evaluate these patients in the medical or the surgical ICU, and we should try to be useful. We have the fortitude to recognize the manifestations of nonconvulsive status epilepticus, impairments of language comprehension and visuospatial perception. We call it *encephalopathy* when there is broad brain dysfunction of any sort. We appreciate that we cannot limit acute encephalopathy to a description of "sleepy, obtunded, drowsy, somnolent," and we recognize that diffuse dysfunction may also have obvious focal manifestations or other neurologic findings. Encephalopathy in clinical practice is primarily a defect of perceptional consciousness (and thus awareness), inattention, distraction, and, yes, drowsiness. The experienced clinician will look for brainstem or lateralizing signs, subtle manifestations of seizures, and features of major toxidromes. Adventitious movements such as multifocal myoclonus (more common with uremia) and asterixis (more common with liver failure) are good markers of a metabolic derangement, albeit nonspecific. Severe muscle rigidity with clonus should raise suspicion for serotonin syndrome or neuroleptic malignant syndrome, and when accompanied by high fever, malignant hyperthermia should cross one's mind. Table 38.1

TABLE 38.1 Differential Diagnoses in ICU Patients With Encephalopathy

Diagnosis	Signs	Test	Intervention
Meningitis	Neck rigidity Kernig sign Brudzinski sign	Lumbar puncture	Antimicrobials
Encephalitis	± lateralizing signs ± seizures	Lumbar puncture	Acyclovir if HSV Gancyclovir if CMV Antiepileptic drugs if seizures Supportive care otherwise
Status epilepticus	Abnormal eye movements Rhythmic movements in the extremities Facial automatisms Staring	EEG	Antiepileptic drugs
Ischemic stroke	Lateralizing signs (right parietal, multifocal) Brainstem signs (basilar artery occlusion)	Neuroimaging	Reperfusion if acute Evaluate mechanism Secondary prevention
Intracranial hemorrhage	Lateralizing signs	Neuroimaging	Consider neurosurgery consult
Cerebral Venous Thrombosis	Lateralizing signs	CTV, MRV	Anticoagulation Consider endovascular therapy when worsening
Fat embolism syndrome	Acute agitation Conjunctival ecchymoses ± lateralizing signs	Neuroimaging	Supportive Avoid manipulating the fracture Evaluate for patent foramen ovale
Neuroleptic malignant syndrome	Extreme rigidity Fever Autonomic instability	Serum CK	Stop antidopaminergics Consider dantrolene

(Continued)

TABLE 38.1 **Continued**

Diagnosis	Signs	Test	Intervention
Serotonin syndrome	Rigidity, tremor Hyperreflexia, clonus Mydriasis Autonomic instability	Serum CK	Stop serotonergic drugs Consider cyproheptadine
Malignant hyperthermia[a]	Extremely high fever Autonomic instability Severe rigidity Hyporeflexia	Arterial blood gas Lactic acid Serum CK	Aggressive control of fever Treatment of acidosis Dantrolene
Anticholinergic toxicity	Mydriasis Skin dry, erythematous Dry tongue and mucosa Tachycardia Ileus		Removal of culprit drug
Alcohol withdrawal[b]	Tremor Diaphoresis Tachycardia ± seizures		Benzodiazepines Thiamine Electrolyte replacement
Uremic encephalopathy	Prominent multifocal myoclonus Tremor Hyperreflexia (if no severe peripheral neuropathy)	BUN	Dialysis if necessary
Hepatic encephalopathy	Prominent asterixis Tremor	Serum ammonia	Lactulose, rifaximin
Posterior reversible encephalopathy syndrome	Cortical blindness, seizures, stupor	MRI (or CT scan)	Blood pressure control Hold immunosuppressants

TABLE 38.1 Continued

Diagnosis	Signs	Test	Intervention
ICU delirium	Nothing specific		Minimize sedatives and opiates Haloperidol or atypical antipsychotics for agitation General supportive care

[a] Only within 30 minutes to 24 hours after exposure to inhalational anesthesia or succinylcholine.
[b] Presented as an example of drug withdrawal syndrome.
BUN, blood urea nitrogen; CK, creatine kinase; CT, computed tomography; CTV, computed tomography venography; CMV, cytomegalovirus; EEG, electroencephalogram; HSV, herpes virus simplex; MRI, magnetic resonance imaging; MRV, magnetic resonance venography.

lists diagnoses to consider when evaluating "encephalopathic" patients in general ICUs.

We call it delirium if there is inattention and confusion, especially with agitation or other manifestations of bewilderment, understanding that agitated patients in a delirium are innately encephalopathic. We have summarized our approach to the evaluation of patients with ICU delirium in Table 38.2. Briefly, after reviewing the history and examining the patient, we try to answer the following questions:

- Do I have a diagnosis?
- Should the patient have more blood tests?
- Should the patient have neuroimaging including vascular studies?
- Should the patient have a lumbar puncture?
- Should the patient have an electroencephalogram? If so, is there a need for continuous monitoring?
- Should I reduce or stop any medications?
- Do I need to recommend specific treatment for agitation?

In the case presented, we found that the patient had a delirium with multifocal myoclonus, but normal brainstem reflexes and no lateralizing signs on examination. Muscle tone was normal. He had decreased deep tendon reflexes in the legs, consistent with his long history of diabetes. He had no meningeal signs or clinical manifestations of seizures. We requested a serum ammonia level, which was normal, and decided to follow

TABLE 38.2 **Approach to the Patient With ICU Delirium**

Evaluation	Indication
History (including preadmission functional and cognitive status)	All patients
Physical examination	All patients
Blood tests	Metabolic panel including BUN, liver transaminases, and serum ammonia in all cases CK level if rigidity Lactic acid if sepsis or acidosis Toxicological screen in any case of coma or delirium at presentation with no known cause
Brain imaging	If lateralizing signs, brainstem signs
Lumbar puncture	Unexplained fever/sepsis Meningeal signs
Electroencephalogram	Rhythmic abnormal movements Staring, not tracking finger Consider in any case of unexplained coma

his clinical course without recommending further testing. We did ask the primary team to stop the infusion of midazolam and to use intravenous haloperidol (2–5 mg every 4 hours) for the patient's episodic agitation. We also insisted on stopping the infusion of fentanyl that the patient had been receiving since surgery. With these simple changes, the patient began to improve despite further increase in his blood urea nitrogen for 2 more days (to reach a peak of 58 mg/dL) before it started to decline. Once off sedatives, he was extubated without complications. Upon discharge 2 weeks later, his intellectual function was nearly normal.

The evaluation of delirium may seem overwhelming, but a simple checklist including the questions listed above may help avoid oversights and focus the consultation. We are worried that the thoughtless use of the term delirium - active or hypoactive- may preclude looking for other explanations.

KEY POINTS TO REMEMBER

- ICU delirium is a common complication of medical and surgical critical illness, and it is associated with worse short-term and long-term clinical outcomes.
- Standardized tools, such as the Confusion Assessment Method for the Intensive Care Unit score, are available for the timely recognition of ICU delirium by nursing staff.
- Sedatives (especially benzodiazepines) and opiates worsen delirium; minimize their use whenever possible.
- New onset delirium requires a careful evaluation for acute brain injury or new onset non-convulsive status epilepticus albeit these are rarely present.

Further Reading

Barr, J., G. L. Fraser, K. Puntillo, et al. "Clinical Practice Guidelines for the Management of Pain, Agitation, and Delirium in Adult Patients in the Intensive Care Unit." [In eng]. *Crit Care Med* 41, no. 1 (Jan 2013): 263–306. https://doi.org/10.1097/CCM.0b013e3182783b72.

Ely, E. W., S. K. Inouye, G. R. Bernard, et al. "Delirium in Mechanically Ventilated Patients: Validity and Reliability of the Confusion Assessment Method for the Intensive Care Unit (CAM-ICU)." [In eng]. *Jama* 286, no. 21 (Dec 5 2001): 2703–10. https://doi.org/10.1001/jama.286.21.2703.

Ely, E. W., B. Truman, A. Shintani, et al. "Monitoring Sedation Status Over Time in ICU Patients: Reliability and Validity of the Richmond Agitation-Sedation Scale (RASS)." [In eng]. *Jama* 289, no. 22 (Jun 11 2003): 2983–91. https://doi.org/10.1001/jama.289.22.2983.

Goldberg, T. E., C. Chen, Y. Wang, et al. "Association of Delirium With Long-Term Cognitive Decline: A Meta-Analysis." [In eng]. *JAMA Neurol* 77, no. 11 (Nov 1 2020): 1373–81. https://doi.org/10.1001/jamaneurol.2020.2273.

Kotfis, K., E. W. Ely, and Y. Shehabi. "Intensive Care Unit Delirium—A Decade of Learning." [In eng]. *Lancet Respir Med* 11, no. 7 (Jul 2023): 584–86. https://doi.org/10.1016/s2213-2600(23)00222-9.

Kress, J. P., A. S. Pohlman, M. F. O'Connor, and J. B. Hall. "Daily Interruption of Sedative Infusions in Critically Ill Patients Undergoing Mechanical Ventilation." [In eng]. *N Engl J Med* 342, no. 20 (May 18 2000): 1471–77. https://doi.org/10.1056/nejm200005183422002.

Pandharipande, P. P., B. T. Pun, D. L. Herr, et al. "Effect of Sedation With Dexmedetomidine vs Lorazepam on Acute Brain Dysfunction in Mechanically

Ventilated Patients: The MENDS Randomized Controlled Trial." [In eng]. *Jama* 298, no. 22 (Dec 12 2007): 2644–53. https://doi.org/10.1001/jama.298.22.2644.

Reade, M. C., and S. Finfer. "Sedation and Delirium in the Intensive Care Unit." [In eng]. *N Engl J Med* 370, no. 5 (Jan 30 2014): 444–54. https://doi.org/10.1056/NEJMra1208705.

Smit, L., A. J. C. Slooter, J. W. Devlin, et al.; EuRIDICE Study Group. "Efficacy of Haloperidol to Decrease the Burden of Delirium in Adult Critically Ill Patients: The EuRIDICE Randomized Clinical Trial." [In eng]. *Crit Care* 27, no. 1 (Oct 30 2023): 413. doi:10.1186/s13054-023-04692-3. PMID: 37904241; PMCID: PMC10617114.

Stollings, J. L., K. Kotfis, G. Chanques, et al. "Delirium in Critical Illness: Clinical Manifestations, Outcomes, and Management." [In eng]. *Intensive Care Med* 47, no. 10 (Oct 2021): 1089–103. https://doi.org/10.1007/s00134-021-06503-1.

Wijdicks, E. F. M., and A. A. Rabinstein. "What Is It Like to Be Delirious?" [In eng]. *Neurocrit Care* 37, no. 1 (Aug 2022): 1–5. https://doi.org/10.1007/s12028-022-01520-4.

Zakhary T, Ahmed I, Luttfi I, Montasser M. Quetiapine Versus Haloperidol in the Management of Hyperactive Delirium: Randomized Controlled Trial. *Neurocrit Care*. 2024 Oct;41(2):550-557. doi: 10.1007/s12028-024-01948-w. Epub 2024 Apr 1.

39 Antibiotic-Associated Toxic Encephalopathy

A 65-year-old woman was admitted with fever, tachycardia, hypotension, and hypoxemic respiratory failure requiring intubation and mechanical ventilation. After fluid resuscitation and norepinephrine infusion improved her perfusion, her initial lactic acidosis resolved. She received treatment for sepsis with broad-spectrum antibiotics including vancomycin, 15 mg/kg every 12 hours, and cefepime, 2 g every 12 hours. Baseline serum estimated glomerular filtration rate (eGFR) was normal. However, she became oliguric on the second day, and her renal function started to deteriorate. By hospital day 3, her eGFR had dropped to 32 mL/kg/1.73 m^2. Her blood urea nitrogen (BUN) was 50 mg/dL. Removed from sedation, the patient remained poorly responsive and started having stereotypic, nonrhythmic mouth and eye-opening movements along with myoclonic jerks in the arms. Head computed tomography (CT) was unremarkable. Her attending physician requested a neurology consultation to evaluate the cause of the abnormal mental status and adventitious movements.

What do you do now?

Sepsis may lead to encephalopathy, conveniently called septic encephalopathy. Of course, this is not a satisfactory characterization because so many factors are at play. We can say *multifactorial encephalopathy* (and add the qualifier toxic to it), but there is a risk we do not carefully look at the probabilities of each factor—in fact, one factor might do it. (The legendary C. Miller Fisher used to say that there is no differential diagnosis, only one correct diagnosis, and the others are wrong.)

One increasingly common factor is toxicity from antibiotics and then predominantly from cefepime administration. Cefepime is a fourth-generation cephalosporin and became listed in the United States in the late 1990s, but case reports of neurotoxicity took much longer to get recognized. It has good bactericidal activity against *Pseudomonas aeruginosa* and *Enterobacteriaceae*, but it covers both gram-positive and gram-negative organisms broadly. This antibiotic is extremely sensitive to changes in renal clearance, and concentrations can build up rapidly.

Generally speaking, drug toxicity is a quite common cause of encephalopathy in the intensive care unit (ICU). While sedatives and opiates are the most frequently implicated agents, other neurotropic medications (such as those with serotonin-enhancing or anticholinergic properties) can also be major culprits. Always, when considering the possibility of drug neurotoxicity, the clinician must consider intercurrent metabolic impairments (especially renal or liver failure) that can reduce drug clearance, and there may be new drug-drug interactions (Figure 39.1). Preexistent brain disease, particularly in patients with less reserve and cognitive impairment, increases the risk of toxic encephalopathy and its severity. Older patients (≥70 years) are far more vulnerable to dose changes and inappropriately high dosing and may have poor renal function, which oftens worsens while in the ICU for sepsis treatment.

We have known for years that beta-lactams, quinolones, and sulfonamides can cause antibiotic-associated encephalopathy. Yet, recognition that cefepime can cause major encephalopathy in the ICU is fairly recent. There are now multiple case reports and case series as well as randomized controlled trial data supporting this. Cefepime neurotoxicity characteristically occurs in patients with renal failure (either acute kidney injury or chronic kidney disease); adjusting the dose according to the degree of impairment of renal function mitigates the risk of encephalopathy—though

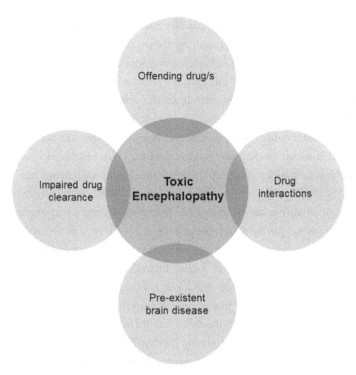

FIGURE 39.1 Causes (and factors) of toxic encephalopathy in sepsis.

it does not eliminate it. With a creatinine clearance of less than or equal to 60 mL/min, we suggest to adjust the dose of cefepime for injection (cefepime hydrochloride) to compensate for the slower rate of renal elimination. Most ICU pharmacists will accept a usual dose of 2 g every 12 hours if creatinine clearance (CrCl) is 30 to 60 mL/min; an appropriate adjustment is 2 g every 24 hours. If CrCl is 11 to 29 mL/min, the correct adjustment is 1 g every 24 hours. For patients receiving continuous renal replacement therapy, a dose less than or equal to 1 g every 12 hours is appropriate. Empirical dosing based on one of these algorithms may not be sufficient to prevent accumulation of cefepime to "toxic" concentrations in certain individuals because extreme pharmacokinetic deviations may exist. Moreover, the risk of encephalopathy may increase in patients receiving cefepime even in the absence of renal failure or despite adequate dose adjustment. Obesity may be a risk factor for the development of beta-lactam neurotoxicity, including cefepime.

Patients with cefepime neurotoxicity have a depressed level of consciousness, though agitation and nonrhythmic abnormal movements is not uncommon. We have noted consistent abnormal movements of facial muscles, such as those described in our case, in patients eventually diagnosed with cefepime neurotoxicity. Myoclonus in the arms or legs is often present. Seizures are much less common, but electroencephalography frequently shows periodic epileptiform discharges. Nonconvulsive status epilepticus is rare and difficult to diagnose or interpret on electroencephalography, but we have seen patients perk up after administering antiseizure medication (along with discontinuation of the antibiotic). Still, we are not convinced that nonconvulsive status epilepticus is common even when one systemic review of cases reported a high prevalence of one in three patients. Certainly, the risk of seizures is much higher with carbapenems and quinolones.

How cefepime suppresses brain function is not known, and one hypothesis is that cefepime enhances inhibitory neurotransmission via concentration-dependent gamma-aminobutyric acid (GABA). In fact, in an induced seizure rat model, it suppressed seizures. Regardless of uncertainties about the underlying mechanism of neurotoxicity, there is now evidence from a randomized controlled trial indicating a higher risk of neurotoxicity with cefepime as compared to piperacillin-tazobactam despite similar risk of renal impairment. Moreover, there might be some indication that rapid infusion time (less than the usual 30 minutes) might increase the chances of neurotoxicity. Cefepime serum levels can be measured but these measurements are not widely available, and more importantly, it is not known how best to interpret the information.

When cefepime neurotoxicity is deemed likely, the only way to find out is to stop the drug. Discontinuation of the drug and replacement with another antibiotic typically improves the encephalopathy within 2 to 3 days—not immediately. There might be pushback against stopping an effective drug, but we prefer to stop the medication rather than reduce the dose even when the dose may have been too high for the current renal function.

Our patient switched from cefepime to piperacillin-tazobactam, and within 48 hours, her encephalopathy and abnormal movements began to subside. Four days after discontinuing cefepime, her level of consciousness had almost returned to normal. Her renal function gradually improved, and she had no neurological sequalae upon discharge. This positive outcome won us friends in the medical ICU. But after we diagnosed multiple cases of neurotoxicity from cefepime in various medical and surgical ICUs over the years, our colleague intensivists are aware of this possibility and even switch to another antibiotic on their own—will they keep consulting us?

KEY POINTS TO REMEMBER

- Toxic exposure, often to medications, is one of the most prevalent causes of acute encephalopathy in the ICU.
- Toxic encephalopathy can manifest with reduced level of alertness or with agitation.
- Seeking a cause for toxic encephalopathy, the first consideration to bear in mind should be the dosing of drugs. Remember that appropriate dosing mey become inappropriate when there has been no adjustment of dose with changing metabolic condition.
- Cefepime can cause acute encephalopathy with a movement disorder, particularly in patients with impaired renal function who receive the antibiotic without appropriate dose adjustment. These abnormal movements can be sleep-jerk like myoclonus, reflex myoclonus or more poorly differentiated adventitious movements.
- Cefepime neurotoxicity resolves within days of discontinuation of the drug. We can exclude this diagnosis if the encephalopathy does not improve within 3 to 5 days of stopping the medication.

Further Reading

Abdul-Aziz, M. H., N. E. Hammond, S. J. Brett, et al. "Prolonged vs Intermittent Infusions of β-Lactam Antibiotics in Adults With Sepsis or Septic Shock: A Systematic Review and Meta-Analysis." [In eng]. *JAMA* 332, no. 8 (Aug 27 2024): 638–48. doi:10.1001/jama.2024.9803.

Amakhin, D. V., I. V. Smolensky, E. B. Soboleva, et al. "Paradoxical Anticonvulsant Effect of Cefepime in the Pentylenetetrazole Model of Seizures in Rats." [In eng]. *Pharmaceuticals (Basel)* 13, no. 5 (2020): 80. doi: 10.3390/ph13050080. PMID: 32357511; PMCID: PMC7281561.

Behal, M. L., J. K. Thomas, M. L. Thompson Bastin, et al. "Cefepime Induced Neurotoxicity Following a Regimen Dose-Adjusted for Renal Function: Case Report and Review of the Literature." [In eng]. *Hosp Pharm* 57, no. 3 (2022): 385–91. https://doi.org/10.1177/00185787211046856.

Bhattacharyya, S., R. R. Darby, P. Raibagkar, et al. "Antibiotic-Associated Encephalopathy." [In eng]. *Neurology* 86, no. 10 (2016): 963–71. https://doi.org/10.1212/wnl.0000000000002455.

Fugate, J. E., E. A. Kalimullah, S. E. Hocker, et al. "Cefepime Neurotoxicity in the Intensive Care Unit: A Cause of Severe, Underappreciated Encephalopathy." [In eng]. *Crit Care* 17, no. 6 (2013): R264. https://doi.org/10.1186/cc13094.

Haddad, N. A., D. J. Schreier, J. E. Fugate, et al. "Incidence and Predictive Factors Associated With Beta-Lactam Neurotoxicity in the Critically Ill: A Retrospective Cohort Study." [In eng]. *Neurocrit Care* 37, no. 1 (2022): 73–80. https://doi.org/10.1007/s12028-022-01442-1.

Maan, G., K. Keitoku, N. Kimura, et al. "Cefepime-Induced Neurotoxicity: Systematic Review." [In eng]. *J Antimicrob Chemother* 77, no. 11 (2022): 2908–21. https://doi.org/10.1093/jac/dkac271.

Payne, L. E., D. J. Gagnon, R. R. Riker, et al. "Cefepime-Induced Neurotoxicity: A Systematic Review." [In eng]. *Crit Care* 21, no. 1 (2017): 276. https://doi.org/10.1186/s13054-017-1856-1.

Qian, E. T., J. D. Casey, A. Wright, et al. "Cefepime vs Piperacillin-Tazobactam in Adults Hospitalized With Acute Infection: The ACORN Randomized Clinical Trial." [In eng]. *Jama* 330, no. 16 (2023): 1557–67. https://doi.org/10.1001/jama.2023.20583.

Singh, T. D., J. C. O'Horo, C. N. Day, et al. "Cefepime Is Associated With Acute Encephalopathy in Critically Ill Patients: A Retrospective Case-Control Study." [In eng]. *Neurocrit Care* 33, no. 3 (2020): 695–700. https://doi.org/10.1007/s12028-020-01035-w.

Stratton, K., and K. W. Davis. "Case Report: Cefepime Induced Neurotoxicity Following a Change in Infusion Time." [In eng]. *Hosp Pharm* 59, no. 4 (Aug 2024): 411–14. doi:10.1177/00185787241237142.

40 Alcohol Withdrawal With Extreme Agitation

A 52-year-old man presented after a fall from a barstool and hitting the back of his head. He lost consciousness and after regaining alertness, he became confused and rapidly belligerent. In the emergency department, he underwent intubation to allow for a noncontrast head computed tomography (CT) scan, which showed traumatic subarachnoid hemorrhage and a thin subdural hemorrhage. His serum ethanol concentration was 350 mg/dL, which, in a less experienced drinker, could lead to inability to walk without assistance and even lapsing into stupor. Admitted to the medical intensive care unit (ICU), he remained sedated on propofol infusion overnight. The following morning, upon discontinuation of sedation, he was intermittently drowsy and restless. Repeat head CT showed no interval changes. Over the next 36 hours, his agitation worsened, and he developed sustained sinus tachycardia, increased pulse pressure, tachypnea, and diaphoresis. He was tremulous and appeared to have visual hallucinations. When stimulated, he would thrash his arms and legs violently.

What do you do now?

We should consider acute alcohol intoxication and subsequent withdrawal a medical emergency. Altered consciousness, seizures, and extreme agitation are the main neurological manifestations. Yet, fewer than 5% of patients with a serious alcohol use disorder ever have a grand mal seizure during withdrawal (usually on day 2 but occasionally hours after admission to the ICU). It is equally uncommon to present with a severe agitated confusion (delirium tremens). Multiple intercurrent systemic complications (dehydration, cardiac dysrhythmias, and aspiration pneumonia, among others) can also occur in these patients, who already may have profound alcohol-associated morbidity, such as pancreatitis. All these factors increase mortality rates and so their management is more complex than most other types of delirium discussed in Chapter 38.

Upon learning that our patient drank excessively and and had done so for years, we anticipated a delirium with or without seizures within 24 hours of admission. We now know more about how alcohol affects brain chemistry. In addition to stimulating gamma-aminobutyric acid receptors, alcohol enhances the release of opioid peptides that are not only rewarding but also associated with dopamine release, which potentially contributes to craving. Ethanol also selectively inhibits N-methyl-D-aspartate (NMDA) receptors that transmit the excitatory effects of the neurotransmitter glutamate. The depressive effect of alcohol on NMDA receptors results in compensatory upregulation of these receptors and consequently brain hyperexcitability that emerges upon the withdrawal of alcohol.

Patients with acute alcohol intoxication often appear in the emergency department after traumatic brain injury, which can be severe due to tumbling down stairs or even a fall from standing height. There are three clinical scenarios. First, these patients may have an acute subdural hematoma that needs immediate evacuation (based on CT scan findings and not so much on the neurologic examination confounded by intoxication). Second, the findings on CT may be minimal, but the effects of alcohol confound their examination and, in particular, their state of consciousness; often these patients appear "clinically worse than their head CT" because of the strong central nervous system–depressant effects of alcohol. Third, these are patients who appear stable and less injured, but they can have a delayed development or worsening of intracranial contusions or subdural hematoma, sometimes facilitated by alcohol-related coagulopathy; this complication may be difficult to recognize at the bedside or characterized by a new arm drift or reduction of speech output. Follow-up neuroimaging is therefore obligatory.

Seizures are not common with acute ethanol intoxication but may be the first manifestation of withdrawal syndrome. Recurrence of seizures and even status epilepticus may ensue, particularly if there are delays in initiating antiseizure medication. We treat these patients with alcohol withdrawal seizures with appropriate doses of benzodiazepines and a loading dose of levetiracetam; they do not usually require administration of second- or third-line agents. Also, coexistent head trauma may indicate the need for a week of an antiseizure medication such as levetiracetam.

As illustrated by our patient, delirium from alcohol withdrawal can manifest with extreme agitation (delirium tremens). Benzodiazepines are the first-line therapy for control of psychomotor agitation from alcohol withdrawal. We recommend using a validated monitoring tool, such as the Clinical Institute Withdrawal Assessment of Alcohol (CIWA), its simplified revised version (CIWA-Ar), or the Glasgow Modified Alcohol Withdrawal Scale, to guide the administration of benzodiazepines, but it should not replace clinical judgment. These tools are less dependable in intubated patients or patients otherwise unable to verbalize responses.

The overall approach is to take initiative. "Front-loading" therapy may be preferable to the traditional "symptom-triggered therapy" in patients with previous episodes of delirium tremens or coexistent cardiovascular disease (who may not tolerate prolonged tachycardia and hypertension).

Dexmedetomidine can control agitation and the hyperadrenergic features of alcohol withdrawal, but patients who are already mildly hypotensive (e.g., decompensated cirrhosis) do not tolerate it well. Gabapentin reduces the risk of withdrawal syndrome in patients with alcohol use disorder; however, it is not effective to treat severe delirium when alcohol withdrawal is already present. Though antidopaminergics (haloperidol, quetiapine, olanzapine) are the mainstay of therapy for other forms of agitation, we avoid administering them to patients with alcohol withdrawal because these drugs can increase the risk of ventricular tachyarrhythmias, particularly if administered before adequate correction of hypokalemia and hypomagnesemia, which are very prevalent in alcohol use disorder. In intubated patients, propofol is an option until other strategies work. It is no exaggeration that the introduction of IV phenobarbital has been a revolutionary change and is greatly effective. We use intravenous boluses of 5 mg/kg not exceeding 15 mg/kg over 24 hours (though arguably intubated patients can receive higher doses). Table 40.1 summarizes the pharmacological options for the treatment of alcohol withdrawal delirium.

TABLE 40.1 **Pharmacological Options for the Treatment of Delirium Tremens**

Drug	Usual Dose	Advantages	Disadvantages
Diazepam	5–10 mg IV per dose		Excessive sedation Respiratory depression
Lorazepam[a]	2–4 mg IV per dose	Antiseizure effect	Excessive sedation Respiratory depression
Phenobarbital	5 mg/kg IV boluses (up to 15 mg/kg)	Can work in cases refractory to BDZ Antiseizure effect	Prolonged sedation Respiratory depression Liver toxicity
Dexmedetomidine	0.2–1.5 mcg/ kg/h	Good control of hyperadrenergic features No liver toxicity	May require intubation at high doses No antiseizure properties
Propofol	20–80 mcg/ kg/min	Effective even in recalcitrant cases Antiseizure effect No liver toxicity	Always requires intubation Risk of propofol infusion syndrome at prolonged high doses (>100 mg/ kg/min for >48 hours)

[a] We prefer lorazepam over diazepam in patients with seizures because it has a longer intracerebral half-life and therefore longer antiepileptic effect. Doses of diazepam or lorazepam can be repeated every 15–20 minutes until the agitation is controlled.
BDZ, benzodiazepine.

Diligent supportive care will minimize complications. We begin rehydration, electrolyte replacement, and thiamine supplementation before giving any glucose. We initiate enteral nutrition as soon as feasible to compensate for the increased metabolic demand caused by the agitation. We administer lactulose for hyperammonemia.

We loaded our patient with a total of 10 mg/kg of intravenous phenobarbital in addition to higher doses of lorazepam. His agitation gradually improved, and he was extubated the following day. We referred him to psychiatry to arrange a plan for detoxification. Alcohol delirium is not the only neurological risk to the patient with excessive alcohol use. We will discuss other acute serious neurologic complications of alcohol abuse in the next chapter.

KEY POINTS TO REMEMBER

- Patients admitted with acute ethanol intoxication can develop withdrawal syndrome rapidly after hospitalization.
- Benzodiazepines are the preferred medications for the treatment of alcohol withdrawal seizures and delirium with agitation.
- When benzodiazepines do not suffice, intravenous phenobarbital is an excellent alternative and often most effective.
- While we usually recommend symptom-triggered protocols for the management of alcohol withdrawal syndrome, a more aggressive, preemptive approach (front-loading) may be preferable in patients deemed to have elevated risk for developing delirium tremens.

Further Reading

Alexiou, A., and T. King. "Alcohol Withdrawal." [In eng]. *Bmj* 381 (2023): 951. https://doi.org/10.1136/bmj.p951.

Alwakeel, M., D. Alayan, T. Saleem, et al. "Phenobarbital-Based Protocol for Alcohol Withdrawal Syndrome in a Medical ICU: Pre-Post Implementation Study." [In eng]. *Crit Care Explor* 5 (2023): e0898. https://doi.org/10.1097/cce.0000000000000898.

Deveau, R., A. Wong, M. Eche, T. Yankama, and C. R. Fehnel. "Safety of Phenobarbital Versus Benzodiazepines for Alcohol Withdrawal in Critically Ill Patients With Primary Neurologic Injuries." [In eng]. *Ann Pharmacother* (Aug 20 2024): 10600280241271156. doi:10.1177/10600280241271156.

Dixit, D., J. Endicott, L. Burry, et al. "Management of Acute Alcohol Withdrawal Syndrome in Critically Ill Patients." [In eng]. *Pharmacotherapy* 36 (2016): 797–22. https://doi.org/10.1002/phar.1770.

Murphy, J. A., B. M. Curran, W. A. Gibbons, 3rd, and H. M. Harnica. "Adjunctive Phenobarbital for Alcohol Withdrawal Syndrome: A Focused Literature Review." [In eng]. *Ann Pharmacother* 55 (2021): 1515–24. https://doi.org/10.1177/106002802 1999821.

Schmidt, K. J., M. R. Doshi, J. M. Holzhausen, et al. "Treatment of Severe Alcohol Withdrawal." [In eng]. *Ann Pharmacother* 50 (2016): 389–401. https://doi.org/10.1177/1060028016629161.

Tidwell, W. P., T. L. Thomas, J. D. Pouliot, et al. "Treatment of Alcohol Withdrawal Syndrome: Phenobarbital vs CIWA-Ar Protocol." [In eng]. *Am J Crit Care* 27 (2018): 454–60. https://doi.org/10.4037/ajcc2018745.

41 Acute Alcohol-Related Neurologic Complications

A 43-year-old male with alcohol use disorder was reportedly discovered unconscious. He moves about and restlessly moans but then suddenly says "I love you" to his mother. His eyes are mostly closed and he actively tries to keep them closed when they are pried open. He has dysarthria with spastic features. There is a near-full ophthalmoparesis and some ptosis. The overall tone is normal. There are no other extrapyramidal signs. There is no evidence of myoclonus or startle myoclonus. Subsequent magnetic resonance imaging (MRI) showed restricted diffusion on bilateral dorsal medial thalami, mammilary bodies, periaqueductal gray matter, and the pons, concerning for both Wernicke-Korsakoff syndrome and central pontine myelinolysis (CPM) (Figure 41.1). He was given aggressive thiamine and magnesium replacement with further correction of his malnutrition guided by a dietitian. He remained significantly impaired with moderate to severe nonaphasic cognitive communication deficits and mild to moderate dysarthria and dysphagia.

What do you do now?

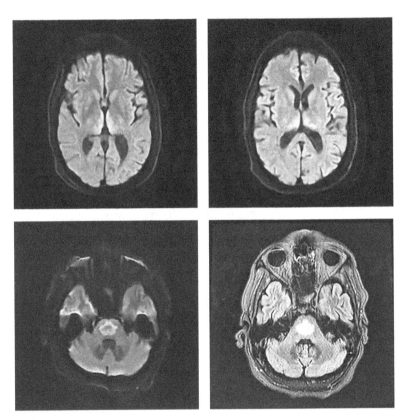

FIGURE 41.1 MRI showed restricted diffusion on bilateral dorsal medial thalami, periaqueductal gray matter, and the pons, concerning for Wernicke-Korsakoff syndrome and central pontine myelinolysis.

When consumed in excess and over several years, alcohol takes a damaging toll on the central and peripheral nervous systems. Alcohol can cause a direct toxic effect in the brain, possible reversible injury associated with chronic malnutrition, and brain dysfunction and structural damage due to a failing liver. Too frequently, alcohol intoxication leads to traumatic brain injury, with severe and permanently incapacitating injury. Some people die from anoxic-ischemic brain injury after binges when nocturnal breathing drive becomes seriously depressed and vomiting obstructs the airway. We have already seen what a single event of alcohol withdrawal and seizures can do in Chapter 40, where we reviewed the adverse effects of repeated episodes of alcohol withdrawal on attention and executive function; this chapter looks at other serious complications from alcohol.

Both CPM and Wernicke-Korsakoff syndrome were first described in long-standing alcoholism with malnutrition. We rarely see both at the same time. Both disorders have also eventually become linked with other medical conditions. We cannot be surprised if nonneurologists fail to recognize these disorders; MRIs are seldom performed in these patients, and other urgent medical problems demand the physician's immediate attention. Both disorders can cause severe injury. While full reversibility is not that common, improvement is possible even in initially severe cases. (We also need to mention the exceptionally rare Marchiafava-Bignami disease with manifestation of a corpus callosal disconnection syndrome.

Neurologists Raymond Adams and Maurice Victor and psychiatrist Elliott Lee Mancall first coined the name "central pontine myelinolysis." They found demyelination at the base of the pons, but later descriptions noted occasional extension into the tegmentum. Later, CPM was frequently linked to rapid correction of severe hyponatremia, but CPM remains very much associated with severe debilitating disease, such as chronic alcoholism. CPM has also been described in patients with major osmolality fluctuations, such as severely burned patients and post–liver transplant patients, again suggesting that osmotic changes affect the brainstem preferentially. The clinical manifestations of CPM can be diverse, but pseudobulbar palsy, facial weakness, inability to swallow or speak, and quadriplegia are prominent. The central location in the pons typically excludes neuro-ophthalmologic signs (and in our patient were caused by associated Wernicke -Korsakoff syndrome). CPM progression to a locked-in syndrome with, as expected, only blinking and vertical eye movements as a means of communication has been noted but is quite unusual. Computed tomographic (CT) scanning may later yield clearly distinctive abnormalities, often with a big hole in the pons, but MRI has facilitated the diagnosis of CPM antemortem and has carefully allowed characterization of the disorder. A symmetrical oval or round area on T1- or T2-weighted images is typical, but lesions in the base of the pons may also be trident or bat shaped because of preferential involvement of horizontal tracts and sparing of vertical tracts. No correlation exists between persistent MRI findings and subsequent potential for recovery. Bulbar dysfunction, truncal and gait ataxia, and spastic quadriparesis remain sources of impairment. Possible pathophysiological considerations are the "grid" phenomenon, suggesting strangulation of myelinated fibers by surrounding edema in the pons, and "osmotic endothelial injury," which implies rapid osmotic changes of endothelial cells in the gray matter release of myelotoxic factors. Not surprisingly, recent data found the syndrome difficult to prove, and sometimes unrelated to rapid sodium correction.

Recommendations on prevention and management are variable. The 2013 U.S. guidelines limit sodium correction to 8 mEq/L for patients at elevated risk (<105 mEq/L; hypokalemia, alcoholism, malnutrition, and advanced liver disease) and 10 to 12 mEq/L for patients at normal risk with chronic severe hyponatremia (<120 mEq/L). The 2014 European guidelines recommend limiting the maximum 24-hour correction rate to 10 mEq/L in patients with moderately symptomatic hyponatremia. In practice, clinicians set the rates of sodium correction to less than 0.5 mEq/L/h or even lower, but a sodium correction rate less than 6 mEq/L per 24 hours was associated with higher mortality in a recent study. It is good to be cautious when correcting symptomatic hyponatremia, but even when correction is too fast, the risk of osmotic demyelination is extremely low. It was very uncommon (a single case in over 400 cases with correction of hyponatremia to <120 mmol/L) in our review at Mayo Clinic despite more than one in four patients with hyponatremia corrected by more than 10 mmol/L over the first 24 hours. A multicenter cohort study led by MacMillan with over 20,000 patients admitted with hyponatremia at five academic hospitals in Toronto, Canada, found rapid correction (>8 mmol per 24 hours) in 18%. Only nine definitive cases of osmotic demyelination syndrome (0.05%) were diagnosed; they were more common in patients with severe hyponatremia (sodium values <110 mmol/L) but not related to the pace of correction. Furthermore, a recent systematic review and meta-analysis concluded that slow correction (defined as <8 or as 6–10 mEq/L per 24 hours) and very slow correction (<6 mEq/L per 24 hours) of severe hyponatremia were associated with an increased risk of mortality and hospital length of stay when compared to rapid correction (≥8–10 mEq/L per 24 hours). Therefore, it is possible that we have become excessively alarmed by the risk of osmotic demyelination with rapid correction of hyponatremia (Chapter 49). And remember: fast correction of symptomatic hyponatremia is safe with recently developed hyponatremia.

Wernicke-Korsakoff encephalopathy is caused by thiamine deficiency and has a range of presenting features including gait disturbance, altered cognitive state, nystagmus, and major eye movement disorders. Wernicke encephalopathy presents often in the alcohol-dependent population. Wernicke encephalopathy is also well recognized following bariatric surgery, gastrointestinal surgery, anorexia nervosa, inflammatory bowel disease, cancer, and pancreatitis. How common is it? In a 9-year autopsy study in Western Australia, the incidence of Wernicke-Korsakoff encephalopathy was around 3%, but the incidence may be increasing. This study also found markedly deficient nutrition in the majority of cases involving patients with long-standing severe alcohol use disorder. They emphasized that only 20% of the 131 cases studied had been diagnosed clinically; in the majority, it was a surprise finding at autopsy.

Carl Wernicke and Sergei Korsakoff did not publish their eponymous disorder as coauthors, and Korsakoff described a "psycho-polyneuritic syndrome," nearly a decade after Wernicke description. Korsakoff emphasized the "alteration of the memory of recent events" with preservation of older memories, leading to "delirium by fabulation." He suggested that the repeated vomiting, which he attributed to chronic alcoholism, aggravated the patient's cognitive function. But addiction was not the only possible cause; he presented 14 cases without intoxication, which occurred during pregnancy, typhus, diabetes, and tuberculosis. He imagined that the nervous system was "poisoned." We now recognize Korsakoff syndrome as a prototype of diencephalic amnesia characterized by both anterograde and retrograde impairments. There is a major problem with autobiographical (episodic) memory, such that a person cannot reexperience events in any detail.

What has been found experimentally? The earliest biochemical change is the decrease of alpha-ketoglutarate-dehydrogenase activity in astrocytes. Astrocyte dysfunction in thiamine deficiency involves a loss of glutamate transporters. A reduction in the thiamine-dependent activity of trans-ketolase leads to a lower use of glucose and oxidative stress secondary to endothelial cell dysfunction. MRI shows altered signal in limbic regions including the paraventricular regions of the thalamus, hypothalamus, mammillary bodies, periaqueductal region, floor of the fourth ventricle, and midline cerebellum.

The presenting symptom triggering hospitalization was a state of mental confusion. In Victor and Adams's series, patients were admitted to the hospital in a state of "exhaustion or collapse," and most patients had more than one presenting symptom. The most common initial symptom was incoordination of gait or staggering with ocular symptoms worsening in a stepwise manner over a period of several days or weeks. Notably, patients did not complain of diplopia.

Wernicke encephalopathy may be identified in malnourished alcoholic patients who are delirious and have trouble walking. In these patients, the delirium is often caused by thiamine deficiency, which may be erroneously diagnosed as alcohol withdrawal delirium.

If there is a substantial risk of Wernicke encephalopathy, parenteral (intravenous or intramuscular) thiamine, 250 mg once a day for 5 days, is advised. Thiamine depends on magnesium to metabolize glucose in the energy-generating processes of the pentose phosphate pathway and the Krebs cycle. Consequently, thiamine supplementation may be ineffective if existing or developing magnesium deficiencies are not corrected at the same time. In comparison to the ocular signs, the onset of improvement of ataxia is delayed and takes longer for complete improvement to occur. Moreover, recovery from ataxia is incomplete in over half of the patients, who are left with a slow, shuffling, wide-based gait.

These diagnoses are a sterling example of typically overlooked conditions when patients are admitted with other pressing medical needs. They are truly hidden in the shadows.

KEY POINTS TO REMEMBER

- Wernicke-Korsakoff syndrome may become apparent after delirium subsides.
- CPM and osmotic demyelination syndrome are rare and not always associated with rapid correction or overcorrection of hyponatremia.
- Morbidity of both disorders is still substantial, but recovery over time is possible even in patients with severe presentations.
- In patients with Wernicke syndrome, rapid administration of high-dose intravenous thiamine is needed to succesfully treat ophthalmoparesis, but gait difficulties often remain improve.

Further Reading

Adams, R. D., M. Victor, and E. L. Mancall. "Central Pontine Myelinolysis: A Hitherto Undescribed Disease Occurring in Alcoholic and Malnourished Patients." [In eng]. *AMA Arch Neurol Psychiatry* 81, no. 2 (Feb 1959): 154–72.

Ayus, J. C., Moritz, M. L., Fuentes, N. A., et al. Correction Rates and Clinical Outcomes in Hospitalized Adults With Severe Hyponatremia: A Systematic Review and Meta-Analysis. *JAMA Intern Med.* 2024 Nov 18:e245981. doi: 10.1001/jamainternmed.2024.5981. Epub ahead of print.

Brunner, J. E., J. M. Redmond, A. M. Haggar, et al. "Central Pontine Myelinolysis and Pontine Lesions After Rapid Correction of Hyponatremia: A Prospective Magnetic Resonance Imaging Study." [In eng]. *Ann Neurol* 27, no. 1 (Jan 1990): 61–66. https://doi.org/10.1002/ana.410270110.

Buis, C. I., and E. F. Wijdicks. "Serial Magnetic Resonance Imaging of Central Pontine Myelinolysis." [In eng]. *Liver Transpl* 8, no. 7 (Jul 2002): 643–45. https://doi.org/10.1053/jlts.2002.34023.

Endo, Y., M. Oda, and M. Hara. "Central Pontine Myelinolysis. A Study of 37 Cases in 1,000 Consecutive Autopsies." [In eng]. *Acta Neuropathol* 53, no. 2 (1981): 145–53. https://doi.org/10.1007/bf00689995.

Geoghegan, P., A. M. Harrison, C. Thongprayoon, et al. "Sodium Correction Practice and Clinical Outcomes in Profound Hyponatremia." [In eng]. *Mayo Clin Proc* 90, no. 10 (Oct 2015): 1348–55.

Graff-Radford, J., J. E. Fugate, T. J. Kaufmann, et al. "Clinical and Radiologic Correlations of Central Pontine Myelinolysis Syndrome." [In eng]. *Mayo Clin Proc* 86, no. 11 (Nov 2011): 1063–67.

Harper, C. "The Incidence of Wernicke's Encephalopathy in Australia—A Neuropathological Study of 131 Cases." [In eng]. *J Neurol Neurosurg Psychiatry* 46, no. 7 (Jul 1983): 593–98. https://doi.org/10.1136/jnnp.46.7.593.

Harper, C. G. "Confusion, Coma, and Death From a Preventable Disease." [In eng]. *Med J Aust* 2, no. 5 (1981): 219–21. https://doi.org/https://doi.org/10.5694/j.1326-5377.1981.tb100928.x. https://onlinelibrary.wiley.com/doi/abs/10.5694/j.1326-5377.1981.tb100928.x.

Loeber, S., T. Duka, H. Welzel Márquez, et al. "Effects of Repeated Withdrawal From Alcohol on Recovery of Cognitive Impairment Under Abstinence and Rate of Relapse." [In eng]. *Alcohol Alcohol* 45, no. 6 (Nov–Dec 2010): 541–47. https://doi.org/10.1093/alcalc/agq065.

MacMillan, T. E., S. Shin, J. Topf, et al. "Osmotic Demyelination Syndrome in Patients Hospitalized With Hyponatremia." [In eng]. *NEJM Evidence* 2, no. 4 (2023): EVIDoa2200215. https://doi.org/doi:10.1056/EVIDoa2200215. https://evidence.nejm.org/doi/abs/10.1056/EVIDoa2200215.

Messert, B., W. W. Orrison, M. J. Hawkins, and C. E. Quaglieri. "Central Pontine Myelinolysis. Considerations on Etiology, Diagnosis, and Treatment." [In eng]. *Neurology* 29, no. 2 (Feb 1979): 147–60. https://doi.org/10.1212/wnl.29.2.147.

Rasiah, R., C. Gregoriano, B. Mueller, A. Kutz, and P. Schuetz. "Hospital Outcomes in Medical Patients With Alcohol-Related and Non-Alcohol-Related Wernicke Encephalopathy." [In eng]. *Mayo Clin Proc* 99, no. 5 (May 2024): 740–53. doi:10.1016/j.mayocp.2023.07.021.

Singh, T. D., J. E. Fugate, and A. A. Rabinstein. "Central Pontine and Extrapontine Myelinolysis: A Systematic Review." [In eng]. *Eur J Neurol* 21, no. 12 (Dec 2014): 1443–50.

Victor, M., R. D. Adams, and G. H. Collins. *The Wernicke-Korsakoff Syndrome and Related Neurologic Disorders Due to Alcoholism and Malnutrition*. Philadelphia, PA: F. A. Davis Company; 1989.

Wallis, W. E., E. Willoughby, and P. Baker. "Coma in the Wernicke-Korsakoff Syndrome." [In eng]. *Lancet* 2, no. 8086 (Aug 19 1978): 400–401. https://doi.org/10.1016/s0140-6736(78)91867-6.

Wijdicks, E. F., P. R. Blue, J. L. Steers, and R. H. Wiesner. "Central Pontine Myelinolysis With Stupor Alone After Orthotopic Liver Transplantation." [In eng]. *Liver Transpl Surg* 2, no. 1 (Jan 1996): 14–16. https://doi.org/10.1002/lt.500020104.

Wijnia, J. W. "A Clinician's View of Wernicke-Korsakoff Syndrome." [In eng]. *J Clin Med* 11, no. 22 (Nov 15 2022): 6755. doi:10.3390/jcm11226755.

Wolfe, M., A. Menon, M. Oto, et al. "Alcohol and the Central Nervous System." [In eng]. *Pract Neurol* 23, no. 4 (Aug 2023): 273–85. https://doi.org/10.1136/pn-2023-003817.

42 Sudden Hypotension and Fever Spike

A 50-year-old man with a history of hypertension, heavy smoking, and alcoholism was admitted with poor-grade subarachnoid hemorrhage. He was intubated to protect his airway. There was no evidence of pulmonary edema on his chest X-ray. Cerebral angiogram showed an anterior communicating artery aneurysm, which was successfully coiled. His condition improved after placement of a ventriculostomy, but in the following days, he showed signs of alcohol withdrawal. Despite treatment with benzodiazepines and dexmedetomidine, he had frequent episodes of agitation, diaphoresis, hyperthermia, and tachycardia. He remained intubated and mechanically ventilated. Serial transcranial Doppler measurements showed progressively increasing velocities in the anterior and middle cerebral arteries from day 6 onward. This was confirmed by computed tomography (CT) angiogram, although CT perfusion showed no abnormalities. However, on day 10 after ictus, he suddenly developed a high fever (40°C) and became abruptly hypotensive and much less responsive.

What do you do now?

edical complications are likely in any mechanically ventilated patient with an acute brain injury, and they occur suddenly. New-onset acute fever and hypotension should always trigger prompt activation of the sepsis management protocol. Delays can be very problematic, especially in patients with compromised cerebral perfusion. Sepsis treatment is currently guided by the recommendations of the *Surviving Sepsis Campaign*, which provides international guidelines for management of sepsis and septic shock, with the most recent update published in 2021 (Box 42.1). The general principles of management of septic shock do apply to patients with acute brain injury, but in critically ill neurological patients, certain aspects of care should be adjusted (Box 42.2).

Fluid resuscitation with IV crystalloid solution should be started emergently. It is common practice to infuse with 1000 to 2000 mL of crystalloids over 30 minutes. Yet, a more moderate approach to IV fluid resuscitation may be associated with decreased sepsis mortality. Fluid responsiveness can be assessed with a 250 ml fluid bolus or a passive leg-raise maneuver increasing blood return to the right ventricle. In patients with cerebral edema, normal saline is preferable to lactated Ringer to avoid fluids with lower tonicity. The usual set target in sepsis treatment is a mean arterial pressure (MAP) of 65 mmHg, but a higher target may be necessary in patients at risk for cerebral ischemia. Serum lactate should be measured quickly, and it is an important indicator of severity. A serum lactic acid level greater than 4 mmol/L indicates tissue hypoperfusion and calls for aggressive hemodynamic support. The patient's urinary output must be closely monitored for the development of oliguria (<20 mL/h). Goal-directed therapy protocols within the first 6 hours (aiming for a central venous oxygen saturation ≥70%) offer no added benefit as long as adequate support is otherwise provided, and these protocols may result in overtreatment.

Norepinephrine is the initial vasopressor of choice. It may be supplemented with low-dose vasopressin (0.04 units per minute) if the blood pressure target is not achieved. Epinephrine and dopamine are reasonable options. However, the pure alpha-adrenergic agonist phenylephrine is undesirable in septic shock because it can reduce cardiac output by increasing afterload without providing inotropic support, and patients with sepsis may already have myocardial dysfunction. In fact, these patients should have an urgent echocardiogram. If shock persists and the left ventricular ejection fraction is

> **BOX 42.1 Strong Recommendations From the Surviving Sepsis Campaign (International Guidelines for Management of Sepsis and Septic Shock 2021)**
>
> For adults with sepsis or septic shock, use crystalloids as first-line fluid for resuscitation. (Weaker recommendation for the administration of at least 30 mL/kg of IV crystalloid fluid within the first 3 hours of resuscitation.)
>
> For adults with septic shock on vasopressors, initial target MAP of 65 mmHg over higher MAP targets.
>
> For adults with possible septic shock or a high likelihood for sepsis, we recommend administering antimicrobials immediately, ideally within 1 hour of recognition.
>
> For adults with septic shock, use norepinephrine as the first-line agent over other vasopressors.
>
> For adults with sepsis-induced ARDS use a low-tidal-volume ventilation strategy (6 mL/kg) over a high-tidal-volume strategy (>10 mL/kg) and an upper limit goal for plateau pressures of 30 cmH_2O over higher plateau pressures.
>
> With recruitment maneuvers, no incremental PEEP titration/strategy.
>
> For adults with sepsis-induced severe ARDS, use prone ventilation for >12 hours daily.
>
> For adults with sepsis or septic shock, use a restrictive (over liberal) transfusion strategy.
>
> For adults with sepsis or septic shock, use pharmacologic venous thromboembolism prophylaxis unless a contraindication to such therapy exists and use low-molecular-weight heparin over unfractionated heparin.
>
> For adults with sepsis or septic shock, initiate insulin therapy at a glucose level of ≥180 mg/dL (10 mmol/L).
>
> ARDS, acute respiratory distress syndrome; MAP, mean arterial pressure; PEEP, positive end-expiratory pressure.

reduced, dobutamine, an inotropic agent, should be started. After successful resuscitation, we administer fluids conservatively (i.e., fluid balance even to negative) to prevent fluid-overload complications (principally related to capillary leak leading to pulmonary edema and anasarca). However, fluid administration should be adjusted depending on the acute neurological disease we are treating. In patients with brain edema, maintaining a negative fluid balance is preferable. However, patients with symptomatic cerebral vasospasm can become ischemic if they develop intravascular volume contraction.

BOX 42.2 Treatment of Septic Shock With Special Considerations in Neurocritically Ill Patients

Start aggressive fluid resuscitation immediately

    1–2 L of 0.9% NaCl

Define resuscitation goal

A MAP goal higher than the usual 65 mmHg may be necessary in neurocritical patients with compromised cerebral perfusion

Start vasopressor if MAP is below target after fluid challenge

    Norepinephrine, low-dose vasopressin or epinephrine

    (Phenylephrine should be avoided)

Obtain echocardiogram and assess systolic function

    Start dobutamine if decreased left ventricular ejection fraction

Conservative fluid strategy after resuscitation goal is achieved

    Can use diuretics if MAP is stable and there is evidence of cerebral edema or raised ICP

Find infectious source

    Panculture (blood cultures, urinalysis with culture and sensitivity, sputum sample)

    Culture CSF

Start broad-spectrum antibiotics as soon as possible

    Vancomycin 25 mg/kg IV loading followed by 15 mg/kg every 12 hours plus

    Piperacillin/tazobactam 4.5 g IV every 6 hours or cefepime 2 g IV every 8–12 hours

Consider hydrocortisone if vasopressor dependence

    Hydrocortisone 50–100 mg IV every 6–8 hours

Administer blood products

    Consider red blood cell transfusion to keep hemoglobin >8 g/dL if cerebral perfusion is compromised

    Platelet transfusion to keep platelet count >50,000 if recent ICH or neurosurgery

    FFP to correct coagulopathy if recent ICH or neurosurgery

Adjust mechanical ventilation

    Careful titration of PEEP if raised ICP

> Reassess sedation and analgesia
>> Sedation holidays
>> Minimize use of opiates if possible
> Control glucose
>> Maintain blood sugars between 100 and 180 mg/dL
>
> CSF, cerebrospinal fluid; FFP, fresh frozen plasma; ICH, intracranial hemorrhage; ICP, intracranial pressure; MAP, mean arterial pressure; PEEP, positive end expiratory pressure.

Patients with refractory septic shock may be treated with hydrocortisone. Corticosteroids may reduce vasopressor dependency but do not appear to improve survival. Their use should not be a problem in critically ill neurological patients.

Early initiation of broad-spectrum antibiotics is crucially important. Ideally, they should be started within the first hour of the diagnosis of septic shock. Pan cultures are obtained before the first antibiotic dose, if possible, but cannot delay the start of antibiotics. Nosocomial meningitis may be associated with early sepsis; thus, cultures should include a cerebrospinal fluid sample in any patient with cerebrospinal fluid diversion devices (ventriculostomy, lumbar drain) or previous neurosurgical procedures.

Septic shock guidelines generally recommend transfusion of red blood cells only when the hemoglobin concentration drops below 7 g/dL. Some practitioners believe that critically ill neurological patients with compromised cerebral perfusion and recent or persistent hypotension should be exceptions to this rule. Large clinical trials (HEMOTION in patients with severe traumatic brain injury and SAHARA in patients with subarachnoid hemorrhage) showed no benefit from liberal transfusion targeting higher hemoglobin levels of 10 g/dl (see Chapters 3 and 17). Thus, we do not order transfusions in our patients with acute brain injury unless the hemoglobin is below 7–8 g/dl.

Glucose management should also be more cautious in patients with acute brain injury. Cerebral microdialysis studies have shown that neuroglycopenia and anaerobic metabolism can occur with glycemia levels between 60 and 80 mg/dL, levels often considered acceptable in other patients. We use insulin infusions in hyperglycemic patients, but cautiously. Our target is generally to keep serum glucose between 100 and 180 mg/dL, avoiding too-tight control.

High positive end-expiratory pressure (PEEP) can improve oxygenation in patients with sepsis complicated by acute respiratory distress syndrome. High PEEP is not contraindicated in patients with raised intracranial pressure, but the effect of gradually increased PEEP on the intracranial pressure should be carefully monitored.

Sedation should be guided by a protocol with a clear goal (e.g., a sedation level defined by the Richmond Agitation Sedation Scale) and scheduled drug interruptions. These sedation holidays allow us to follow the neurological examination and reduce the incidence of delirium. Opiates are excellent analgesic agents but will greatly confound the neurological examination. For elderly patients and those with liver or renal failure, the confounding effect of opiates may be quite prolonged.

We promptly resuscitated our patient with fluids and norepinephrine. We started broad-spectrum antibiotics within 30 minutes of the onset of hypotension. The source of sepsis was eventually recognized to be ventilator-associated pneumonia. Despite rapid control of the hypotension and adequate treatment of the infection, the brief hypotension proved too much for him. He remained stuporous, and a repeat head CT scan 4 days later showed multifocal brain infarctions. This case illustrates how exquisitely sensitive the brain is to ischemia, particularly after a major initial insult such as subarachnoid hemorrhage in our case.

Fever is ubiquitous in critically ill patients, and central fever is common in patients with acute brain injury. Yet, when fever is accompanied by hypotension, patients should promptly receive treatment for early sepsis following a comprehensive protocol. Any delay in reversing the situation may cause additional brain injury. Some have used the Sequential Organ Failure Assessment (SOFA) Score to detect systemic infection in critically ill patients, but the usefulness of SOFA in neurocritical patients is limited because many of our patients have an abnormal level of consciousness, which is a key component of the score. Repeatedly, we must rely on our own diagnostic skills and focus on the urgency of changed clinical circumstances. These immediate threats to clinical stability often reveal themselves obliquely.

> **KEY POINTS TO REMEMBER**
>
> - Although components of the systemic inflammatory response syndrome (e.g., persistent fever, tachycardia) can be attributed to the brain injury in acute neurological patients, their association with sudden hypotension should activate a septic shock protocol.
> - The standard principles of septic shock management are appropriate in patients with acute brain injury, but there are notable differences.
> - Obtain samples for panculture, including cerebrospinal fluid, immediately.
> - The brain is at risk for additional injury from systemic complications, and critical first measures are swift initiation of isotonic (or hypertonic) fluid resuscitation, vasopressors and inotropes, broad coverage with antibiotics, blood transfusion, and glucose control.

Further Reading

Angus, D. C., A. E. Barnato, D. Bell, et al. "A Systematic Review and Meta-Analysis of Early Goal-Directed Therapy for Septic Shock: The Arise, Process and Promise Investigators." [In eng]. *Intensive Care Med* 41, no. 9 (Sep 2015): 1549–60. https://doi.org/10.1007/s00134-015-3822-1.

Corl KA, Levy MM, Holder AL, Douglas IS, Linde-Zwirble WT, Alam A. Moderate IV Fluid Resuscitation Is Associated With Decreased Sepsis Mortality. *Crit Care Med.* 2024 Nov 1;52(11):e557–e567. doi: 10.1097/CCM.0000000000006394. Epub 2024 Aug 23.

Evans, L., A. Rhodes, W. Alhazzani, et al. "Executive Summary: Surviving Sepsis Campaign: International Guidelines for the Management of Sepsis and Septic Shock 2021." [In eng]. *Crit Care Med* 49, no. 11 (Nov 1 2021): 1974–82. https://doi.org/10.1097/ccm.0000000000005357.

Godoy, D. A., M. Di Napoli, and A. A. Rabinstein. "Treating Hyperglycemia in Neurocritical Patients: Benefits and Perils." [In eng]. *Neurocrit Care* 13, no. 3 (Dec 2010): 425–38. https://doi.org/10.1007/s12028-010-9404-8.

Mayer, N. J. Prescott, H. C. "Sepsis and Septic Shock." (in engl) *N Engl J Med* 2024;391:2133–46. DOI: 10.1056/NEJMra2403213

Rivers, E., B. Nguyen, S. Havstad, et al. "Early Goal-Directed Therapy in the Treatment of Severe Sepsis and Septic Shock." [In eng]. *N Engl J Med* 345, no. 19 (Nov 8 2001): 1368–77. https://doi.org/10.1056/NEJMoa010307.

Robertson, C. S., H. J. Hannay, J. M. Yamal, et al. "Effect of Erythropoietin and Transfusion Threshold on Neurological Recovery After Traumatic Brain Injury: A Randomized Clinical Trial." [In eng]. *Jama* 312, no. 1 (Jul 2 2014): 36–47. https://doi.org/10.1001/jama.2014.6490.

Seethapathy, H., S. Zhao, T. Ouyang, et al. "Severe Hyponatremia Correction, Mortality, and Central Pontine Myelinolysis." *NEJM Evidence* 2, no. 10 (2023): EVIDoa2300107. https://doi.org/doi:10.1056/EVIDoa2300107. https://evidence.nejm.org/doi/abs/10.1056/EVIDoa2300107.

Spasovski, G., R. Vanholder, B. Allolio, et al. "Clinical Practice Guideline on Diagnosis and Treatment of Hyponatraemia." [In eng]. *Nephrol Dial Transplant* 29, no. Suppl 2 (Apr 2014): i1–i39. https://doi.org/10.1093/ndt/gfu040.

Verbalis, J. G., S. R. Goldsmith, A. Greenberg, et al. "Diagnosis, Evaluation, and Treatment of Hyponatremia: Expert Panel Recommendations." [In eng]. *Am J Med* 126, no. 10 Suppl 1 (Oct 2013): S1–42. https://doi.org/10.1016/j.amjmed.2013.07.006.

Wiedemann, H. P., A. P. Wheeler, G. R. Bernard, et al. "Comparison of Two Fluid-Management Strategies in Acute Lung Injury." [In eng]. *N Engl J Med* 354, no. 24 (Jun 15 2006): 2564–75. https://doi.org/10.1056/NEJMoa062200.

Yang, A., J. N. Kennedy, K. M. Reitz, et al. "Time to Treatment and Mortality for Clinical Sepsis Subtypes." [In eng]. *Crit Care* 27, no. 1 (Jun 15 2023): 236. https://doi.org/10.1186/s13054-023-04507-5.

43 When Blood Pressure Is Too High

A 56-year-old man with a history of long-standing, poorly controlled hypertension presents to the emergency department with sudden onset of a speech abnormality and right-sided weakness. Time from symptom onset is 70 minutes. First examination reveals a global aphasia, right hemianopia, right hemiparesis (National Institutes of Health Stroke Scale [NIHSS] score 14). Head computed tomography (CT) scan shows a probable hyperdense dot sign in a Sylvian branch of the left middle cerebral artery with no evidence of acute infarction or hemorrhage. Blood pressure is initially 204/112 mmHg. He responds only briefly to two doses of 10 mg of intravenous labetalol each. The patient is potentially a candidate for intravenous thrombolysis, but after these two doses of labetalol, the blood pressure rebounds to 194/106 mmHg. There are no other clinical or laboratory contraindications for intravenous thrombolysis.

What do you do now?

Three pieces of information are needed to know how—or even when—to treat hypertension in a patient with acute stroke: first, the type of stroke—ischemic or hemorrhagic; second, the time from the onset of symptoms; and third, in acute ischemic stroke, whether the patient is a candidate for thrombolysis (Figure 43.1). Although this is a quite frequent problem, evidence from randomized controlled trials is limited and inconclusive. Blood pressure targets differ depending on the specific clinical situation as summarized in the following sections. However, some general concepts apply to all patients with neurovascular emergencies. Chief among them is that extreme hypertension is dangerous but large blood pressure variability is also very concerning. Regardless of whether a patient presents with acute brain ischemia or hemorrhage, sudden, excessive decreases in blood pressure can cause cerebral (and renal) hypoperfusion. Because the autoregulatory curve of some patients may have shifted to the right, they are at higher risk of ischemia when blood pressure is rapidly lowered. Therefore, take initial blood pressure and history of chronic hypertension into account when deciding the initial targets for blood pressure reduction after stroke. Prehospital reduction of blood pressure was evaluated in the Intensive Ambulance-delivered Blood Pressure Reduction in Hyper-Acute Stroke Trial (INTERACT-4). Blood pressure lowering to a target below 140 mmHg was associated with a decrease in the odds of a poor functional outcome among patients with hemorrhagic stroke, but an increase among patients with ischemic stroke. The results of this trial confirm something we already knew: you need to know what you are treating before deciding how much to reduce the blood pressure in hypertensive patients with acute stroke symptoms.

Orders for blood pressure management require targets to which we must commit. These targets have some rationale and are not entirely coming out of nowhere. Yet, we will be the first ones to admit this is murky territory. We divide our recommendations into (1) the acute phase (first 24 hours) and (2) the time thereafter.

Ischemic Stroke—Candidate for Thrombolysis—First 24 Hours

Patient candidates for thrombolysis must have reliably controlled hypertension to reduce the risk of reperfusion hemorrhage. Expert guidelines recommend reducing the systolic blood pressure below 180 mmHg and the diastolic blood pressure below 100 mmHg before administering the lytic agent.

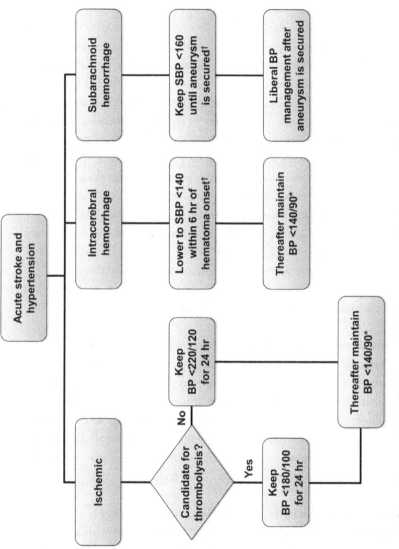

FIGURE 43.1 Recommended algorithm for control of hypertension in patients with acute stroke. * Target should be 130/80 mmHg in patients with diabetes mellitus. Ideal blood pressure less than 120/80 mmHg. † If suspected increased intracranial pressure, then monitor intracranial pressure and maintain cerebral perfusion pressure greater than 60 mmHg. BP, blood pressure.

Guidelines state that if these parameters cannot be reached and consistently maintained, intravenous thrombolysis should not be administered. Yet, there is some evidence challenging this conventional approach and suggesting that blood pressure reduction before thrombolysis may be actually worse than proceeding with thrombolysis without first treating the hypertension. This is a new quandary that might be resolved with a randomized controlled trial.

Following thrombolysis (or mechanical disruption with recanalization), monitor the blood pressure closely (every 15 minutes for the first 2–3 hours, then every 30 minutes for 6 hours, and then hourly for the rest of the first day), again keeping it below 180/100 mmHg. Failure to control hypertension during the first day could result in a cerebral hematoma with rapid neurologic deterioration.

In our patient, we were able to reduce the blood pressure to an acceptable range after initiating an infusion of nicardipine, which was then continued for 24 hours in the neurosciences intensive care unit. The patient received intravenous recombinant tissue plasminogen activator and improved substantially over the following day. On the second hospital day, we restarted his angiotensin-converting enzyme (ACE) inhibitor and started a thiazide. Later, we progressively adjusted the dose of the ACE inhibitor until the blood pressure normalized. His discharge NIHSS score was 3. He only had minor symptoms and no disability 3 months later.

Ischemic Stroke — Treated With Mechanical Thrombectomy

Observational studies have shown that higher blood pressure correlates with worse outcomes after endovascular recanalization. Yet, randomized controlled trials completed thus far indicate that aggressive treatment of hypertension (to systolic targets lower than 180 mmHg) after successful reperfusion is not beneficial and might even be detrimental. Thus, based on available evidence, we treat hypertension after endovascular reperfusion only if systolic blood pressure exceeds 180 mmHg.

Ischemic Stroke — Ineligible for Any Reperfusion Therapy

Hypertension may be a physiological response in patients with acute brain ischemia (as indicated by the spontaneous resolution of hypertension typically seen after successful recanalization). Therefore, when the patient is not a candidate for acute recanalization therapy, it is better not to lower the blood pressure unless it is above 220/120 mmHg. The concept of accepting high blood pressures ("permissive hypertension") is based on the notion that lowering the blood pressure in these patients with persistent vessel occlusion could worsen the brain ischemia by reducing collateral flow. When allowing blood pressure to remain high, we commit ourselves to monitor patients for signs of congestive heart failure, acute kidney injury, and other complications of acute hypertension. In patients with concomitant heart failure, gradual and modest blood pressure reduction under close neurological monitoring is safe.

Ischemic Stroke—After the First 24 Hours

After the first day, we gradually start oral medications (beginning with any prescribed medications the patient had been taking before admission). The goal is to arrive at normotension while avoiding sudden drops in blood pressure. If blood pressure control is not optimal upon discharge, we arrange for close outpatient follow-up until achieving blood pressure normalization.

Intracerebral Hemorrhage—First 24 Hours

Even after two large phase III trials (INTERACT-2 and ATACH-2) comparing systolic blood pressure targets of 140 mmHg vs. 180 mmHg in patients presenting within the first few hours after cerebral hematoma onset, optimal management of hypertension in these patients remains unresolved. Neither of the two trials proved superiority of the more intensive treatment strategy for the primary endpoint, and their pooled results showed that major blood pressure drops (especially >60 mmHg in systolic pressure) correlated with worse functional outcomes. In ATACH-2, patients in the intensive blood pressure–lowering group also had higher risk of acute kidney injury at 1 week. Yet, subsequent guidelines have recommended a systolic blood pressure goal below 140 mmHg while also avoiding large variability of systolic blood pressure and drops below 130 mmHg. Others surveyed their practice and found that patients maintained with a systolic blood pressure less than 140 mmHg were predisposed to adverse events. Acute renal failure occurred in patients who experienced hypotension requiring antihypertensive agent discontinuation or vasopressor initiation. We may use less than 180 mmHg as a target for patients with long-standing hypertension previously treated with multiple antihypertensives.

Intracerebral Hemorrhage—After the First 24 Hours

Similarly to ischemic stroke, we typically initiate oral antihypertensives after the first 24 hours. We then titrate these to achieve progressive normalization of the blood pressure before or shortly following discharge from the hospital.

Aneurysmal Subarachnoid Hemorrhage

No good evidence guides the treatment of hypertension in acute aneurysmal subarachnoid hemorrhage. We prefer to treat hypertension with the goal of maintaining the systolic blood pressure below 180 to 160 mmHg until the aneurysm is secured, but we recognize there is no robust evidence that blood pressure above those values correlates with higher risk of aneurysm rebleeding. Most patients with aneurysmal subarachnoid hemorrhage have elevated blood pressures due to the excessive sympathetic release immediately following the aneurysm rupture. Moreover, in these patients, intracranial hypertension is common, and many patients with abnormal levels of consciousness will need a ventriculostomy. Acutely lowering the blood pressure in patients with intracranial hypertension could compromise cerebral perfusion pressure. When intracranial pressure is known, the cerebral perfusion pressure should be kept above 60 mmHg.

Once the aneurysm is treated by means of clipping or endovascular coiling, we stop antihypertensives except for nimodipine (and low-dose beta-blockers in patients with a history of heart disease previously on beta-blockers), anticipating the need to maintain adequate cerebral perfusion in a narrowed arterial bed from vasospasm.

What Drugs Should You Use?

Although a bolus of labetalol or hydralazine may be a practical first step, we prefer to use continuous infusions to minimize blood pressure swings. Nicardipine and clevidipine, both calcium channel blockers, are safe and effective agents for the acute control of severe hypertension. Optimal titration of antihypertensive drug infusions requires placement of an arterial catheter. We avoid nitrates because their known venodilatory effect can increase intracranial pressure, although we are less certain about the claimed deleterious effect on intracranial pressure with sodium nitroprusside. We also avoid rapid-acting medications, such as sublingual nifedipine, because they can provoke excessive drops in blood pressure.

Clonidine is not a safe option either in the hyperacute phase because the first dose can occasionally cause paradoxical hypertension. Table 43.1 lists the doses of the medications we use most often for the treatment of acute hypertension in ischemic and hemorrhagic stroke.

TABLE 43.1 **Options for the Treatment of Hypertension in Patients With Acute Stroke**

Drug	Usual Dose
Labetalol	10–20 mg IV over 1–2 minutes, may repeat after 10–15 minutes (maximum dose 300 mg over 24 hours) Infusion: 2–8 mg/min
Hydralazine	10–20 mg IV over 1–2 minutes, may repeat after 10–15 minutes
Nicardipine	Start infusion at 5 mg/h, titrate up to 15 mg/h as needed
Clevidipine	Start infusion at 1–2 mg/h, titrate up to 21 mg/h as needed

KEY POINTS TO REMEMBER

- Treatment of hypertension in acute stroke patients depends on the type of stroke and the time from symptom onset.
- Patients with an ischemic stroke receiving thrombolysis need strict and consistent control of hypertension to avoid hemorrhagic complications.
- Patients with an ischemic stroke who are not candidates for reperfusion therapies should have their hypertension managed more conservatively to avoid a decrease in collateral cerebral blood flow.
- In patients with an intracerebral hemorrhage, moderate reduction of blood pressure is safe and may reduce the chances of hematoma expansion.
- In patients with aneurysmal subarachnoid hemorrhage, we favor gradual blood pressure reduction during the first few hours, which we maintain until the aneurysm is treated. Afterwards, hypertension should be permitted to reduce the risk of ischemia if cerebral vasospasm develops.

- Major blood pressure variability (especially major sudden drops in blood pressure) should be avoided in all patients with acute stroke, whether ischemic or hemorrhagic, and particularly in patients with chronic hypertension.

Further Reading

Anderson, C. S., E. Heeley, Y. Huang, et al. "Rapid Blood-Pressure Lowering in Patients With Acute Intracerebral Hemorrhage." [In eng]. *N Engl J Med* 368, no. 25 (2013): 2355–65. https://doi.org/10.1056/NEJMoa1214609.

Bath, P. M., L. Song, G. S. Silva, et al. "Blood Pressure Management for Ischemic Stroke in the First 24 Hours." [In eng]. *Stroke* 53, no. 4 (2022): 1074–84. https://doi.org/10.1161/strokeaha.121.036143.

Greenberg, S. M., W. C. Ziai, C. Cordonnier, et al. "2022 Guideline for the Management of Patients With Spontaneous Intracerebral Hemorrhage: A Guideline From the American Heart Association/American Stroke Association." [In eng]. *Stroke* 53, no. 7 (2022): e282–361. https://doi.org/10.1161/str.0000000000000407.

Hawkes, M. A., C. S. Anderson, and A. A. Rabinstein. "Blood Pressure Variability After Cerebrovascular Events: A Possible New Therapeutic Target: A Narrative Review." [In eng]. *Neurology* 99, no. 4 (2022): 150–60. https://doi.org/10.1212/wnl.0000000000200856.

Hawkes, M. A., and A. A. Rabinstein. "Acute Hypertensive Response in Patients With Acute Intracerebral Hemorrhage: A Narrative Review." [In eng]. *Neurology* 97, no. 7 (2021): 316–29. https://doi.org/10.1212/wnl.0000000000012276.

Hoh, B. L., N. U. Ko, S. Amin-Hanjani, et al. "2023 Guideline for the Management of Patients With Aneurysmal Subarachnoid Hemorrhage: A Guideline From the American Heart Association/American Stroke Association." [In eng]. *Stroke* 54, no. 7 (2023): e314–70. https://doi.org/10.1161/str.0000000000000436.

Leshko, N. A., R. F. Lamore, M. K. Zielke, et al. "Adherence to Established Blood Pressure Targets and Associated Complications in Patients Presenting With Acute Intracerebral Hemorrhage." [In eng]. *Neurocrit Care* 39, no. 2 (2023): 378–85. https://doi.org/10.1007/s12028-023-01679-4.

Li, G., Y. Lin, J. Yang, et al.; INTERACT4 investigators; INTERACT4 Investigators. "Intensive Ambulance-Delivered Blood-Pressure Reduction in Hyperacute Stroke." [In eng]. *N Engl J Med* 390, no. 20 (May 30 2024): 1862–72. doi:10.1056/NEJMoa2314741.

Nam, H. S., Y. D. Kim, J. Heo, et al. "Intensive vs Conventional Blood Pressure Lowering After Endovascular Thrombectomy in Acute Ischemic Stroke: The OPTIMAL-BP Randomized Clinical Trial." [In eng]. *Jama* 330, no. 9 (2023): 832–42. https://doi.org/10.1001/jama.2023.14590.

Powers, W. J., A. A. Rabinstein, T. Ackerson, et al. "Guidelines for the Early Management of Patients With Acute Ischemic Stroke: 2019 Update to the 2018 Guidelines for the Early Management of Acute Ischemic Stroke: A Guideline for Healthcare Professionals From the American Heart Association/American Stroke Association." [In eng]. *Stroke* 50, no. 12 (2019): e344–418. https://doi.org/10.1161/str.0000000000000211.

Qureshi, A. I., Y. Y. Palesch, W. G. Barsan, et al. "Intensive Blood-Pressure Lowering in Patients With Acute Cerebral Hemorrhage." [In eng]. *N Engl J Med* 375, no. 11 (2016): 1033–43. https://doi.org/10.1056/NEJMoa1603460.

Treggiari, M. M., A. A. Rabinstein, K. M. Busl, et al. "Guidelines for the Neurocritical Care Management of Aneurysmal Subarachnoid Hemorrhage." [In eng]. *Neurocrit Care* 39, no. 1 (2023): 1–28. https://doi.org/10.1007/s12028-023-01713-5.

Wardlaw, J. M. "More Reasons Not to Lower High Blood Pressure Early After Ischemic Stroke." [In eng]. *JAMA Netw Open* 7, no. 8 (Aug 1 2024): e2430781. doi:10.1001/jamanetworkopen.2024.30781.

Zonneveld, T. P., Vermeer, S. E., van Zwet, E. W., et al. Safety and efficacy of active blood-pressure reduction to the recommended thresholds for intravenous thrombolysis in patients with acute ischemic stroke in the Netherlands (TRUTH): a prospective, observational, cluster-based, parallel-group study. *Lancet Neurol* 23, no. 8 (Aug 2024): 807–815. doi: 10.1016/S1474-4422(24)00177-7. Epub 2024 May 16.

44 Acute White-Out on Chest X-Ray

A 17-year-old boy traveled at high speed through a dust cloud and collided with a truck. His neurologic examination on arrival was completely normal, and he could clearly describe the sequence of events before and after the accident. Computed tomography (CT) scan of the brain was normal. He had severe pain in his left leg and was found to have a displaced femoral fracture (Figure 44.1A). He was admitted to the orthopedic ward after undergoing fixation. He asked for opioids frequently to control his pain but remained alert and oriented. Three days after the operation, he suddenly developed respiratory distress and very shortly thereafter he became comatose with irregular breathing. His neurologic examination reveals small reactive pupils and intact corneal reflexes, but extensor motor responses. CT scan of the brain is unchanged, but the X-ray of the chest reveals diffuse infiltrates ("white-out" lungs) (Figure 44.1B and C). He is emergently intubated and transferred to the surgical intensive care unit.

What do you do now?

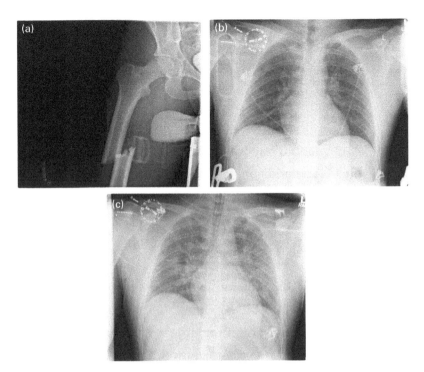

FIGURE 44.1 Note displaced femur fracture. (A) Serial chest X-rays in patient example: (B) normal on admission and (C) diffuse pulmonary edema 12 hours later.

Acute pulmonary distress in a patient after significant trauma has multiple causes. In the acute setting, consider several disorders including pulmonary contusion, aspiration pneumonitis, and the much less common neurogenic pulmonary edema. Pulmonary emboli are usually seen after a considerable time interval, but they may occur after only a few days of immobilization in predisposed patients. In these patients, X-rays are normal, but there is a significant hypoxemia that does not improve with incremental oxygen administration (refractory alveolar-arterial [A-a] gradient) because of a large ventilation-perfusion mismatch. We always exclude pulmonary embolus after neurosurgical procedures, after prolonged bedrest, and in patients with hemiplegia (when the paralyzed leg is at risk for deep venous thrombosis). Helical CT angiogram of the chest has become the standard diagnostic test for pulmonary embolism. Acute respiratory distress in a mechanically ventilated patient may have multiple other causes including acute main bronchus obstruction (mucous plugging), inappropriate ventilator settings, pneumothorax, atelectasis, or dislodgement of the tracheostomy tube.

Flash pulmonary edema in a patient with an acute traumatic brain injury (TBI) is another worrisome situation that immediately will require intubation and high positive end-expiratory pressure (PEEP) to open the collapsed and filled alveoli. We carefully monitor the effects of high PEEP on intracranial pressure in patients with TBI. In hemodynamically unstable patients, high PEEP may reduce cardiac venous return and lead to worsening hypotension. Flash pulmonary edema is usually a result of increased sympathetic activation due to an acute medulla oblongata lesion or due to a rapidly increased intracranial pressure. Pulmonary arterial constriction leads to shunting to other areas that cannot handle pressure, resulting in capillary leak and edema. It can also be seen as a secondary phenomenon of severe stress-induced cardiomyopathy (takotsubo cardiomyopathy). In these patients, there is significant apical ballooning from a major sympathetic outburst associated with acute brain injury, in turn resulting in severe pulmonary edema. Vasodilators and diuretics may relieve pulmonary congestion and reduce ventricular preload. Stress-induced cardiomyopathy requires specific treatment to improve ventricular contractility. Fortunately, surviving patients recover quite quickly with a good prognosis.

In 2023 a new global definition of acute respiratory distress syndrome (ARDS) attempted to address changes in practice that have occurred over the past decade. First, the increasing use of high-flow nasal oxygen (HFNO) delivery was acknowledged with the addition of a minimum HFNO flow rate of 30 liters/min. Second, a move toward less invasive monitoring has led to the addition of SpO_2:FiO_2 (SF ratio) with SpO_2 less than 97% as an alternative to identify and grade hypoxemia. As a result, either an arterial oxygen tension PaO_2/FiO_2 less than 300 or SpO_2/FiO_2 less than 315 (if SpO_2 <97%) identifies hypoxemia. Third, it adds lung ultrasound as an acceptable imaging modality in lieu of chest radiography. The 2023 Global Definition of ARDS requires that all the following criteria are met to diagnose ARDS: (1) respiratory symptoms must be acute, defined as within 7 days from a precipitating event or new or worsening symptoms during the previous week; (2) bilateral opacities consistent with pulmonary edema on chest radiography, CT scan, or lung ultrasound; (3) respiratory failure not fully explained by cardiac failure or fluid overload; and (4) hydrostatic pulmonary edema as primary driver excluded by objective invasive (pulmonary artery catheter) or noninvasive (point-of-care ultrasound, echocardiography) evaluation or by expert opinion.

On paper, this patient had a typical presentation of fat embolism syndrome. Acute coma and respiratory distress in a patient with a recent femur fracture are sufficient clues to arrive at the diagnosis. In practice, this entity is not easily recognized, and reports are infrequently published. Furthermore, the diagnosis is difficult to prove; the "textbook" truncal and axillary petechiae may disappear quickly, fat in bronchial secretions may be suctioned out by bronchoscopy, and fat globules in urine may not be found. (Identifying fat globules requires a special stain such as Sudan red, which is often not readily available.)

Fat embolism syndrome is rare but can be recognized usually about 48 hours after trauma. Gurd's criteria can be used to determine the certainty of the diagnosis (Table 44.1).

The treatment of fat embolism syndrome remains supportive and requires hemodynamic stabilization and adequate oxygenation and ventilation with PEEP. The minimal oxygenation goal should be an arterial PO_2 more than 60 mmHg. Ventilation should maintain plateau pressure below 30 cmH_2O and low tidal volumes (6 mL/kg of ideal body weight) to prevent volutrauma.

Fat emboli to the brain may cause sudden neurologic deterioration from injury to the gray and white matter, which may be severe enough to produce coma. Patients may remain comatose for weeks but then may slowly awaken and go on to recover. Magnetic resonance imaging (MRI)

TABLE 44.1 **Gurd's Criteria for Fat Embolism Syndrome (FES)**

Major Feature	Minor Feature	Laboratory Findings
Petechial rash	Pyrexia	Anemia
Respiratory insufficiency	Tachycardia	Thrombocytopenia
Neurologic involvement	Retinal changes	Elevated sedimentation rate
Renal insufficiency	Jaundice	Fat macroglobulinemia

Diagnosis of FES needs at least two major criteria or one major and four minor criteria or laboratory findings.

abnormalities can be particularly severe, with numerous spotty lesions reminiscent of a "star field" on diffusion-weighted imaging. These abnormalities on repeat MRI look even more dramatic as they become larger and more confluent. Unfortunately, the lesions are often misinterpreted as an indicator of poor outcome.

Our patient had persistent extensor posturing but recovered well with supportive care, and the MRI findings disappeared. This case taught us that fat emboli to the brain resulting in coma may have a good outcome against all odds—even in situations with persistent extensor motor responses for weeks. There were also episodes of paroxysmal sympathetic hyperactivity which are more often associated with poor outcome.

Of course, these conditions are not common, and we should rule out more mundane causes in a trauma patient who develops sudden respiratory distress. Most patients with decreased levels of consciousness cannot handle oral secretions, and pooling of these secretions with a weak cough will lead to bronchial obstruction. Intubation is needed, and

TABLE 44.2 **Acute Pulmonary Conditions After Acute Brain Injury**

Features	Neurogenic Pulmonary Edema	Aspiration	Fat Emboli	Pulmonary Embolus
Onset	Hyperacute	<6 hours	Delayed	Delayed
Clues	SAH, acute Brainstem injury	Intubation, vomiting, seizure	Long bone fracture	Bedrest, fever
Chest X-ray	Flash edema	Lobar/ multilobar	Flash edema in most severe cases	Normal
Therapy	PEEP	Broad-spectrum antibiotics	PEEP	Anticoagulation, IVC filter, IV thrombolysis, endovascular therapy

IVC, inferior vena cava; PEEP, positive end expiratory pressure; SAH, subarachnoid hemorrhage.

bronchoscopy is most helpful in these cases. Neurogenic pulmonary edema is just as rare as fat embolism syndrome. More likely, patients either develop an aspiration pneumonitis evolving into ARDS or have pulmonary emboli. Both conditions have characteristic features, which are easily distinguished on chest X-ray and CT of the chest, each with a specific treatment. The differences between pulmonary complications in acute brain injury are shown in Table 44.2.

KEY POINTS TO REMEMBER

- Acute pulmonary edema after trauma may be due to cardiogenic or neurogenic pulmonary edema, but the pure forms are infrequent. Aspiration is more common, particularly after a seizure, vomiting, and difficult intubation.
- Clinical suspicion of acute pulmonary emboli is based on sudden oxygen desaturation with increased A-a gradient but normal chest X-ray.
- Consider fat emboli in a patient with a recent major long bone fracture who develops sudden respiratory failure and neurological decline.
- Treatment may include broad-spectrum antibiotics (suspected aspiration), high PEEP (flash pulmonary edema), and bronchoscopy.
- Be careful when estimating prognosis in comatose patients with cerebral fat embolism syndrome because they can recover well even after prolonged coma.

Further Reading

Bahloul, M., A. N. Chaari, H. Kallel, et al. "Neurogenic Pulmonary Edema Due to Traumatic Brain Injury: Evidence of Cardiac Dysfunction." *Am J Crit Care* 15, no. 5 (2006): 462–70.

Bulger, E. M., D. G. Smith, R. V. Maier, et al. "Fat Embolism Syndrome: A 10-Year Review." *Arch Surg* 132, no. 4 (1997): 435–39. https://doi.org/10.1001/archs urg.1997.01430280109019.

Busl, K. M., and T. P. Bleck. "Neurogenic Pulmonary Edema." *Crit Care Med* 43, no. 8 (2015): 1710–15. https://doi.org/10.1097/ccm.0000000000001101.

Fontes, R. B., P. H. Aguiar, M. V. Zanetti, et al. "Acute Neurogenic Pulmonary Edema: Case Reports and Literature Review." *J Neurosurg Anesthesiol* 15, no. 2 (2003): 144–50. https://doi.org/10.1097/00008506-200304000-00013.

Gurd, A. R., and R. I. Wilson. "The Fat Embolism Syndrome." *J Bone Joint Surg Br* 56b, no. 3 (1974): 408–16.

Kawakami, D., S. Yoshino, S. Kawakami, et al. "Fat Embolism Syndrome." *Intensive Care Med* 48, no. 6 (2022): 748–49. https://doi.org/10.1007/s00134-022-06664-7.

Kosova, E., B. Bergmark, and G. Piazza. "Fat Embolism Syndrome." *Circulation* 131, no. 3 (2015): 317–20. https://doi.org/10.1161/circulationaha.114.010835.

Kwon, J., and R. Coimbra. "Fat Embolism Syndrome After Trauma: What You Need to Know." [In eng]. *J Trauma Acute Care Surg* (Aug 30 2024). doi:10.1097/ TA.0000000000004434.

Matthay MA, Arabi Y, Arroliga AC, Bernard G, Bersten AD, Brochard LJ, Calfee CS, Combes A, Daniel BM, Ferguson ND, Gong MN, Gotts JE, Herridge MS, Laffey JG, Liu KD, Machado FR, Martin TR, McAuley DF, Mercat A, Moss M, Mularski RA, Pesenti A, Qiu H, Ramakrishnan N, Ranieri VM, Riviello ED, Rubin E, Slutsky AS, Thompson BT, Twagirumugabe T, Ware LB, Wick KD. A New Global Definition of Acute Respiratory Distress Syndrome. *Am J Respir Crit Care Med*. 2024 Jan 1; 209(1):37–47. doi: 10.1164/rccm.202303-0558WS.

Meyer, N. J., L. Gattinoni, and C. S. Calfee. "Acute Respiratory Distress Syndrome." *Lancet* 398, no. 10300 (2021): 622–37. https://doi.org/10.1016/ s0140-6736(21)00439-6.

Mittal, M. K., T. M. Burrus, N. G. Campeau, et al. "Pearls & Oy-sters: Good Recovery Following Cerebral Fat Embolization With Paroxysmal Hyperactivity Syndrome." *Neurology* 81, no. 14 (2013): e107–9. https://doi.org/10.1212/WNL.0b013e318 2a6ca3e.

Rimoldi, S. F., M. Yuzefpolskaya, Y. Allemann, et al. "Flash Pulmonary Edema." *Prog Cardiovasc Dis* 52, no. 3 (2009): 249–59. https://doi.org/10.1016/ j.pcad.2009.10.002.

45 Storming With Sweating, Fever, and Rigid Posturing

A 22-year-old woman rolled over her car while driving without a seatbelt on an icy road. She was comatose at the scene intubated. Initial head computed tomography (CT) scan revealed bifrontal contusions and a small subdural hematoma overlying the right cerebral convexity without significant mass effect. She remained comatose with extensor posturing. Neurosurgery inserted an intraparenchymal pressure monitor. Over the subsequent days, the intracranial pressures ranged mostly between 15 and 25 mmHg, requiring occasional doses of mannitol and hypertonic saline to keep it under control. Repeat head CT scan on day 3 showed the expected evolution of the frontal contusions with progression of the surrounding edema.

A week after the injury, she began to exhibit recurrent episodes of sinus tachycardia, tachypnea, hypertension, hyperthermic, profuse sweating, and shivering and posturing. Blood cultures were negative, and serum lactic acid and creatine kinase levels were normal. When severe, these episodes correlated with transient elevations of intracranial pressure beginning after the onset of the changes in vital signs.

What do you do now?

The clinical presentation illustrated by this case is characteristic of paroxysmal sympathetic hyperactivity (PSH). Frequently PSH remains unrecognized and goes untreated. Physicians unfamiliar with this complication may consider these manifestations a mere epiphenomenon of severe brain injury, may start antibiotics while searching (even obsessively) for an infectious source, or, worse, may treat it as seizures with multiple doses of benzodiazepines and maintenance antiseizure medications. PSH can cause major problems in itself. Because they can happen with any stimulation, they create major challenges for nursing care. Severe PSH episodes produce marked, temporary rises in intracranial pressure. Potentially, when PSH goes untreated, the severity of rigidity and posturing can result in contractures and make later rehabilitation efforts difficult.

These spells, also known colloquially as "sympathetic storms," are frequent in patients with severe acute brain injury. They are most common in young patients with diffuse axonal traumatic brain injury, but we have also seen them after severe anoxic-ischemic encephalopathy, large intraparenchymal hemorrhages, subarachnoid hemorrhage, autoimmune encephalitis (particularly related to anti-N-methyl-D-aspartate receptor antibodies), fat embolism syndrome (Chapter 44), and acute hydrocephalus. Episodes of PSH can begin during the acute phase, typically in comatose patients. PSH can also continue into the subacute phase or become first manifest in this later phase and diagnosed by brain rehabilitation specialists.

There is lack of uniformity in the nomenclature and definition of PSH. The denomination PSH includes the three terms that describe the key features. They are rapid and episodic (i.e., paroxysmal) manifestations of excessive sympathetic activity. Patients become tachycardic, hypertensive (with increased pulse pressure), tachypneic, febrile, and diaphoretic. Often, they develop markedly increased muscle tone, which may result in pseudo dystonic postures. Pupillary dilatation, piloerection, and skin flushing can also be seen. Stimulation often provokes PSH, but the degree of stimulation necessary to trigger the spells can be minimal in the most sensitive patients, and episodes can also occur without apparent provocation. An assessment measure for diagnosing paroxysmal sympathetic hyperactivity is shown in Table 45.1. PSH is likely with a score of 17 or higher.

PSH spells are characteristic, making the diagnosis readily apparent to physicians caring for acute brain injury, but rehabilitation physicians

TABLE 45.1 Assessment Measure for the Diagnosis of Paroxysmal Sympathetic Hyperactivity

Clinical Feature Scale (CFS)	0	1	2	3	Score
Heart rate	<100	100–119	120–139	≥140	
Respiratory rate	<18	18–23	24–29	≥30	
Systolic blood pressure	<140	140–159	160–179	≥180	
Temperature	<37	37–37.9	38–38.9	≥39.0	
Sweating	Absent	Mild	Moderate	Severe	
Posturing during episodes	Absent	Mild	Moderate	Severe	
			CFS Subtotal		

Severity of Clinical Features		Nil	0	
		Mild	1–6	
		Moderate	7–12	
		Severe	≥13	

Diagnosis Likelihood Tool (DLT)

Clinical features occur simultaneously	
Episodes are paroxysmal in nature	
Overreactivity to normally nonpainful stimuli	

(Continued)

TABLE 45.1 **Continued**

Features persist ≥3 consecutive days	
Features persist ≥2 weeks after brain injury	
Features persist despite treatment of differential diagnoses	
Medication administered to decrease sympathetic features	
≥2 episodes daily	
Absence of parasympathetic features during episodes	
Absence of other presumed cause of features	
Antecedent acquired brain injury	
(Score 1 point for each feature present)	DLT Subtotal	

Combined total (CFS + DLT)	

PSH Diagnostic Likelihood	Unlikely	<8	
	Possible	8–16	
	Probable	>17	

may also encounter a fair number of cases. However, it is important to consider other causes of sudden, exaggerated sympathetic response. Early sepsis with bacteriemia (sudden febrile component of PHS) or pulmonary emboli (sudden tachypnea component) are often considered first. However, unlike PSH, pulmonary embolism is distinctly associated with hypoxia and increased alveolar-arterial oxygen gradient. Also, unlike PSH, sepsis does not present with hypertension. Other pertinent conditions to consider are listed in Table 45.2.

What can be done to treat these episodes of PSH? There are effective therapies for this condition but first exacerbating drugs should be avoided. Acutely, the manifestations of PSH respond best to bolus doses of

TABLE 45.2 **Differential Diagnosis of Paroxysmal Sympathetic Hyperactivity**

Consider	Diagnosis Clues and/or Test
Pulmonary embolism	Arterial blood gases CT angiogram of the chest
Sepsis[a]	White blood cell count Blood cultures Serum lactic acid
Seizures	Electroencephalogram
Neuroleptic malignant syndrome	New antipsychotic drug Serum creatine kinase
Serotonin syndrome	Selective serotonin reuptake inhibitors Serum creatine kinase
Alcohol withdrawal	History of alcohol abuse Response to benzodiazepines
Wooden Chest Syndrome	Fentanyl
Cushing response	Head CT scan
Autonomic dysreflexia from spinal cord injury[b]	Spinal cord imaging
Encephalitis	Cerebrospinal fluid analysis
Aneurysmal rebleeding in subarachnoid hemorrhage	Head CT scan

[a] Typically associated with hypotension rather than hypertension.
[b] Typically associated with bradycardia rather than tachycardia.

morphine sulfate (2.5–5 mg intravenously). This favorable response is not related to the analgesic effect of opiates but rather to modulation of central pathways responsible for the autonomic dysfunction. The response to morphine is rapid and quite dependable in aborting spells of PSH, but occasionally we have encountered patients who required much larger doses than usual (up to 10–15 mg). In these patients, a continuous opiate infusion may be helpful. For us, the impressive response to IV morphine qualifies as a diagnostic test. Once PSH is diagnosed, preventive treatment should be initiated. Gabapentin, an agent that binds GABA receptors and voltage-gated calcium channels in the dorsal horn of the spinal cord, is our drug of choice. We typically start it at 300 mg three times daily and titrate it every 3–5 days until we achieve adequate control of the PSH episodes. High doses may be needed, and it often, results in dramatic improvement of intensity and frequency of the spells.

Other effective medications for the treatment of PSH include noncardioselective beta-blockers (such as propranolol), clonidine (a central alpha-2 receptor agonist), dexmedetomidine (another central alpha-2 receptor agonist), bromocriptine (a dopamine D2 receptor agonist), baclofen (a $GABA_B$ receptor agonist), benzodiazepines ($GABA_A$ receptor agonists). In our experience, beta-blockers and clonidine are useful in controlling the tachycardia and hypertension but less so for the rigidity. Baclofen and benzodiazepines (especially diazepam) relax muscles but may not improve the other hypersympathetic features. We have not been impressed by the efficacy of bromocriptine. Antidopaminergic drugs, such as haloperidol, and sympathetic agonists need to be avoided (Table 45.3). In the published literature the most frequently prescribed medication classes are β-blockers, opioids, α-2 agonists, gabapentin, benzodiazepines, and baclofen.

Choosing the right medication to treat the spells is not enough, and other aspects of management are equally important. These patients sweat profusely, and fluid intake should be adjusted to compensate for this marked increase in insensible losses and to prevent volume contraction. Use cooling measures to treat fever aggressively because it has a negative impact on the acutely injured brain. It is best to minimize patient stimulation.

How did we manage our patient? We treated her acutely with boluses of morphine, and she responded well. Her tachycardia and hypertension improved on low doses of propranolol. We also started her on gabapentin

TABLE 45.3 Pharmacological Options for the Treatment of Paroxysmal Sympathetic Hyperactivity

Medication	Usual Dose	Usefulness	Side Effects
Morphine sulfate	2.5–5 mg IV bolus	Abortive	Sedation Respiratory depression Hypotension Ileus Raised intracranial pressure (rare)
Gabapentin	Start 300 mg every 8 hours by enteral route and titrate up to 1800–3600 mg/d	Preventive	Mild sedation
Propranolol	20–60 mg every 4–8 hours by enteral route	Preventive control of tachycardia and hypertension	Bradycardia Hypotension Bronchospasm Negative inotropism
Clonidine	0.1–0.3 mg every 6–8 hours by enteral route	Preventive control of tachycardia and hypertension	Bradycardia Hypotension Sedation Rebound hypertension with abrupt withdrawal
Dexmedetomidine	0.2–1.5 mcg/kg/h	Preventive	Bradycardia Hypotension Sedation
Baclofen[a]	5–10 mg every 8 hours (up to 60–80 mg/d) by enteral route	Control of increased muscle tone	Sedation Increased muscle weakness Hepatotoxicity Increased respiratory secretions
Diazepam	50–10 mg IV every 4–8 hours	Control of increased muscle tone	Sedation Hypotension Respiratory depression

[a] Intrathecal baclofen can be useful in refractory cases with extreme posturing.

with a target dose of 1800 mg/d. Ten days later, her episodes of PSH had become much milder and infrequent.

PSH often correlates severe brain injury and thus poor neurologic outcome but not always. This is because it is often seen in young individuals with traumatic brain injury who can recover well. The manifestations excessively increase the metabolic demand, risk increase in intracranial pressure, and may cause long-term complications. Because it is a common and treatable complication clinicians need to be aware of it and start effective therapy. The response of the patient to the right drugs is surprising and rewarding.

KEY POINTS TO REMEMBER

- PSH is common, especially in young patients with severe traumatic brain injury.
- The differential diagnosis is broad but can be sorted out quickly by a focused evaluation. When the clinical signs are not characteristic, consider pulmonary embolism, early sepsis, and seizures.
- Failure to recognize PSH can lead to major complications, such as intracranial hypertension, dehydration, prolonged fever, refractory surges of hypertension, and muscle contractures.
- Boluses of morphine sulfate are highly effective in aborting the episodes.
- Propranolol and clonidine can help control the tachycardia and hypertension.
- Baclofen and diazepam can improve the increased muscle tone.
- Gabapentin is useful in achieving persistent control of the sympathetic dysfunction.

Further Reading

Baguley, I. J., R. E. Heriseanu, J. A. Gurka, et al. "Gabapentin in the Management of Dysautonomia Following Severe Traumatic Brain Injury: A Case Series." *J Neurol Neurosurg Psychiatry* 78, no. 5 (2007): 539–41. https://doi.org/10.1136/jnnp.2006.096388.

Baguley, I. J., I. E. Perkes, J. F. Fernandez-Ortega, et al. "Paroxysmal Sympathetic Hyperactivity After Acquired Brain Injury: Consensus on Conceptual Definition, Nomenclature, and Diagnostic Criteria." *J Neurotrauma* 31, no. 17 (2014): 1515–20. https://doi.org/10.1089/neu.2013.3301.

Hughes, J. D., and A. A. Rabinstein. "Early Diagnosis of Paroxysmal Sympathetic Hyperactivity in the ICU." *Neurocrit Care* 20, no. 3 (2014): 454–59. https://doi.org/10.1007/s12028-013-9877-3.

Jerousek, C. R., and J. P. Reinert. "The Role of Dexmedetomidine in Paroxysmal Sympathetic Hyperactivity: A Systematic Review." *Ann Pharmacother* (2023): 10600280231194708. https://doi.org/10.1177/10600280231194708.

Meyfroidt, G., I. J. Baguley, and D. K. Menon. "Paroxysmal Sympathetic Hyperactivity: The Storm After Acute Brain Injury." *Lancet Neurol* 16, no. 9 (2017): 721–29. https://doi.org/10.1016/s1474-4422(17)30259-4.

Ott, J. L., and T. K. Watanabe. "Evaluation and Pharmacologic Management of Paroxysmal Sympathetic Hyperactivity in Traumatic Brain Injury." [In eng]. *J Head Trauma Rehabil* (May 24 2024). doi:10.1097/HTR.0000000000000960. Epub ahead of print.

Podell, J. E., S. S. Miller, M. N. Jaffa, et al. "Admission Features Associated With Paroxysmal Sympathetic Hyperactivity After Traumatic Brain Injury: A Case-Control Study." *Crit Care Med* 49, no. 10 (2021): e989–1000. https://doi.org/10.1097/ccm.0000000000005076.

Rabinstein, A. A. "Paroxysmal Sympathetic Hyperactivity in the Neurological Intensive Care Unit." *Neurol Res* 29, no. 7 (2007): 680–82. https://doi.org/10.1179/016164107x240071.

Scott, R. A., and A. A. Rabinstein. "Paroxysmal Sympathetic Hyperactivity." *Semin Neurol* 40, no. 5 (2020): 485–91. https://doi.org/10.1055/s-0040-1713845.

Tu, J. S. Y., J. Reeve, A. M. Deane, et al. "Pharmacological Management of Paroxysmal Sympathetic Hyperactivity: A Scoping Review." *J Neurotrauma* 38, no. 16 (2021): 2221–37. https://doi.org/10.1089/neu.2020.7597.

46 Common Cardiac Arrhythmias

An 86-year-old patient with a prior history of hypertension, hyperlipidemia, and atrial fibrillation presents with difficulty speaking and right-sided numbness. On examination, she has apraxia of speech and right hemiparesis. Magnetic resonance imaging (MRI) shows a left internal carotid occlusion with acute ischemic change in the left cerebral hemisphere. Systolic blood pressure fluctuates and, at times, rises to 130 mmHg. Her speech problems also fluctuate, and providers assume a link between worsening aphasia and relative hypotension. The providers decide to discontinue atenolol to maintain a higher blood pressure. Within 12 hours, the patient develops a rapid ventricular response to her atrial fibrillation with a pulse up to 140 beats per minute. Serum troponin has increased to 0.16 ng/mL. The electrocardiogram (ECG) shows rate-related repolarization changes (Figure 46.1). The neurosciences intensive care unit (ICU) accepts the patient for acute management.

What do you do now?

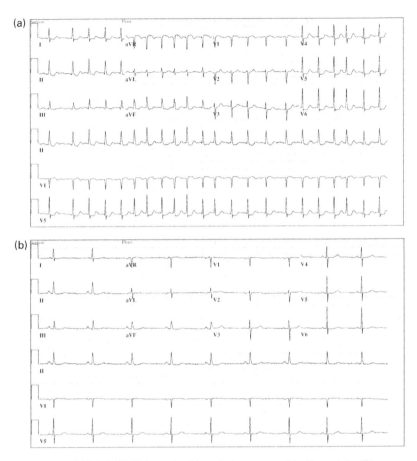

FIGURE 46.1 ECG: Atrial fibrillation and rapid ventricular response (A) with resolution (B).

Cardiac arrhythmias and ECG changes are quite common in patients with critical neurologic illness, often needing more than cursory attention, and management may become complex. In acute brain injury, cardiac arrhythmias often present as brief periods of premature beats, sinus bradycardia, or, as in our case, atrial fibrillation with rapid ventricular response.

After an acute ischemic stroke, patients may have a low to normal blood pressure, which may be partly due to relative dehydration. "Low" systolic blood pressure (<155 mmHg) correlates with increased mortality after a stroke, but the nature of the relationship remains unexplained. This provides a motivation to allow permissive hypertension in the acute stage to provide better perfusion in collaterals and reduce the ischemic area. Thus, we often withhold vasodilators including beta-blockers. However, stopping rate-control medication in patients with atrial fibrillation may result in tachycardia from a rapid ventricular response, leading to demand ischemia, a potentially severe complication in patients with coronary artery disease. This occurred in our case example as demonstrated by an increase in serum troponin. In retrospect, we should have continued the drug in a lower (e.g., half) dose. Cardiologists also consider switching metoprolol to nadolol, which induces less hypotension. In other situations atrial fibrillation with a sustained rapid ventricular rate may be triggered by a sympathetic response enhancing the atrioventricular node conduction (sympathetic drive from acute brain injury or any other major illness). In addition, we always check for undiagnosed hyperthyroidism.

The treatment for atrial fibrillation with rapid ventricular rate is to slow the atrioventricular conduction with intravenous calcium channel blockers (diltiazem), beta-blockers (esmolol), or amiodarone. These drugs all control ventricular rate successfully, but amiodarone induces less hypotension and has higher frequency of converting patients with new-onset atrial fibrillation into normal sinus rhythm. Thus, cardiologists consider it the preferred first-line drug. We start with 5 mg of metoprolol up to three bolus doses. Then we start amiodarone or short-acting diltiazem. Amiodarone starts with 150 mg intravenously (IV) over 1 hour, followed by 1 mg/min IV over 6 hours, followed by half the dose for 18 hours. Additional bolus doses of 150 mg can be administered up to six doses in 24 hours. We also give additional magnesium and calcium. Amiodarone requires intact liver synthetic function. Alternatively, diltiazem is used with 0.25 mg/kg bolus over 2 minutes, followed by repeat bolus of 0.35 mg/kg if rate control is not adequate after 15 minutes. We use a continuous infusion, 5 to 10 mg/h, titrating up to a maximum of 15 mg/h. If that fails, we start a digoxin load with a maintenance dose, as long as renal function remains stable and there is no hypokalemia. We rarely attempt cardioversion, either electrical or chemical, in acute stroke because (1) conversion to sinus rhythm carries a risk of cardioembolism, (2) hypotension might be deleterious, and (3) patients are unlikely to stay in sinus rhythm with prior long-standing atrial fibrillation. After achieving control of the ventricular response, we administer oral doses of beta-blockers (e.g., metoprolol) or calcium channel blockers (typically diltiazem) to maintain rate control. Atrial fibrillation is common in all ICU settings, and in a recent international cohort, which included 1423 noncardiac ICU patients, the incidence of atrial fibrillation was 15.6% and associated with history of hypertension, prior paroxysmal atrial fibrillation, sepsis, and disease severity. In this large cohort, amiodarone, beta-1 selective blockers, and digoxin were the most used interventions.

While cardiac arrhythmias are prevalent in the neurosciences ICU, they can be transient and without any consequence. We need to consider drug-induced arrhythmias. Drugs such as antidepressants, antipsychotics, ondansetron, quinolones, macrolides, fosphenytoin, nicardipine, and famotidine may prolong the QT interval, similarly to electrolyte abnormalities (hypocalcemia, hypokalemia, hypomagnesemia). Although torsade de pointes is uncommon, patients with severe acute brain injury can have QT prolongation, and we should avoid exacerbating medications in these cases. Lacosamide prolongs the PR interval (Chapter 33), and must avoid its use in combination with atrioventricular blockers (beta-blockers, calcium channel blockers).

New cardiac arrhythmia could indicate new-onset sepsis, pulmonary emboli, or sudden blood loss. We may see brief cardiac arrhythmias in patients with a deep peripherally inserted central catheter and recent position change of the patient. Finally, acute myocardial ischemia with new cardiac arrhythmias may occur in any patient with a recent neurosurgical procedure.

Another frequently asked question is whether the acute neurologic injury causes the ECG changes. Morphological ECG changes are common in traumatic brain injury and subarachnoid hemorrhage (typically ST-segment sagging, prolonged QT interval, and symmetrically peaked T waves, often referred to as cerebral T waves), and patients with ischemic strokes affecting the insula appear to be more prone to cardiac arrhythmias. However, it is not wise to categorically attribute cardiac rhythm changes to the acute brain injury—even if it remains the cardiologist's favorite explanation. Further cardiac evaluation (echocardiography, set of troponins) is often necessary in these patients. We do interpret the results of these evaluations with caution. Acute echocardiographic changes may be due to stress-induced

TABLE 46.1	**Guidance for the Treatment of Common Cardiac Arrhythmias**
Arrhythmia	Therapy
Sinus tachycardia	Fluids, esmolol
Sinus bradycardia	Atropine, cardiac pacing
Atrial fibrillation	Metoprolol, amiodarone, diltiazem
Multifocal atrial tachycardia	Verapamil or metoprolol, oxygen
Atrioventricular block	Cardiac pacing
Ventricular tachycardia	Cardioversion
Torsades de pointes	Magnesium sulfate

cardiomyopathy rather than myocardial ischemia—even if the pattern of wall motion abnormalities is not the typical apical ballooning.

We offer a general guideline for treatment of cardiac arrhythmias in Table 46.1. In most cases, the neurointensivist is the first person to diagnose and treat cardiac arrhythmias in patients with acute brain injury. We seek help from cardiologists when suspecting primary cardiac disease requiring specific therapy and often curbside them with complex cardiac arrhythmias.

KEY POINTS TO REMEMBER

- Sudden discontinuation of antiarrhythmic drugs can lead to rapid ventricular response in patients with known atrial fibrillation.
- Metoprolol can usually control atrial fibrillation with rapid ventricular response. Amiodarone infusion may be necessary.
- ST-segment sagging, prolonged QT interval, and peaked T waves may be due to acute brain injury, but cardiac evaluation may be necessary to exclude acute cardiac disease.
- New ECG changes in critically ill neurologic patients could indicate systemic complications, such as pulmonary emboli or sepsis.

Further Reading

Ahmed, T., S. H. Lodhi, P. J. Haigh, and V. L. Sorrell. "The Many Faces of Takotsubo Syndrome: A Review." [In eng]. *Curr Probl Cardiol* 49, no. 3 (Mar 2024): 102421. doi:10.1016/j.cpcardiol.2024.102421.

Barnes, B. J., and J. M. Hollands. "Drug-Induced Arrhythmias." [In eng]. *Crit Care Med* 38, no. 6 Suppl (2010): S188–97. https://doi.org/10.1097/CCM.0b013e318 1de112a.

Battaglini, D., C. Robba, A. Lopes da Silva, et al. "Brain-Heart Interaction After Acute Ischemic Stroke." [In eng]. *Crit Care* 24, no. 1 (2020): 163. https://doi.org/10.1186/s13054-020-02885-8.

Bosch, N. A., J. Cimini, and A. J. Walkey. "Atrial Fibrillation in the ICU." [In eng]. *Chest* 154, no. 6 (2018): 1424–34. https://doi.org/10.1016/j.chest.2018.03.040.

Chen, Z., P. Venkat, D. Seyfried, et al. "Brain-Heart Interaction: Cardiac Complications After Stroke." [In eng]. *Circ Res* 121, no. 4 (2017): 451–68. https://doi.org/10.1161/circresaha.117.311170.

Finsterer, J., and K. Wahbi. "CNS-Disease Affecting the Heart: Brain-Heart Disorders." [In eng]. *J Neurol Sci* 345, no. 1–2 (2014): 8–14. https://doi.org/10.1016/j.jns.2014.07.003.

Martindale, J. L., I. S. deSouza, M. Silverberg, et al. "β-Blockers Versus Calcium Channel Blockers for Acute Rate Control of Atrial Fibrillation With Rapid Ventricular Response: A Systematic Review." [In eng]. *Eur J Emerg Med* 22, no. 3 (2015): 150–54. https://doi.org/10.1097/mej.0000000000000227.

Oppenheimer, S. "Cerebrogenic Cardiac Arrhythmias: Cortical Lateralization and Clinical Significance." [In eng]. *Clin Auton Res* 16, no. 1 (2006): 6–11. https://doi.org/10.1007/s10286-006-0276-0.

Samuels, M. A. "The Brain-Heart Connection." [In eng]. *Circulation* 116, no. 1 (2007): 77–84. https://doi.org/10.1161/circulationaha.106.678995.

Wetterslev, M., M. Hylander Møller, A. Granholm, et al. "Atrial Fibrillation (AFIB) in the ICU: Incidence, Risk Factors, and Outcomes: The International AFIB-ICU Cohort Study." [In eng]. *Crit Care Med* 51, no. 9 (2023): 1124–37. https://doi.org/10.1097/ccm.0000000000005883.

47 Dysautonomia in Guillain-Barré Syndrome

A 73-year-old man was admitted with progressive weakness and inability to stand unassisted. The patient initially noted tingling in all his limbs followed a day later by rapid onset of weakness lasting for 4 days. Initially, he had no swallowing difficulties, double vision, or shortness of breath, but he gradually became short-winded and could not swallow liquids well. On admission, he had a flaccid quadriplegia with generalized areflexia but also had marked tachypnea requiring intubation and mechanical ventilation. On examination, there was bifacial diplegia with limited eye movements. He was not breathing over the set ventilator rate and had a weak cough with tracheal suctioning. The patient was treated with intravenous immunoglobulin, but on the fourth admission day, he developed marked blood pressure fluctuations. At some point, his systolic blood pressure was 240 mmHg and then suddenly dropped to 70 mmHg, which recovered with Trendelenburg positioning. In the subsequent days, these blood pressure fluctuations continued, often with episodes of hypertensive surges.

What do you do now?

Managing a patient with severe Guillain-Barré syndrome (GBS) involves more than just providing intravenous immunoglobulin or plasma exchange but also adequate supportive intensive care unit care. Patients with GBS are rapidly at risk for ventilator-associated pneumonia, urinary tract infection and sepsis, decubitus ulcers, and gastrointestinal hemorrhages due to the stress of mechanical ventilation. Deep venous thrombosis must be prevented with intermittent pneumatic compression devices plus subcutaneous heparin injections. Important early management considerations are shown in Box 47.1.

Treatment of acute autonomic failure, usually observed in more severe cases, is the most critical part of management. Dysautonomia in GBS is manifested by blood pressure fluctuations, cardiac arrhythmias, bladder dysfunction, gastrointestinal dysfunction, bronchial smooth muscle dysfunction, and exaggerated drug responses. The possible systemic effects in GBS are shown in Figure 47.1. Most common, as exemplified by our patient, is the need to treat blood pressure fluctuations. Paroxysmal or sustained hypertension occurs in about one in four patients with a rapid onset of GBS. Systolic blood pressures can rise substantially and reach values that not only challenge ventricular function but also even predispose the patient to posterior reversible encephalopathy syndrome

---

BOX 47.1 **Early Management of Guillain-Barré Syndrome**

IVIG (0.4 g/kg for 5 consecutive days)[a]
PLEX (5 plasma volumes in 5–10 days)[a]
Prevent early complications
    Subcutaneous heparin 5000 U three times a day or subcutaneous enoxaparin 40 mg/day
    PPI for GI protection
    Decubitus protection (special beds)
    NG tube feeding, consider early PEG in intubated patients, watch for ileus
    Tracheostomy in severely affected patients

GI, gastrointestinal; IVIG, intravenous immunoglobulin; NG, nasogastric; PEG, percutaneous gastrostomy; PLEX, plasma exchange; PPI, proton pump inhibitor.

[a] Treatments of equal efficacy; repeat treatments have not resulted in substantial improvement and may have additional risks such as deep venous thrombosis and pulmonary emboli.

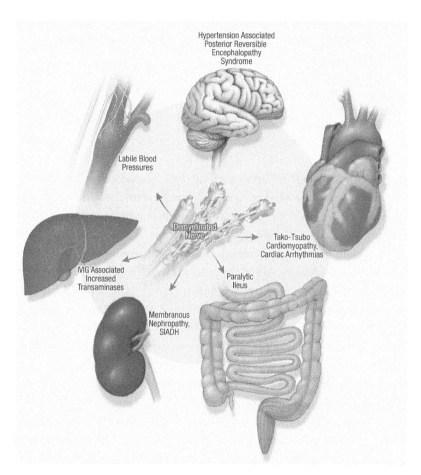

FIGURE 47.1 The other syndrome of GBS.

(PRES). In some situations, these hyperadrenergic responses can also cause stress-induced cardiomyopathy.

Why these blood pressure fluctuations occur is not fully understood, but a baroreflex dysfunction has been postulated. Baroreceptor sensitivity might change because of vagal nerve demyelination (sympathetic nerves have less myelin), resulting in sympathetic overdrive. Dysfunction of afferent input from atrial stretch receptors could also play a role in the origin of these blood pressure surges.

Marked hypertension requires treatment, but the treatment must avoid creating a marked hypotension. This could be due to exaggerated

> **BOX 47.2 Management of Blood Pressure Fluctuation and Cardiac Arrhythmias in GBS**
>
> Low doses of IV morphine
> Labetalol, clonidine, or nicardipine
> Avoid bradycardia with suctioning
> Consider pacemaker

drug sensitivity in GBS. Drugs such as clonidine, sodium nitroprusside, or a calcium channel blocker such as nicardipine or clevidipine can treat severe hypertension, but in our experience, simply controlling these responses with doses of intravenous morphine is just as effective and perhaps safer because of decreased risk of hypotension—though opiates may cause ileus. Many GBS patients have a baseline sinus tachycardia as another manifestation of increased sympathetic output. In addition, patients may develop so-called vagal spells, typically after tracheal suctioning. These bradycardic spells may create a brief asystole. A pacemaker may be considered if these episodes are symptomatic and recurrent. In some patients, atrioventricular block, or other more benign arrhythmias (e.g., bigeminy) become apparent. In hypotensive patients, echocardiography can detect stress-induced cardiomyopathy (Box 47.2). Dysautonomia remains a well-documented feature of severe GBS, and dysautonomia may cause sudden deaths (severe bradycardia followed by asystole). Clinical manifestations of autonomic failure include sinus node dysfunction, sinus arrest, and refractory hypotensive shock. There are no solid recommendations for placing a temporary or permanent pacemaker in GBS dysautonomia.

Bronchial function may be impaired in GBS because vagal and sympathetic innervation control bronchoconstriction and bronchodilatation. Impaired bronchoconstriction and dilation due to abnormal innervation of bronchial smooth muscle may profoundly impair clearing of secretions and, in turn, lead to atelectasis of large lung segments.

Examining patients for adynamic ileus, which occurs in about 1 in 10 patients with severe GBS, should be part of dysautonomia screening. Clues include loss of abdominal sounds, expansion of the abdominal girth, tympanic sound to percussion, and clearly demonstrable enlarged colonic loops on abdominal X-ray (Figure 47.2). Perforation of the colon

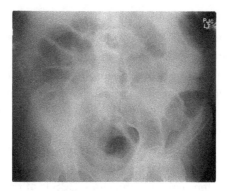

FIGURE 47.2 Marked dilated colonic loops on abdominal X-ray.

is a serious complication that can substantially change the outcome of a recoverable neurological illness and can even lead to in-hospital death.

Treatment of patients with adynamic ileus is stopping enteral feeding, rectal (red rubber) catheter and oral suction tube, and, in more severe cases, a therapeutic decompressive colonoscopy. If ileus is present, opiates should be replaced. The use of erythromycin is an option for patients with gastroparesis, but its side effects (cardiac arrhythmias) in patients with severe dysautonomia make it a less favorable choice. We discourage the use of metoclopramide as a promotility agent because of its association with asystole in GBS. Similarly, neostigmine should be used cautiously (if at all) because it can induce severe bradycardia. Methylnaltrexone or naloxegol can be used when opiates may have contributed to the pathogenesis of the ileus.

Placing our patient on a mechanical ventilator made administration of multiple doses of intravenous morphine much safer, and we could control his blood pressure within the set parameters of 100 and 140 mmHg systolic. Nursing staff were particularly careful with tracheal suctions, trying to avoid multiple passages and straining that could lead to bradycardia and hypotension. The blood pressure swings became less apparent in the following weeks, with gradual disappearance over time.

Acute autonomic failure in GBS usually resolves before improvement in motor function. Marked orthostatic hypotension may persist during the recovery phase. Whether this is due to persistent autonomic failure or long-standing bedrest is undetermined.

KEY POINTS TO REMEMBER

- Acute autonomic failure is common in severe presentations of GBS. Marked blood pressure fluctuations and sustained hypertension are the most concerning manifestations.
- Hypertensive surges can be treated with morphine, clonidine, or, if necessary, an infusion of a calcium channel blocker, such as nicardipine or clevidipine.
- Vagal spells may lead to prolonged episodes of asystole, and a transcutaneous pacemaker might be needed.
- Every bedridden patient with severe GBS is at risk of developing severe adynamic ileus, and treatment is urgent.

Further Reading

Abbas, Z., and Z. Sardar. "Use of Pacemaker in GBS Dysautonomia." [In eng]. *BMJ Case Rep* 14, no. 10 (Oct 13 2021): e242464. doi:10.1136/bcr-2021-242464.

Chakraborty, T., C. L. Kramer, E. F. M. Wijdicks, and A. A. Rabinstein. "Dysautonomia in Guillain-Barré Syndrome: Prevalence, Clinical Spectrum, and Outcomes." [In eng]. *Neurocrit Care* 32, no. 1 (Feb 2020): 113–20. https://doi.org/10.1007/s12 028-019-00781-w.

Cortese, I., V. Chaudhry, Y. T. So, et al. "Evidence-Based Guideline Update: Plasmapheresis in Neurologic Disorders: Report of the Therapeutics and Technology Assessment Subcommittee of the American Academy of Neurology." [In eng]. *Neurology* 76, no. 3 (Jan 18 2011): 294–300. https://doi.org/10.1212/ WNL.0b013e318207b1f6.

Fugate, J. E., E. F. Wijdicks, G. Kumar, and A. A. Rabinstein. "One Thing Leads to Another: GBS Complicated by PRES and Takotsubo Cardiomyopathy." [In eng]. *Neurocrit Care* 11, no. 3 (Dec 2009): 395–97. https://doi.org/10.1007/s12 028-009-9279-8.

Hughes, R. A., E. F. Wijdicks, R. Barohn, et al. "Practice Parameter: Immunotherapy for Guillain-Barré Syndrome: Report of the Quality Standards Subcommittee of the American Academy of Neurology." [In eng]. *Neurology* 61, no. 6 (Sep 23 2003): 736–40. https://doi.org/10.1212/wnl.61.6.736.

Hughes, R. A., E. F. Wijdicks, E. Benson, et al. "Supportive Care for Patients With Guillain-Barré Syndrome." [In eng]. *Arch Neurol* 62, no. 8 (Aug 2005): 1194–98. https://doi.org/10.1001/archneur.62.8.1194.

Leonhard, S. E., M. R. Mandarakas, F. A. A. Gondim, et al. "Diagnosis and Management of Guillain-Barré Syndrome in Ten Steps." [In eng]. *Nat Rev Neurol* 15, no. 11 (Nov 2019): 671–83. https://doi.org/10.1038/s41582-019-0250-9.

Lizarraga, A. A., K. J. Lizarraga, and M. Benatar. "Getting Rid of Weakness in the ICU: An Updated Approach to the Acute Management of Myasthenia Gravis and Guillain-Barré Syndrome." [In eng]. *Semin Neurol* 36, no. 6 (Dec 2016): 615–24. https://doi.org/10.1055/s-0036-1592106.

McDaneld, L. M., J. D. Fields, D. N. Bourdette, and A. Bhardwaj. "Immunomodulatory Therapies in Neurologic Critical Care." [In eng]. *Neurocrit Care* 12, no. 1 (Feb 2010): 132–43. https://doi.org/10.1007/s12028-009-9274-0.

Mukerji, S., F. Aloka, M. U. Farooq, et al. "Cardiovascular Complications of the Guillain-Barré Syndrome." [In eng]. *Am J Cardiol* 104, no. 10 (Nov 15 2009): 1452–55. https://doi.org/10.1016/j.amjcard.2009.06.069.

Netto, A. B., N. Chandrahasa, S. S. Koshy, and A. B. Taly. "Hyponatremia in Guillain-Barre Syndrome: A Review of Its Pathophysiology and Management." [In eng]. *Can J Neurol Sci* (Feb 16 2024): 1–11. doi:10.1017/cjn.2024.27. Epub ahead of print.

Walgaard, C., B. C. Jacobs, H. F. Lingsma, et al. "Second Intravenous Immunoglobulin Dose in Patients with Guillain-Barré Syndrome With Poor Prognosis (SID-GBS): A Double-Blind, Randomised, Placebo-Controlled Trial." [In eng]. *Lancet Neurol* 20, no. 4 (Apr 2021): 275–83. https://doi.org/10.1016/s1474-4422(20)30494-4.

Wijdicks, E. F., and C. J. Klein. "Guillain-Barré Syndrome." [In eng]. *Mayo Clin Proc* 92, no. 3 (Mar 2017): 467–79. https://doi.org/10.1016/j.mayocp.2016.12.002.

Zaeem, Z., Z. A. Siddiqi, and D. W. Zochodne. "Autonomic Involvement in Guillain-Barré Syndrome: An Update." [In eng]. *Clin Auton Res* 29, no. 3 (Jun 2019): 289–99. doi:10.1007/s10286-018-0542-y. Epub 2018 Jul 17.

Zochodne, D. W. "Autonomic Involvement in Guillain-Barré Syndrome: A Review." [In eng]. *Muscle Nerve* 17, no. 10 (Oct 1994): 1145–55. https://doi.org/10.1002/mus.880171004.

48 Difficult Ventilator Weaning in Myasthenia Gravis

A 60-year-old man with a recent diagnosis of myasthenia gravis developed shortness of breath and trouble keeping his head up. In the following days, he developed difficulty swallowing. He was admitted to an outside hospital, where he received three infusions of intravenous immunoglobulin (IVIG) but was found "unresponsive" on the fourth day with an arterial PCO_2 greater than 110 mmHg and a pH of 6.8 and required emergency intubation. He awakened quickly after arterial PCO_2 correction but was profoundly weak. Chest X-ray showed only minor atelectasis. He was transferred to our neurosciences intensive care unit, where we started him on oral prednisone and plasma exchange. After three exchanges, his muscle strength significantly improved, and coughing appeared strong. After extubation, he maintained good oxygenation for several hours; however, during the day, he became increasingly tachypneic and was placed on bilevel positive airway pressure (BiPAP) ventilation.

His neurological examination shows good neck flexion, hoarseness, and a weak cough. Muscle strength is good in all extremities with no hint of fatigable weakness. However, he barely tolerates BiPAP and has trouble with pooling of secretions. Arterial PCO_2 has climbed to 55 mmHg, requiring reintubation. Chest X-ray shows marked atelectasis of the left lung (Figure 48.1).

What do you do now?

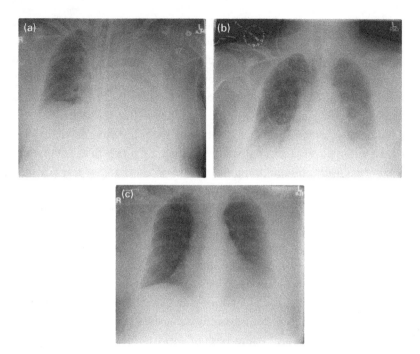

FIGURE 48.1 Hypersecretion and neuromuscular respiratory failure in myasthenia gravis. Serial X-rays of the chest show marked left atelectasis from a mucous plug (A) and gradual improvement after intubation and bronchoscopy (B, C).

Management of myasthenic crisis with neuromuscular respiratory failure remains poorly defined and largely empirical. Published experiences often span decades with changes in practice preferences over time. There is simply no consensus on how to manage intubated patients after a myasthenic crisis. Once intubated, patients need ventilation for several days, and up to one in four will fail extubation or require tracheostomy. A large multicenter observational study reported extubation failure in 43% of cases after a first extubation attempt. How do we safely get our patient with a recent flare-up of myasthenia gravis off the ventilator and keep him off?

Weaning from the ventilator becomes a priority after the patient has improved substantially—meaning good ventilatory and oropharyngeal muscle strength, little if any ptosis or ophthalmoplegia, and no marked limb weakness. Liberating myasthenic patients from the ventilator, however, remains frustrating for most clinicians. Moreover, a pulmonary infection or atelectases can make weaning even more challenging.

There are some prerequisites to consider for physicians attempting to liberate patients from the ventilator. The priority remains satisfactory treatment of the myasthenic symptoms. This may be best accomplished with plasma exchange (PLEX) in the acute phase. PLEX may have a more rapid onset of action than IVIG, but—at least in the more severe cases— we have no prospective comparative studies to prove that assumption. Treatment with immunosuppressive drugs should be started, and usually this includes prednisone 60 mg daily. To prevent recurrent crises, additional immune therapy is advisable. Traditional options include azathioprine and mycophenolate mofetil. A host of newer options have also proven beneficial to improve control of the disease and reduce the need for rescue therapies, including eculizumab, efgartigimod, ravulizumab, rozanolixizumab, zilucoplan, batoclimab or low-dose intravenous rituximab (single dose 500 mg in recent onset myasthenia). Yet, none of these medications have been extensively studied in patients coming out of a crisis.

Most neurologists will try to find an adequate dose of pyridostigmine that improves muscle strength and oropharyngeal function and could assist in weaning the patient off the ventilator. However, at the same time, we must find a dose of pyridostigmine that does not cause abundant secretions. Thick secretions will predispose the patient to sudden mucous plugs, which, as it was in our case, may occlude a large bronchial branch. Multiple bronchoscopies may be necessary to clear secretions from the bronchial tree, and often an infection requiring specific antibiotic treatment becomes apparent. Only after the secretions and infection are under control can the patient be considered for weaning.

Success of extubation is difficult to predict clinically, and we have not found a good way to do it. Some of the extubation parameters described in neuromuscular respiratory failure and their predictive values are shown in Table 48.1. Oropharyngeal function is hard to assess in an intubated patient, and weakness of neck flexion or shoulder shrug does not reliably predict failure. Often the patient is extubated and seems to do well for a couple of hours, only to deteriorate with increased work of breathing (recognized by tachypnea over 30 breaths per minute), shallow breathing, and gradual rise in arterial PCO_2. We need to appreciate that many patients

TABLE 48.1 Predictors for Successful Extubation Parameters in Myasthenia Gravis

Test	Predictive Value
Secretion volume	Good
T-piece trials (with assessment of rapid shallow breathing)	Good
Normal chest X-ray	Good
Neurological examination (oropharyngeal function, head-flexion strength)	Uncertain
White-card test	Uncertain
Pulmonary function tests	Poor

may deny they are tiring out and it may be their impaired judgment with hypercapnea.

Several recently developed tests might be useful in assessing the probability of successful extubation. One unconfirmed study proposed the use of a so-called white-card test. This white card is placed 1 to 2 cm from the end of the endotracheal tube, and any moisture present on the card following two to three coughs is considered a positive test. The patient is positioned with the head of the bed at 30 to 45 degrees and coached to cough maximally. It is unclear whether this test is a better predictor than a simple clinical assessment of cough strength. Another possibility is to place the patient on a spontaneous breathing trial and observe respiratory frequency and tidal volume for about an hour. We recommend following extubation with noninvasive BiPAP ventilation, which augments airflow and maintains positive airway pressure in the inhalation and exhalation phases.

Some patients just cannot tolerate BiPAP or may have more secretions than we anticipated. A humidified high-flow nasal canula is a possible alternative (starting at 45 L/min and an FIO_2 of 0.25–0.30) and does reduce some work of breathing through dead-space washout, reduction of nasopharyngeal resistance, positive pharyngeal pressure, and alveolar recruitment. Despite that, a high-flow nasal cannula may not provide sufficient support to the breathing muscles affected by neuromuscular disease and is most preferable in patients with hypoxemia from other causes.

The strongest risk factor for extubation failure in myasthenic patients remains the presence of atelectasis on chest X-ray. Patients may also fail extubation if there is a significant secretion volume (an arbitrary judgment), evidence of a recent yet not sufficiently treated pneumonia, and pulmonary edema prior to extubation. The diaphragm should be sufficiently strong; thus, reinstitution of pyridostigmine is key. It is very difficult— and probably too stressful for the patient—to try weaning from the ventilator without pyridostigmine. Simply said, breathing is unsustainable if the bellows don't work.

Finally, patients may also develop postextubation stridor. One recently noted complication is that vocal cord abduction paralysis may occur in the anti-muscle-specific kinase (MuSK) variant of myasthenia gravis. Of note, myasthenic patients with anti-MuSK antibodies have greater risk of developing crises and probably greater risk of extubation failure than patients with anti-acetylcholine receptor antibodies.

How did we proceed with our patient? How could we get the infected secretions under control and wean the patient from the ventilator safely? We decided to place a tracheostomy, and after a week, cultures came back with a multiresistant *Pseudomonas*, which we treated with aerosolized colistin. The patient gradually improved, after multiple bronchoscopies to clear the secretions. A gradual decrease in pyridostigmine may have also contributed to the decreased secretions. Eventually, the patient was transitioned—in incremental steps—to pressure support and then to spontaneous breathing trials.

Treatment of myasthenia gravis with acute neuromuscular respiratory failure takes time; once intubated, the average time on mechanical ventilation is usually 10 to 11 days. We were able to dismiss the patient from the hospital after about 6 weeks. Patients with myasthenia gravis who have difficulty getting off the ventilator often have had prior episodes of severe exacerbations, and unfortunately, we must anticipate prolonged hospitalization. Prolonged intubation carries an added risk of ventilator-associated pneumonia. Yet, while it is just better to get the patient off the ventilator as soon as possible, rushing extubation is ill-advised.

KEY POINTS TO REMEMBER

- Reintubation is common in myasthenia gravis, especially in patients with bronchial hypersecretion and atelectasis.
- Long-term management with placement of a tracheostomy may be needed after reintubation.
- Immuno-modulating therapy (usually with PLEX or at times IVIG) is necessary in myasthenic patients with severe neuromuscular respiratory muscle weakness.
- Do not attempt weaning from mechanical ventilation without having the patient on pyridostigmine.
- Finding an optimal dose of pyridostigmine after treatment of myasthenic crisis is difficult. There is a fine line between minimizing secretions and optimizing the strength of oropharyngeal and respiratory muscles.
- Biological agents (such as the FcRn inhibitor efgartigimod) are novel effective options for the treatment of myasthenia gravis. While their effect is sort of rapid, they have not been tested in patients with myasthenic crisis.

Further Reading

Bedlack, R. S., and D. B. Sanders. "How to Handle Myasthenic Crisis: Essential Steps in Patient Care." [In eng]. *Postgrad Med* 107, no. 4 (2000): 211–14, 220–12. 10.3810/pgm.2000.04.1003

Claytor, B., S. M. Cho, and Y. Li. "Myasthenic Crisis." [In eng]. *Muscle Nerve* 68, no. 1 (2023): 8–19.

Dhawan, P. S., B. P. Goodman, C. M. Harper, et al. "IVIG Versus PLEX in the Treatment of Worsening Myasthenia Gravis: What Is the Evidence?: A Critically Appraised Topic." [In eng]. *Neurologist* 19, no. 5 (2015): 145–48. https://doi.org/10.1097/nrl.0000000000000026.

Díaz-Lobato, S., M. A. Folgado, A. Chapa, and S. Mayoralas Alises. "Efficacy of High-Flow Oxygen by Nasal Cannula With Active Humidification in a Patient With Acute Respiratory Failure of Neuromuscular Origin." [In eng]. *Respir Care.* 58, no. 12 (Dec 2013): e164–67. https://doi.org/10.4187/respcare.02115.

Frutos-Vivar, F., N. D. Ferguson, A. Esteban, et al. "Risk Factors for Extubation Failure in Patients Following a Successful Spontaneous Breathing Trial." [In eng]. *Chest* 130, no. 6 (2006): 1664–71. https://doi.org/10.1378/chest.130.6.1664.

Gilhus, N. E. "Myasthenia Gravis." [In eng]. *N Engl J Med* 375, no. 26 (2016): 2570–81. https://doi.org/10.1056/NEJMra1602678.

Khamiees, M., P. Raju, A. DeGirolamo, et al. "Predictors of Extubation Outcome in Patients Who Have Successfully Completed a Spontaneous Breathing Trial." [In eng]. *Chest* 120, no. 4 (2001): 1262–70. https://doi.org/10.1378/chest.120.4.1262.

Mandawat, A., A. Mandawat, H. J. Kaminski, et al. "Outcome of Plasmapheresis in Myasthenia Gravis: Delayed Therapy Is Not Favorable." [In eng]. *Muscle Nerve* 43, no. 4 (2011): 578–84. https://doi.org/10.1002/mus.21924.

Neumann, B., K. Angstwurm, C. Dohmen, et al.; Initiative of German NeuroIntensive Trial Engagement (IGNITE). "Weaning and Extubation Failure in Myasthenic Crisis: A Multicenter Analysis." [In eng]. *J Neurol* 271, no. 1 (Jan 2024): 564–74. doi:10.1007/s00415-023-12016-2.

Pasnoor, M., G. I. Wolfe, and R. J. Barohn. "Myasthenia Gravis." [In eng]. *Handb Clin Neurol* 203 (2024): 185–203. doi:10.1016/B978-0-323-90820-7.00006-9.

Piehl, F., A. Eriksson-Dufva, A. Budzianowska, et al. "Efficacy and Safety of Rituximab for New-Onset Generalized Myasthenia Gravis: The RINOMAX Randomized Clinical Trial." [In eng]. *JAMA Neurol* 79, no. 11 (2022): 1105–12. https://doi.org/10.1001/jamaneurol.2022.2887.

Rabinstein, A. A., and E. F. Wijdicks. "Weaning From the Ventilator Using BiPAP in Myasthenia Gravis." [In eng]. *Muscle Nerve* 27, no. 2 (2003): 252–53. https://doi.org/10.1002/mus.10329.

Seneviratne, J., J. Mandrekar, E. F. Wijdicks, et al. "Predictors of Extubation Failure in Myasthenic Crisis." [In eng]. *Arch Neurol* 65, no. 7 (2008): 929–33. https://doi.org/10.1001/archneur.65.7.929.

Sylva, M., A. J. van der Kooi, and W. Grolman. "Dyspnoea Due to Vocal Fold Abduction Paresis in Anti-MuSK Myasthenia Gravis." [In eng]. *J Neurol Neurosurg Psychiatry* 79, no. 9 (2008): 1083–84. https://doi.org/10.1136/jnnp.2007.135319.

Vakrakou, A. G., E. Karachaliou, E. Chroni, et al. "Immunotherapies in MuSK-Positive Myasthenia Gravis; An IgG4 Antibody-Mediated Disease." [In eng]. *Front Immunol* 14 (Jul 26 2023): 1212757. doi:10.3389/fimmu.2023.1212757.

49 Decreasing Serum Sodium

A 46-year-old woman with a history of smoking and hypertension developed a thunderclap headache associated with emesis but no loss of consciousness. On arrival to the emergency department, she was mildly confused but had no focal neurological deficits. Head computed tomography scan showed subarachnoid hemorrhage (SAH) with aneurysmal pattern and mildly dilated ventricles. Her admission serum sodium level was 140 mmol/L. An anterior communicating artery aneurysm was found and was coiled. She remained well over the following days but developed increasing polyuria and a progressive decline in serum sodium. On day 4, we noticed subtle new cognitive difficulties. Repeat transcranial Doppler showed that the mean blood flow velocities in the anterior cerebral arteries and the right middle cerebral artery had increased by 30% to 40% from prior. Her fluid balance had been negative by 1.5 L over the preceding 24 hours. Her serum sodium level declined to 128 mmol/L from 135 mmol/L 8 hours earlier.

What do you do now?

Depending on its definition, hyponatremia can occur in approximately 30% to 50% of cases of aneurysmal SAH. We consider hyponatremia clinically relevant if it drops below 130 mmol/L and certainly if the decline is more than 10 mmol/L over 24 hours. Serum sodium may decline at any time between 3 and 14 days after aneurysm rupture but, more commonly, before the onset of cerebral vasospasm. Symptoms from hyponatremia are generally not severe. However, acute confusion, increased drowsiness, and even seizures can occur when sodium levels decline precipitously. Hyponatremia does not cause focal deficits. The appearance of hyponatremia in SAH should be considered a warning sign indicating the possibility of intravascular volume contraction, which can be particularly concerning in the setting of cerebral vasospasm (and which causes focal deficits).

Hyponatremia and volume contraction go hand in hand because the main cause of hyponatremia in SAH is cerebral salt-wasting syndrome. This is a disorder characterized by excessive secretion of natriuretic peptides, leading to increased urinary sodium loss. In turn, the increased sodium in the urine drags water with it. The consequences are polyuria and intravascular volume depletion. Theoretically, patients with SAH may also have the syndrome of inappropriate secretion of antidiuretic hormone (SIADH), which produces excessive retention of free water at the tubular level and results in dilutional hyponatremia. The problem is that readily available tests of the blood and urine are not useful for differentiating SIADH (associated with normal or mildly expanded intravascular volume) from cerebral salt wasting (associated with intravascular volume contraction—Figure 49.1 and Figure 49.2). Cerebral salt wasting typically predominates, as reflected by the frequent improvement of hyponatremia after infusion of isotonic saline in these patients (isotonic fluid administration worsens SIADH-associated hyponatremia).

Determining the volume status of the intravascular compartment in SAH is extremely difficult and often can only be roughly estimated. Thus, since there are no ideal ways to gauge the volume status, it is most prudent to assume that sudden polyuria followed by worsening hyponatremia will result in volume contraction.

When treating patients with SAH, we must therefore replace fluid volume and sodium. Hypertonic saline can achieve this goal. We often start with 1.5% sodium chloride but resort to 3% solution if the hyponatremia

Variable	CSW	SIADH
Extracellular fluid volume	↓	↑
Body weight	↓	↑
Fluid balance	Negative	Negative
Urine volume	↔ or ↑	↔ or ↓
Tachycardia	+	−
Hematocrit	↑	↔
Albumin	↑	↔
Serum bicarbonate	↑	↔ or ↓
Blood urea nitrogen	↑	↔ or ↓
Serum uric acid	↔ or ↓	↓
Urinary sodium	↑	↑
Sodium balance	Negative	Neutral or +
Central venous pressure	↓ (<6 cm H_2O)	↔ or slightly ↑ (6-10 cm H_2O)

FIGURE 49.1 Differential diagnosis between cerebral salt wasting (CSW) and syndrome of inappropriate secretion of antidiuretic hormone (SIADH).

is severe or fails to improve with lower concentration of sodium replacement. If hyperchloremic acidosis develops, we switch to sodium acetate, adjusting the concentration to maintain the same tonicity. Our therapeutic goal is to correct the hyponatremia and, most importantly, to maintain euvolemia. Using 3% saline is not without risks because about 10% of patients develop excessive correction due to unanticipated emergence of a water diuresis. Similar unpredictability of overcorrection occurs with vasopressin antagonists. Some have suggested combining it with desmopressin, but this is an unsafe practice. It is simply better to avoid these drugs altogether.

Some patients with SAH become extremely polyuric, and this tends to occur at the peak of cerebral vasospasm. In these situations, it is all too common to get stuck in a vicious cycle of giving more crystalloid fluids to compensate for the unrelenting fluid and sodium loss. One must scale back

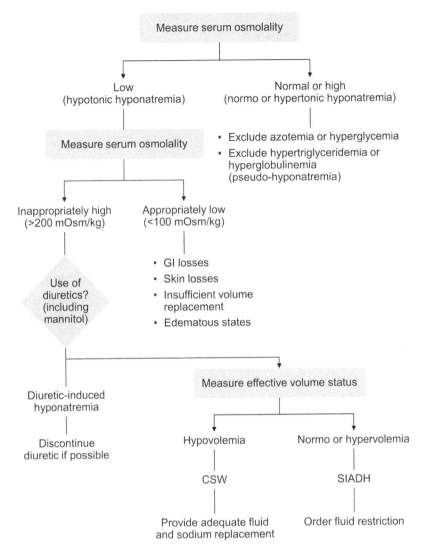

FIGURE 49.2 Algorithm for the evaluation and management of hyponatremia in a critically ill neurological patient. CSW, cerebral salt wasting; SIADH, syndrome of inappropriate secretion of antidiuretic hormone.

fluid administration to avoid complications such as pulmonary edema or renal medullary washout.

Mineralocorticoids are useful to prevent or ameliorate excessive urinary excretion and hyponatremia in patients with SAH. Only early initiation (within 72 hours of aneurysm rupture) has been formally tested and proven effective. In placebo-controlled studies, fludrocortisone correlated with fewer side effects than hydrocortisone, which may cause glucocorticoid activity–related hyperglycemia, but neither medication increased the risk of congestive heart failure. In our practice, we start fludrocortisone, 0.2 mg twice daily, early in most patients with SAH with any signs of cerebral salt wasting. Patients on fludrocortisone typically require potassium replacement.

Hypotonic intravenous fluids (Table 49.1) should be avoided in patients with SAH, not only because hyponatremia is so frequent but also because of the increased risk of intracranial hypertension. In alert patients tolerating an oral diet, the tonicity and sodium concentration of ingested fluids should also be regulated. These patients usually get thirsty as they become polyuric, and abundant ingestion of water may exacerbate the hyponatremia. In these cases, we have patients only drink fluids enriched with high concentrations of sodium. And it is a common mistake among health care providers to confuse free water restriction (indicated for SIADH and possible without

TABLE 49.1 **Sodium Content in Common Intravenous Fluid Solutions**

Intravenous Fluid	Sodium Content (mmol/L)
5% dextrose[a]	0
0.45% sodium chloride[a]	77
Ringer's lactate[a]	130
0.9% sodium chloride[b]	154
1.5% sodium chloride[b]	256
3% sodium chloride[b]	513

[a] Not recommended for use in aneurysmal subarachnoid hemorrhage.
[b] Recommended for use in aneurysmal subarachnoid hemorrhage.

restricting overall fluid intake) with fluid restriction (which should be avoided in SAH).

We treated our patient with fludrocortisone and increased volume with 1.5% sodium chloride infusion. Her sodium level improved progressively despite persistent polyuria and returned to normal range 48 hours later. She also developed fluctuating alertness, which we attributed to diffuse cerebral vasospasm, and which resolved with hemodynamic augmentation therapy (i.e., norepinephrine infusion). She was discharged home after 15 days of hospital stay and returned to work 5 weeks later.

Hyponatremia is a common concern in patients with SAH, and its pathophysiology is fairly well understood. It is an indicator of volume contraction, and its treatment is hypertonic saline. Fludrocortisone can help prevent this complication. Fluid restriction may substantially increase the risk of cerebral infarction in patients with hyponatremia and cerebral vasospasm and should be avoided. There is a salt-wanting physiologic state with salt-wasting.

KEY POINTS TO REMEMBER

- Hyponatremia is common after aneurysmal SAH, and it is often associated with intravascular volume contraction.
- Treatment of the polyuric, hyponatremic patient should include replacement of sodium and fluid volume.
- The goals of fluid management in cases of aneurysmal SAH are maintenance of normonatremia and euvolemia.
- One must replace volume effectively but be careful not to induce fluid overload.
- Fludrocortisone is useful to ameliorate urinary sodium loss and hyponatremia.

Further Reading

Adrogué, H. J., and N. E. Madias. "The Syndrome of Inappropriate Antidiuresis." [In eng]. *N Engl J Med* 389, no. 16 (2023): 1499–509. https://doi.org/10.1056/NEJMcp 2210411.

Adrogué, H. J., B. M. Tucker, and N. E. Madias. "Diagnosis and Management of Hyponatremia: A Review." [In eng]. *Jama* 328, no. 3 (2022): 280–91. https://doi. org/10.1001/jama.2022.11176.

Audibert, G., G. Steinmann, N. de Talancé, et al. "Endocrine Response After Severe Subarachnoid Hemorrhage Related to Sodium and Blood Volume Regulation." [In eng]. *Anesth Analg* 108, no. 6 (2009): 1922–28. https://doi.org/10.1213/ane.0b013 e31819a85ae.

Brimioulle, S., C. Orellana-Jimenez, A. Aminian, et al. "Hyponatremia in Neurological Patients: Cerebral Salt Wasting Versus Inappropriate Antidiuretic Hormone Secretion." [In eng]. *Intensive Care Med* 34, no. 1 (2008): 125–31. https://doi.org/10.1007/s00134-007-0905-7.

Busl, K. M., and A. A. Rabinstein. "Prevention and Correction of Dysnatremia After Aneurysmal Subarachnoid Hemorrhage." [In eng]. *Neurocrit Care* 39, no. 1 (2023): 70–80. https://doi.org/10.1007/s12028-023-01735-z.

Hasan, D., K. W. Lindsay, E. F. Wijdicks, et al. "Effect of Fludrocortisone Acetate in Patients With Subarachnoid Hemorrhage." [In eng]. *Stroke* 20, no. 9 (1989): 1156–61. https://doi.org/10.1161/01.str.20.9.1156.

Knepper, M. A., T. H. Kwon, and S. Nielsen. "Molecular Physiology of Water Balance." [In eng]. *N Engl J Med* 372, no. 14 (2015): 1349–58. https://doi.org/10.1056/NEJMra1404726.

Maesaka, J. K., and L. J. Imbriano. "Cerebral Salt Wasting Is a Real Cause of Hyponatremia: PRO." [In eng]. *Kidney360* 4, no. 4 (Apr 1 2023): e437–e440. doi:10.34067/KID.0001422022. Epub 2022 Jun 2.

Sterns, R. H., and H. Rondon-Berrios. "Cerebral Salt Wasting Is a Real Cause of Hyponatremia: CON." [In eng]. *Kidney360* 4, no. 4 (Apr 1 2023): e441–e444. doi:10.34067/KID.0001412022. Epub 2022 Jun 2.

Wijdicks, E. F., M. Vermeulen, A. Hijdra, et al. "Hyponatremia and Cerebral Infarction in Patients With Ruptured Intracranial Aneurysms: Is Fluid Restriction Harmful?" [In eng]. *Ann Neurol* 17, no. 2 (1985): 137–40. https://doi.org/10.1002/ana.410170206.

Wijdicks, E. F., M. Vermeulen, J. A. ten Haaf, et al. "Volume Depletion and Natriuresis in Patients With a Ruptured Intracranial Aneurysm." [In eng]. *Ann Neurol* 18, no. 2 (1985): 211–16. https://doi.org/10.1002/ana.410180208.

Wijdicks, E. F. M. "Duck or Rabbit? Cerebral Salt Wasting and SIADH in Acute Brain Injury." [In eng]. *Neurocrit Care* 39, no. 1 (2023): 260–63. https://doi.org/10.1007/s12028-022-01622-z.

50 Increasing Serum Sodium

A 40-year-old woman underwent evaluation for recurrent suprasellar pilocytic astrocytoma causing worsening headaches, visual loss, and hydrocephalus (Figure 50.1A). Previously, she underwent debulking of the tumor and radiation. She took cabergoline to control her excessive prolactin production, levothyroxine for her hypothyroidism, and dexamethasone for treatment of tumor swelling. Until a couple of months previously, she used low dose desmopressin acetate (DDAVP) to manage central diabetes insipidus, but her physicians discontinued this medication after she developed hyponatremia. As a first step, she underwent ventriculoperitoneal shunt placement with improvement of her symptoms. Six weeks later, she underwent tumor resection. The surgical approach was interhemispheric, transcallosal, and transventricular and tumor removal was successful (Figure 50.1B). The tumor had infiltrated the pituitary infundibulum. Within hours of the surgery, the patient developed marked polyuria (1.4 L over 90 minutes). Her serum sodium level increased to 146 mmol/L from 138 mmol/L. Serum osmolality was 297 mOsm/kg, urine osmolality was 113 mOsm/kg, and urine specific gravity was 1.003.

What do you do now?

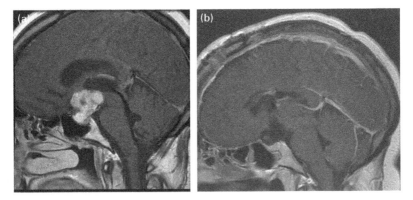

FIGURE 50.1 (A) Preoperative MRI scan shows a large suprasellar enhancing mass with associated obstructive hydrocephalus. (B) Postoperative MRI scan shows complete resection of the previously observed suprasellar mass. (Both images are gadolinium-enhanced sagittal T1 sequences.)

A neurosurgical procedure in the region of the pituitary gland often causes deficiency of arginine vasopressin (AVP) secretion and central diabetes insipidus (DI), which manifests with polyuria and hypernatremia (Box 50.1). AVP increases the water permeability of the renal cells lining the distal tubules and medullary-collecting ducts. With AVP deficiency, patients cannot reabsorb water and excrete large quantities of diluted urine. Patients can become rapidly dehydrated and develop severe hypertonic hypernatremia if their water intake is insufficient to compensate for the loss (more water loss than electrolytes increases tonicity). Ambulatory patients get thirsty, and their fluid intake may maintain a balance if they drink enough (polydipsia). Critically ill and neurosurgical patients depend entirely on the health care team to administer sufficient fluids. A severe disturbance requires full replacement of AVP (as an aside there is a strong push to change the name diabetes insipidus into *AVP-Deficiency* (cranial DI) and *AVP-Resistance* (nephrogenic DI)).

When evaluating a neurological patient with polyuria (defined as 24-hour urinary excretion >50 mL/kg of body weight), the first necessary piece of information is the serum sodium concentration. If the patient is markedly hypernatremic and the hypernatremia is not iatrogenic (e.g., after large

> **BOX 50.1 Causes of Central Diabetes Insipidus in the Neurosciences ICU**
>
> **Brain tumors[a]**
>> Pituitary adenoma
>>
>> Craniopharyngioma
>>
>> Pilocytic astrocytoma
>>
>> Meningioma
>>
>> Hypothalamic hamartoma
>>
>> Metastasis
>>
>> Lymphoma
>
> **Transsphenoidal neurosurgery[a]**
>
> **Brain death[a]**
>
> **Traumatic brain injury[a]**
>
> **Aneurysmal subarachnoid hemorrhage**
>
> **Sheehan syndrome (postpartum ischemic pituitary necrosis)**
>
> **Other rare disorders**
>> Langerhans cell histiocytosis
>>
>> Erdheim-Chester disease (non–Langerhans cell histiocytosis)
>>
>> Sarcoidosis
>>
>> Granulomatosis with polyangiitis
>
> [a] Common causes in the neurosciences ICU.

doses of hypertonic saline or mannitol), the diagnosis of DI is likely. Hypotonic urine despite hypertonic serum (urine osmolality <300 mOsm/kg, urine specific gravity <1.010) supports this diagnosis. Moreover, the major improvement in urine concentration that follows the administration of DDAVP clinches the diagnosis.

The management of DI is more complicated than appreciated. Physicians need to follow the changes in serum sodium concentration and fluid balance very closely. The management of hypertonic hypernatremia from DI starts by maximizing adequate water replacement. One must administer enough fluids to prevent or correct hypovolemia. Sodium chloride 0.9% is often quite hypotonic in relation to serum sodium concentration in these patients, and we use this intravenous solution first unless the degree of hypernatremia becomes dangerously high (>160 mmol/L). Always maintain caution about administering hypotonic intravenous solutions to patients at risk of postoperative brain swelling; we favor a less aggressive replacement of the free water deficit in these patients.

Calculating the free water deficit is useful to adequately treat patients with central DI. The formula for this calculation is:

$$\text{Free water deficit} = \text{Normal TBW} - \text{Current TBW}$$

where normal TBW (total body water) is 60% of lean body weight in kilograms in men and 50% in women. Calculate current TBW as follows:

$$\text{Current TBW} = \text{Normal TBW} \times (140/\text{current serum sodium level})$$

Once the free water deficit is known, one can calculate the amount of fluid to give depending on the fluid tonicity:

$$\text{Replacement fluid volume(in liters)} = \text{Free water deficit} \times (1/1 - X)$$

where X = replacement fluid sodium concentration - isotonic fluid sodium concentration. (See also the patient discussed in Chapter 34 and Table 34.1 for information on sodium concentration in commonly used intravenous fluids.)

These formulas fail to tell us how the serum sodium concentration changes as we replace the fluid. Therefore, we have found the following alternative formula to be useful in practice:

$$\text{Change in serum Na} = \text{replacement fluid Na} - \text{serum Na}/\text{normal TBW} + 1$$

This formula indicates the amount by which the serum sodium concentration will change after the retention of 1 L of the replacement fluid.

Avoid rapid swings in serum sodium concentration. The risk of osmotic demyelination or central pontine myelinolysis is unknown when correcting hypernatremia compared to hyponatremia, but we still prefer to reduce hypernatremia by less than or equal to 10 mmol/L/d. In addition, and most importantly, patients with postoperative brain swelling may worsen when correcting a high serum sodium level too quickly. In such patients, lowering the sodium but maintaining a more moderate degree of hypernatremia is a better target.

Oral intake and enteral administration (via gastric tube) of free water are safe. We have seen patients in whom small volumes of intravenous hypotonic fluids were detrimental, while large volumes of free water given by nasogastric tube were not. Therefore, we prefer gastric free water administration for the gradual correction of hypernatremia in neurocritical patients.

We start desmopressin when the polyuria is severe (>500 mL/h for 2 consecutive hours or an average of >300 mL/h over 4 hours) and when the serum sodium concentration is rising fast. We often start with a low dose of desmopressin (e.g., 0.5–1 μg intravenously). Typically, the urinary output begins to slow down within 15 to 20 minutes. If the response is insufficient after 60 minutes, we repeat with a higher dose (1–2 μg). Monitoring of urinary output and serial serum sodium measurements should guide the timing of the next dose. Because gastric absorption may be poor in these patients, we prefer intravenous administration until we are confident that we have defined a daily requirement, and the situation is stable. At that point, we may switch to nasal (or oral) formulations. Chlorpropamide (sometimes combined with a thiazide) can be used to treat central DI, but we rarely administer this medication because it can provoke severe hypoglycemia.

Patients with aneurysmal subarachnoid hemorrhage who develop central DI represent another challenge. Although uncommon, DI may present early after rupture of a midline aneurysm and mostly in patients who present with poor clinical grade. The onset is sudden, and the hypernatremia can be quite severe, but the duration is short and followed by cerebral salt wasting. Use desmopressin and hypotonic intravenous fluids very cautiously in these patients, as they may lead to severe hyponatremia.

After resection of sellar tumors, particularly craniopharyngiomas, it is quite frequent to see a triphasic response of DI–SIADH–recurrent DI that can occur at a dizzying pace. One study found that the pituitary stalk transection group demonstrated a postoperative pattern of initially high, then low, and finally high urine output and high serum sodium values in 40% of patients, and this pattern occurred in only 1% when the stalk was preserved. Although in the immediate postoperative phase patients in the infundibular preservation group demonstrated high urine output and serum sodium values, these normalized without a subsequent period of concerning elevation. (Infundibular preservation is debated by neurosurgeons, as maximal resection decreases recurrence rates but causes hypopituitarism.) This shift from hypernatremia to hyponatremia can also occur in patients with traumatic brain injury, but the change is slower. Finally, DI may be an initial sign that a patient is meeting criteria for brain death. Usually, hypotension accompanies the development of polyuria and hypernatremia.

We treated our patient with a combination of crystalloids (a combination of 0.9% and 0.45% sodium chloride), free water flushes, and desmopressin (first intravenously and then orally after several days). We extended her stay in the neuro intensive care unit by a week to closely monitor her labile DI. Eventually, she recovered well except for short-term memory deficits, due to fornix injury. Six months later, her urinary production and serum sodium levels were stable on oral desmopressin (0.4 mg twice daily). As was the case in our patient, patients with brain tumors or brain trauma or after neurosurgery typically need long-term treatment with desmopressin. These patients also need a comprehensive endocrine evaluation for possible panhypopituitarism. In fact, even in the absence of signs of pituitary apoplexy, consider investigation of adrenal and thyroid function in any patient with central DI. Box 50.2 offers a protocol to treat diabetes insipidus.

BOX 50.2 **Protocol to Treat Diabetes Insipidus**

Stable hypernatremia (≤50 mmol/L)

Monitor polyuria and match with fluid intake.

Consider free water (250 mL) flushes through nasogastric tube.

Monitor body weight, urine specific gravity.

Rising or severe hypernatremia (>150 mmol/L)

Start desmopressin 0.5–1 mcg IV and repeat if inadequate response (maximal 4 mcg/d in divided doses).

Start 0.45% sodium chloride or 5% dextrose and calculate infusion rate (see text).

Monitor serum sodium every 2–4 hours.

Monitor urine specific gravity.

KEY POINTS TO REMEMBER

- Postoperative polyuria after surgery for a suprasellar tumor should promptly raise suspicion of DI.
- DI can be a component of panhypopituitarism in patients with brain tumor, brain trauma, and infiltrating granulomatous diseases.
- DI in a catastrophically injured patient may be one of the first signs of brain death.
- Diagnosis of DI is based on the presence of polyuria associated with hypernatremia, serum hyperosmolality, and urine hypoosmolality.
- Management of central DI consists of aggressive rehydration and intravenous administration of desmopressin.
- Be wary of giving hypotonic intravenous fluids to patients with brain swelling. Lowering serum sodium to a more moderate degree of hypernatremia, primarily by administering free water through the gastric tube, is a safer strategy.

Further Reading

Adrogué, H. J., and N. E. Madias. "Hypernatremia." [In eng]. *N Engl J Med* 342, no. 20 (2000): 1493–99. https://doi.org/10.1056/nejm200005183422006.

Arima H, Cheetham T, Christ-Crain M, Cooper D, Drummond J, Gurnell M, Levy M, McCormack A, Newell-Price J, Verbalis JG, Wass J. Changing the name of diabetes insipidus: a position statement of the working group to consider renaming diabetes insipidus. *Clin Endocrinol (Oxf)*. 2024 Nov;101(5):443–445. doi: 10.1111/cen.14819. Epub 2022 Oct 14.

Busl, K. M., and A. A. Rabinstein. "Prevention and Correction of Dysnatremia After Aneurysmal Subarachnoid Hemorrhage." [In eng]. *Neurocrit Care* 39, no. 1 (2023): 70–80. https://doi.org/10.1007/s12028-023-01735-z.

de Vries, F., D. J. Lobatto, M. J. T. Verstegen, et al. "Postoperative Diabetes Insipidus: How to Define and Grade This Complication?" [In eng]. *Pituitary* 24, no. 2 (2021): 284–91. https://doi.org/10.1007/s11102-020-01083-7.

Fountas, A., A. Coulden, S. Fernández-García, G. Tsermoulas, J. Allotey, and N. Karavitaki. "Central Diabetes Insipidus (Vasopressin Deficiency) After Surgery for Pituitary Tumours: A Systematic Review and Meta-Analysis." [In eng]. *Eur J Endocrinol* 191, no. 1 (Jul 2 2024): S1–S13. doi:10.1093/ejendo/lvae084.

Jane, J. A., Jr., M. L. Vance, and E. R. Laws. "Neurogenic Diabetes Insipidus." [In eng]. *Pituitary* 9, no. 4 (2006): 327–29. https://doi.org/10.1007/s11102-006-0414-7.

Krahulik, D., J. Zapletalova, Z. Frysak, et al. "Dysfunction of Hypothalamic-Hypophysial Axis After Traumatic Brain Injury in Adults." [In eng]. *J Neurosurg* 113, no. 3 (2010): 581–84. https://doi.org/10.3171/2009.10.Jns09930.

Kristof, R. A., M. Rother, G. Neuloh, et al. "Incidence, Clinical Manifestations, and Course of Water and Electrolyte Metabolism Disturbances Following Transsphenoidal Pituitary Adenoma Surgery: A Prospective Observational Study." [In eng]. *J Neurosurg* 111, no. 3 (2009): 555–62. https://doi.org/10.3171/2008.9.Jns08191.

Lopez, D. C., J. P. Almeida, A. A. Momin, et al. "Triphasic Response After Endoscopic Craniopharyngioma Resection and Its Dependency on Infundibular Preservation or Sacrifice." [In eng]. *J Neurosurg* 139, no. 3 (Feb 3 2023): 790–97.

Nemergut, E. C., A. S. Dumont, U. T. Barry, et al. "Perioperative Management of Patients Undergoing Transsphenoidal Pituitary Surgery." [In eng]. *Anesth Analg* 101, no. 4 (2005): 1170–81. https://doi.org/10.1213/01.ane.0000166976.61650.ae.

Patel, N., D. Patel, S. S. Farouk, et al. "Salt and Water: A Review of Hypernatremia." [In eng]. *Adv Kidney Dis Health* 30, no. 2 (2023): 102–9. https://doi.org/10.1053/j.akdh.2022.12.010.

Singh, T. D., N. Valizadeh, F. B. Meyer, et al. "Management and Outcomes of Pituitary Apoplexy." [In eng]. *J Neurosurg* 122, no. 6 (2015): 1450–57. https://doi.org/10.3171/2014.10.Jns141204.

Woodmansee, W. W., J. Carmichael, D. Kelly, et al. "American Association of Clinical Endocrinologists and American College of Endocrinology Disease State Clinical Review: Postoperative Management Following Pituitary Surgery." [In eng]. *Endocr Pract* 21, no. 7 (2015): 832–38. https://doi.org/10.4158/ep14541.Dscr.

51 Rising Serum Ammonia in Liver Cirrhosis

A 38-year-old female with alcohol-associated liver cirrhosis (grade 3–4) was admitted with hyperammonemia and progressive decline in attention, which was diagnosed as hepatic encephalopathy. She was found to be a heterozygote for carbamoylphosphate synthetase I but with a normal amino acid profile. Her clinical course progressed with deepening coma with paratonia, disconjugate downward gaze, jactitations, and forceful repetitive eye blinking. These clinical signs coincided with extensive hypodensities and swelling on serial computed tomography (CT) scan (Figure 51.1).

After admission, she immediately received lactulose and rifaximin, but her severe hyperammonemia (>200 µg/dL) did not decrease for 6 days, which prompted initiation of a molecular absorbent recirculating system, continuous venovenous hemofiltration, and, eventually, endovascular inferior mesenteric vein/ inferior vena cava shunt closure. Some change was noted, and she started to open her eyes. However, despite the decrease in serum ammonia, awakening stalled, and she remained minimally conscious for months.

What do you do now?

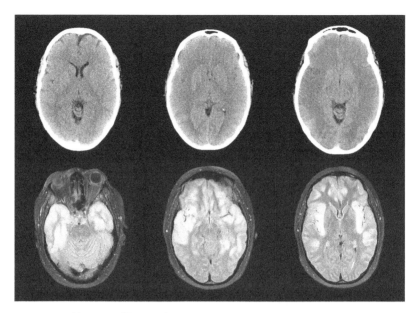

FIGURE 51.1 Upper row: CT scans of the brain with progressive cortical hypodensities and early swelling. Lower row: MRI (fluid-attenuated inversion recovery) confirms the significant (toxic) cortical injury.

This case brought us back to a fundamental question—what happens to the brain when serum ammonia rises exponentially and stays high? How does this relate to the clinical signs of hepatic encephalopathy? Are we right to say, "Just correct the ammonia, and signs and symptoms will resolve"? Do we dance around the subject?

Clinically, hepatic encephalopathy has been categorized in clinical stages of stepwise worsening. The description of each stage varies in the literature, but the differences across progressive stages are clear enough to be helpful in clinical practice because they represent major jumps in neurologic severity and responsiveness. Motor responses do fluctuate over time but usually closely correlate with the depth of coma. We may see restless tossing and multifocal myoclonus. With worsening stupor, we note rigidity in the extremities and neck muscle, and resistance to passive movements (paratonia or *gegenhalten*). Extensor posturing, which often suggests structural injury, characteristically manifests in late stages of this encephalopathy but may be completely reversible after correction of hyperammonemia.

Grasp reflexes were common in other reports but we have not seen them. Oculocephalic responses remain intact but may become quite easy to elicit, leaving the impression that the eyes are perched on rollers. Eyes may move in all directions and even stay in a lateral or vertical gaze. Sometimes disconjugate or fixed disconjugate gaze appears but then disappears after serum ammonia levels decrease. These eye movements are often misinterpreted as an indication of seizures. The pupillary reaction becomes sluggish (admittedly, an imprecise term) only in end-stage encephalopathy and, because of diffuse cerebral edema, eventually disappears as a consequence of progressive central brain tissue and brainstem displacement.

In our patient, the unusual appearance of the CT scan on sequential studies prompted a magnetic resonance imaging (MRI) scan, which showed far more extensive T2 signal prolongation and prominent cytotoxic cortical edema in the anterior temporal lobes and insula on diffusion-weighted imaging and apparent diffusion-coefficient mapping. We now wondered whether the condition was reversible or a permanent toxic effect of prolonged hyperammonemia. We do not order routine MRIs (or even serial CT scans) in patients with liver cirrhosis. But this time we did because the CT findings were highly unusual. We do a routine electroencephalogram to exclude seizures, but we see triphasic waves most of the time.

So how do the underlying molecular mechanisms of this disease state work? Pivotal in the mechanism of hepatic encephalopathy, ammonia may tip the balance between excitatory and inhibitory neurotransmitters. Failed liver clearance impairs conversion of ammonia to urea and glutamine and, consequently, creates a surfeit of glutamate. As a result of the linkage of ammonia with glutamate, formation of gamma-aminobutyric acid produces an inhibitory action after depolarization through the opening of chloride channels. Profound hyperammonemia, though much less with cirrhosis than with acute de novo fulminant hepatic failure, causes rapid diffuse brain edema due to the properties of glutamine, which is a water-attracting osmolyte. Ammonia diffuses through the bloodstream barrier, and glutamine synthetase, present in astrocytes, increases glutamine (synthesized from ammonia and glutamate).

We can conclude that increased ammonia causes brain injury by acting as a damaging (direct or indirect) neurotoxin or interrupting (reversibly) brain metabolism. We expect a greater degree of structural injuries to lead to poor neurologic outcome. In a few cases that went to autopsy we saw on microscopy necrotic red neurons typical for hypoxic-ischemic brain injury (although the patients never had a cardiac arrest or refractory hypotension). This brain injury pattern is known in neonatal and pediatric metabolic disorders but is much less recognized in adults with chronic liver disease, again likely due to underutilization of MRI in these patients. CT scan may show some cerebral edema in the affected areas, but it is not similar to fulminant hepatic failure, and very few case examples of substantial brain swelling in cirrhotic patients have been reported in the literature.

Lactulose with or without rifaximin is sufficient to treat hyperammonemia in most patients with decompensated cirrhosis. Emergency treatment of severe hyperammonemia may include continuous hemofiltration as well as intravenous administration of sodium phenylacetate and sodium benzoate, supplemented by arginine, citrulline, and carnitine. Molecular adsorption recirculation systems (MARS) lowers serum ammonia and it is a good option in intractable cases. Dextromethorphan or other competitive inhibitors (e.g., kynurenic acid) are therapeutic options. A search for a portosystemic shunt may be needed, which could lead to coil-assisted retrograde transvenous obliteration.

Prolonged hyperammonemic encephalopathy leads to substantial parenchymal brain injury, and surviving patients have impaired cognitive function. Takanashi et al. have classified MRI findings in acute hyperammonemic encephalopathy into four important groups: (1) diffuse cerebral edema followed by diffuse cerebral atrophy; (2) extensive, infarct-like abnormality often presenting as acute hemiplegia; (3) ischemic lesions in cerebral vascular territory; and (4) potentially reversible, symmetric, cortical involvement of the cingulate gyri, temporal lobes, and insular cortex with sparing of the perirolandic cortex. In the present patient, the changes on MRI resembled those of the fourth group but were more extensive and diffuse. A number of these major MRI abnormalities have been shown in patients with urea cycle disorders, including late-onset deficiencies. Curiously, our patient was a heterozygote for carbamoylphosphate synthetase I, which should not be symptomatic.

We should set this case apart from the clinical manifestations of fulminant hepatic failure. When liver failure is profound and acute in a previously healthy patient, the excitotoxicity of the neuronal glutamate receptors is a more pertinent explanation. The formation of glutamate results in production of nitric oxide, which leads to cerebral vasodilatation, increased cerebral blood volume, cerebral edema, and increased intracranial pressure. Astrocyte-detoxified ammonia synthesized through glutamine also acts as an osmolyte, causing osmotic stress and brain swelling. Cerebral edema must be immediately treated with osmotic agents in patients with acute hepatic failure, but liver transplantation remains the only solution for many. The success of organ transplantation directly correlates with aggressive control of brain edema and, thus, intracranial pressure.

Our patient improved, but we do not know if her cognitive dysfunction will improve substantially, and more serious systemic complications are expected down the line. It was not so well known to us that hyperammonemia in chronic liver cirrhosis could cause havoc, resulting in intensive care unit admission and prolonged mechanical ventilation. It behooves us to take this matter seriously and persuade the hepatologist to lower the serum ammonia levels quickly.

KEY POINTS TO REMEMBER

- Hyperammonemia can rapidly become toxic.
- Hyperammonemia in chronic liver disease can damage the brain structurally.
- Once brain injury occurs, recovery is uncertain.
- Efforts to reduce ammonia must be aggressive and could include obliteration of portocaval shunts.
- Massive brain edema is only seen in fulminant hepatic failure and generally not with established cirrhosis.

Further Reading

Butterworth, R. F. "Hepatic Encephalopathy in Cirrhosis: Pathology and Pathophysiology." [In eng]. *Drugs* 79, no. Suppl 1 (Feb 2019): 17–21.

Denk CH, Kunzmann J, Maieron A, et al. Histopathological examination of characteristic brain MRI findings in acute hyperammonemic encephalopathy: A case report and review of the literature. *Neuroradiol J.* 2024 Oct;37(5):630–635. doi: 10.1177/19714009231212370. Epub 2023 Nov 1.

McKinney, A. M., B. D. Lohman, B. Sarikaya, et al. "Acute Hepatic Encephalopathy: Diffusion-Weighted and Fluid-Attenuated Inversion Recovery Findings, and Correlation With Plasma Ammonia Level and Clinical Outcome." [In eng]. *AJNR Am J Neuroradiol* 31, no. 8 (Sep 2010): 1471–79. https://doi.org/10.3174/ajnr.A2112.

Takanashi, J., A. J. Barkovich, S. F. Cheng, et al. "Brain MR Imaging in Acute Hyperammonemic Encephalopathy Arising From Late-Onset Ornithine Transcarbamylase Deficiency." [In eng]. *AJNR Am J Neuroradiol* 24, no. 3 (Mar 2003): 390–93.

Takanashi, J., A. J. Barkovich, S. F. Cheng, et al. "Brain MR Imaging in Neonatal Hyperammonemic Encephalopathy Resulting from Proximal Urea Cycle Disorders." [In eng]. *AJNR Am J Neuroradiol* 24, no. 6 (Jun–Jul 2003): 1184–87.

U-King-Im, J. M., E. Yu, E. Bartlett, et al. "Acute Hyperammonemic Encephalopathy in Adults: Imaging Findings." [In eng]. *AJNR Am J Neuroradiol* 32, no. 2 (Feb 2011): 413–18. https://doi.org/10.3174/ajnr.A2290.

Wijdicks, E. F. "Hepatic Encephalopathy." [In eng]. *N Engl J Med* 375, no. 17 (Oct 27 2016): 1660–70. https://doi.org/10.1056/NEJMra1600561.

SECTION 4

PRINCIPLES OF PROGNOSTICATION

52 Prognostication After Severe Traumatic Brain Injury

A 34-year-old woman was the seatbelt-restrained driver in a rollover accident at highway speed. After a 20-minute extrication from the vehicle, she was unconscious with reactive pupils and spontaneous decorticate posturing. Blood pressure at the scene was 97/68 mmHg and oxygen saturation was 99%. She was intubated and sedated by emergency medical services and, on arrival at the emergency department, was treated as a Level 1 trauma case. No extracranial injuries were identified on primary or secondary surveys. Glucose was 186 mg/dL and hemoglobin was 11.6 g/dL. After sedation and neuromuscular blockade cleared, she remained comatose. Pupils were reactive. There was no eye opening to painful stimulus, and she had extensor posturing to nociceptive stimulation. A noncontrast head computed tomography (CT) scan showed multiple contusions and traumatic subarachnoid hemorrhage (Figure 52.1). Associated cranial injuries included a complex skull fracture in the skull base and bilateral temporal bone fractures. An intraparenchymal intracranial pressure (ICP) monitor was placed with initial reading of 25 mmHg. On hospital day 2, she developed refractory intracranial hypertension, which was medically managed with head-of-the-bed elevation, sedation, and osmotic therapy, but it persisted through hospital day 10, after which her ICPs steadily settled below 15 mmHg and the ICP monitor was removed. However, she remained comatose, and her family wondered when she would "wake up" and how she would be.

What do you do now?

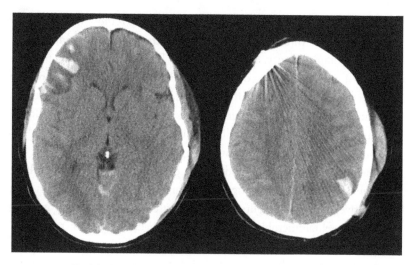

FIGURE 52.1 CT of the brain shows scattered subarachnoid hemorrhage and hyperattenuation at the gray-white junction in the frontal and parietal lobes from contusions. There is also a large left parietal scalp hematoma. There is a streak artifact from the ICP monitor.

The stone-cold fact that traumatic brain injury (TBI) is a condition with highly variable and unpredictable outcomes will undermine any attempt to predict outcome. Of course, physicians are as eager as family members to know a patient's outcome, and (even if true) they cannot respond with "time will tell" each time family members ask about the days ahead. More specifics would be appreciated. So where do we go from here?

There are multiple clinical and radiological prediction models, scales, and scores in TBI but no hard or fast rules. The largest database of TBI (International Mission for Prognosis and Analysis of Clinical Trials in Traumatic Brain Injury [IMPACT]) uses admission characteristics to estimate prognosis. Factors included are age, motor response, pupil responses, presence of hypoxia and hypotension, Marshall's CT categorization of lesion severity and mass effect, presence of traumatic subarachnoid hemorrhage, and epidural and subdural hematoma with mass effect. An extended model adds serum glucose and hemoglobin levels (calculator at http://www.tbi-impact.org). Using the extended model, our patient's predicted 6-month mortality score by IMPACT is 64%. Prediction of unfavorable outcome at 6 months (death, vegetative state, and severe disability) using the extended model is 84%.

The second largest database, Corticosteroid Randomization After Significant Head Injury (CRASH) expands the equation to incorporate major extracranial injury, more detailed CT findings, and the patient's country of residence to account for different medical care resources in developing countries (calculator at http://www.trialscoordinatingcentre.lshtm.ac.uk/). The CRASH model provides a somewhat different prediction for our patient—a 7% probability of mortality at 14 days and a 40% likelihood of unfavorable outcome at 6 months.

None of these prognostic models have explored the potential usefulness of magnetic resonance imaging (MRI), and emerging data suggest that quantitative, diffusion-weighted MRI and susceptibility-weighted imaging (detecting cerebral microbleeds) in patients with TBI may predict outcome. Moreover, with diffuse axonal injury, the presence of lesions that extend into the corpus callosum, brainstem, and thalamus bodes poorly for recovery. Clinicians, often doubt whether the changes found on MRI are meaningful; some persistently comatose patients in the neurosciences intensive care unit (ICU) may have relatively unaffected white and cortical matter on initial MRIs only to show diffuse cerebral atrophy months later. Nonetheless, the combination of MRI findings (such as diffuse axonal injury and subarachnoid hemorrhage) and diffusion tensor imaging metrics may improve prognostication at 3 months after injury. Most of us agree that the information is insufficiently determinative for use in clinical practice.

Decisions in neurocritical care are based on probabilities, but we recognized that in acute neurology and critical care medicine high probability rarely reaches about 50% to 60% (and not the proverbial "95%"). The same applies to low probability, which may still be close to 10%. Prediction scores are therefore deceiving. Most neurorehabilitation experts involved with long-term care of TBI know that we can never be that certain; indeed, prediction in young comatose patients with intact brainstem reflexes is nothing more than a roll of the dice.

One could assume that large databases encompassing thousands of patients are superior to any individual physician's cumulative experience. Still, we must advise extreme caution when applying these prediction models to individual patients; they represent probabilities only applicable to a large cohort of cases and cannot provide any level of certainty regarding an individual patient's outcome. Extrapolating from findings in large cohorts to individual cases is problematic because we cannot know how patients were treated or whether they were given a chance. Also, as illustrated by our case, different prognostic scores can suggest a markedly different chance of poor outcome.

All that said, we do know that the most significant determinants of outcome include the age of the patient; severity of the injury, as evidenced by presence or absence of pupillary reactivity, motor response, and CT findings; and associated systemic insults (Table 52.1). Neurosurgical intervention also affects outcome, and many would encourage evacuation of large intraparenchymal, epidural, or subdural hematomas. The Transforming Research and Clinical Knowledge in Traumatic Brain Injury (TRACK-TBI) found that prior TBI increases cerebral vulnerability to subsequent injuries and could increase mortality but not morbidity or unfavorable outcomes 12 months after injury.

ICP as a prognostic indicator in trauma has been evaluated in several studies. The presence of refractory intracranial hypertension is strongly predictive of mortality and (albeit much less strongly) of morbidity. Some studies have found that refractory ICP increases the risk of poor outcome by sixfold. Knowing the ICP is useful for prognosis, but estimations of long-term prognosis obviously should not be made solely based on ICP or its refractoriness. Also, the value of decompressive craniectomy as a treatment for refractory increased ICP has been questioned. A large clinical trial (conducted in Latin American hospitals with limited resources

TABLE 52.1 **Data Points in Prognostication of Traumatic Brain Injury**

Patient characteristics	Age, ethnic origin, socioeconomic status, medical history
Clinical severity	Pupil reactivity, motor score
Secondary insults	Hypoxemia, hypotension, refractory increased intracranial pressure
Structural abnormalities	Compressed or obliterated cisterns, midline shift, subarachnoid hemorrhage, presence of a mass lesion
Acute neurosurgical intervention	Acute subdural hematoma, acute epidural hematoma, swollen and hemorrhagic contusions

and no previous regular use of ICP monitoring) found that care based on monitoring did not change outcome compared with care based on imaging and clinical examination.

Biomarkers are new tools for prognostication. Two such biomarkers—glial fibrillary acidic protein (GFAP), a structural protein found in astrocytes, and ubiquitin C-terminal hydrolase L1 (UCH-L1), an enzyme found abundantly in neurons—have generated interest. A recent study found that day-of-injury GFAP and UCH-L1 concentrations predict unfavorable outcome and death at 6 months with good to excellent discriminative ability. However, these biomarkers do not accurately predict incomplete recovery. Their predictive ability is modest at best in alert or drowsy patients with TBI but stronger in stuporous and comatose patients with TBI. The reproducibility of these findings is not yet known, and thus it cannot be broadly adopted in the clinical setting.

More recently, machine learning has been evaluated in TBI, and in one study, an imaging model performed well for predicting long-term outcomes when compared with the predictions of attending neurosurgeons and IMPACT. Errors were made when predictions were based on emergency department information. This does not include the ICU course of the patient, which can go either way. Making rational decisions based on this information would require special serial MRI studies and serum biomarkers, which take time to process. Careful clinical assessment over time remains the best approach, and auxiliary information should be regarded cautiously.

After a 24-day hospital course, our patient was transferred to an inpatient rehabilitation facility. On the day of discharge, she was opening her eyes spontaneously, tracking people and objects inconsistently, initiating purposeful movements of the upper extremities, and smiling occasionally, but she did not yet follow commands. She required total assistance for all activities of daily living and depended on tube feeding. Six weeks after the TBI, she was eating on her own, ambulating, and speaking clearly in full sentences. At 3-month follow-up, she was reading, writing, and living at home with her family. However, she still requires 24-hour supervision, struggles with planning, and needs standby assistance for ambulation.

In young patients with TBI, substantial recovery can occur over many months even in the most severe cases. Long periods of neurorehabilitation are often needed. Unfortunately, and lurking insidiously beneath the radar, many of these patients may have cognitive dependence despite being physically independent after discharge from acute rehabilitation. Cognitive rehabilitation may improve the executive aspects of attention and everyday functioning, but attentional deficits and emotional lability remain. This also increases patients' propensity to develop addictions.

Having beaten the odds, our patient has a reasonable chance to continue to improve. We know this because years later several patients with comparable injuries have returned to our neuro-ICU to say hello—looking quite good.

KEY POINTS TO REMEMBER

- The heterogeneity of TBI limits prognostication, and prognostication is particularly challenging in young patients.
- Half of comatose patients with severe TBI improve significantly over 6 months.
- The impact of ICP monitoring on the outcome of TBI is uncertain.
- Cognitive impairment, depression, agitation, and addictions are a major cause of decreased functional independence after severe TBI.

Further Reading

Bonds, B., A. Dhanda, C. Wade, et al. "Prognostication of Mortality and Long-Term Functional Outcomes Following Traumatic Brain Injury: Can We Do Better?" [In eng]. *J Neurotrauma* 38, no. 8 (Apr 15 2021): 1168–76. https://doi.org/10.1089/neu.2014.3742.

Goostrey, K., and S. Muehlschlegel. "Prognostication and Shared Decision Making in Neurocritical Care." [In eng]. *Bmj* 377 (Apr 7 2022): e060154. https://doi.org/10.1136/bmj-2021-060154.

"Guidelines for the Management of Severe Traumatic Brain Injury." [In eng]. *J Neurotrauma* 24, no. Suppl 1 (2007): S1–106. https://doi.org/10.1089/neu.2007.9999.

Korley, F. K., S. Jain, X. Sun, et al. "Prognostic Value of Day-of-Injury Plasma GFAP and UCH-L1 Concentrations for Predicting Functional Recovery After Traumatic Brain Injury in Patients From the US Track-TBI Cohort: An Observational Cohort Study." [In eng]. *Lancet Neurol* 21, no. 9 (Sep 2022): 803–13. https://doi.org/10.1016/s1474-4422(22)00256-3.

Lingsma, H. F., B. Roozenbeek, E. W. Steyerberg, et al. "Early Prognosis in Traumatic Brain Injury: From Prophecies to Predictions." [In eng]. *Lancet Neurol* 9, no. 5 (May 2010): 543–54. https://doi.org/10.1016/s1474-4422(10)70065-x.

Maas, A. I., A. Marmarou, G. D. Murray, et al. "Prognosis and Clinical Trial Design in Traumatic Brain Injury: The Impact Study." [In eng]. *J Neurotrauma* 24, no. 2 (Feb 2007): 232–38. https://doi.org/10.1089/neu.2006.0024.

Pease, M., D. Arefan, J. Barber, et al. "Outcome Prediction in Patients With Severe Traumatic Brain Injury Using Deep Learning From Head CT Scans." [In eng]. *Radiology* 304, no. 2 (Aug 2022): 385–94. https://doi.org/10.1148/radiol.212181.

Rath, J. F., J. N. McGiffin, H. Glubo, et al. "Cognitive Dependence in Physically Independent Patients at Discharge From Acute Traumatic Brain Injury Rehabilitation." [In eng]. *Arch Phys Med Rehabil* 103, no. 9 (Sep 2022): 1866–69. https://doi.org/10.1016/j.apmr.2022.01.160.

Richter, S., S. Winzeck, E. N. Kornaropoulos, et al. "Neuroanatomical Substrates and Symptoms Associated With Magnetic Resonance Imaging of Patients With Mild Traumatic Brain Injury." [In eng]. *JAMA Netw Open* 4, no. 3 (Mar 1 2021): e210994. https://doi.org/10.1001/jamanetworkopen.2021.0994.

Wijdicks, E. F. M. *Communicating Prognosis.* Core Principles of Acute Neurology. New York: Oxford University Press; 2014.

Yue, J. K., L. L. Etemad, M. M. Elguindy, et al. "Prior Traumatic Brain Injury is a Risk Factor for In-Hospital Mortality in Moderate to Severe Traumatic Brain Injury: A TRACK-TBI Cohort Study." [In eng]. *Trauma Surg Acute Care Open* 9, no. 1 (Jul 24 2024): e001501. doi:10.1136/tsaco-2024-001501. PMID: 39081460.

53 Prognostication After Acute Ischemic Stroke and Cerebral Hemorrhage

A 68-year-old woman with history of hypertension, heart failure with preserved ejection fraction, chronic kidney disease stage 3b, and medically complicated obesity (body mass index 53) suddenly became poorly responsive. When paramedics arrived, they found her stuporous, unable to speak, and weak on the left side. Her blood pressure was 212/105 mmHg. She was brought to the emergency department, where she had to be intubated for airway protection. A head computed tomography (CT) scan showed a right thalamic hemorrhage (estimated volume 18 mL) with intraventricular extension and early hydrocephalus (Figure 53.1). Her intracerebral hemorrhage score was 2. Her blood pressure was treated with intravenous clevidipine, and she was admitted to the neurosciences intensive care unit (neuro ICU), where a right frontal ventriculostomy catheter was placed. Follow-up head CT was stable. After stopping sedation, the patient did not awaken and had no motor responses to pain in the left arm or leg. Her family was anxious to hear about her chances of recovery.

What do you do now?

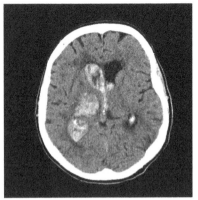 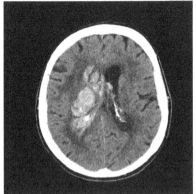

FIGURE 53.1 Head CT shows a right thalamic hemorrhage with intraventricular extension and hydrocephalus.

Major strokes whether ischemic or hemorrhagic, have similarities in presentation and prognosis according to their natural history. Prognosis depends on what is destroyed and what cannot come back. However, treatment of these two disorders differs substantially, which obviously has implications for outcome prediction. While reperfusion therapy can dramatically change the prognosis of a patient with a severe acute ischemic stroke, there is no major, prognosis-changing medical treatment for intracerebral hemorrhage. Despite that, there are enough commonalities between ischemic and hemorrhagic strokes that their prognosis can be discussed in a single chapter. Similar brain structures are often involved; in fact, it is common to diagnose a ganglionic hemorrhage as a large-vessel occlusion (and call a stroke alert for potential thrombolysis or endovascular retrieval) before CT shows a more accurate picture.

Myriad scores attempt to predict the outcome of patients with acute ischemic stroke or intracerebral hemorrhage; only some have been validated, and very few are commonly used in practice. The intracerebral hemorrhage score (Table 53.1) is probably the exception because its documentation in the medical records has become a metric for certifying bodies in the United States, forcing health care providers to use it whether they like it or not. The maximal score of 6 predicts a 100% mortality risk and an inflection point was found between 2 and 3 (26% vs 72% risk). These numbers are rarely used for prediction. We must not forget that the

TABLE 53.1 ICH Score (Developed to Predict 30-Day Mortality)

Variable	Points
GCS sum score at presentation	
3–4	2
5–12	1
13–15	0
ICH volume on initial scan	
≥30 cm^3	1
<30 cm^3	0
Intraventricular extension of ICH	
Yes	1
No	0
Infratentorial origin of ICH	
Yes	1
No	0
Age	
≥80 years	1
<80 years	0

GCS, Glasgow Coma Scale; ICH intracerebral hemorrhage.

information provided in outcome prediction scores applies to populations rather than individuals. Therefore, it is inadvisable to use these scores to estimate prognosis on an individual basis. The ICH score is simple but too simplistic (for sure, for practicing neurointensivists) and does not measure brainstem reflexes or other possible important determinants such as shift, anticoagulation reversal, initial use of osmotic agents, blood pressure control, and early neurosurgical interventions.

The site of intracerebral hematoma is important in prognostication. Ganglionic hemorrhages often extend into the ventricular system, and the development of hydrocephalus together with coma significantly increases the chance of early (30-day) mortality. Patients with a cerebellar hematoma do very well even with troubling presentations as long as the neurosurgeon evacuates the hematoma. Recovery is possible in these cases because compression rather than destruction is the main mechanism. Pontine hemorrhages are often devastating because they destroy the most vital region of the brain—the brainstem.

Older age, previous functional status, and greater severity of neurological condition at presentation are major indicators of worse prognosis for survival and neurological recovery after both acute ischemic stroke and intracerebral hemorrhage. The neurologic examination must be assessed at several time points. The degree of brainstem involvement in acute supratentorial lesions has always been the most important determinant. Multiple other factors correlate with lower likelihood of good functional recovery (Table 53.2). For ischemic stroke, the extent of involved arterial territory and final infarct volume are important determinants of prognosis. For intracerebral hemorrhage, location and final volume of the hematoma and presence of associated intraventricular hemorrhage are major prognostic factors.

In patients presenting with severely disabling acute ischemic stroke from a large-vessel occlusion, clinical improvement after successful reperfusion with intravenous thrombolysis or endovascular therapy can markedly improve their chances of regaining functional independence. (Of note, improvement after reperfusion treatment is often not included in the scores

TABLE 53.2 **Main Factors Associated With Worse Prognosis in Stroke**

Ischemic Stroke	Intracerebral Hemorrhage
Baseline disability	Baseline disability
Older age	Older age
Higher initial NIHSS score/decreased level of alertness	Stupor or coma
Early neurological decline	Early neurological decline
Larger area of infarcted tissue	Expansion and large final hematoma volume
Longer onset to treatment time	Brainstem involvement
Failure to reperfuse a large-vessel occlusion	Intraventricular extension
Acute and persistent hyperglycemia	Anticoagulant use (or overuse) at onset

NIHSS, National Institutes of Health Stroke Scale.

for predicting recovery after ischemic stroke.) For intracerebral hemorrhage, instead, no specific medical treatment has been shown to improve the chances of good recovery. Various clinical trials have investigated reduction of hematoma expansion with antihypertensives (INTERACT-2 and ATACH-2), tranexamic acid (TICH-2), and hemostatic therapy (SPOTLIGHT/STOP-IT) based on the "spot sign" (a sign of ongoing extravasation into the hematoma; see Chapter 1). Although these interventions sometimes decreased total clot volumes, they did not improve what matters: the functional outcomes. Other forms of invasive treatment (hemicraniectomy for hemispheric brain infarctions, suboccipital craniectomy for large cerebellar infarcts or hematomas, hematoma evacuation for selected cases of lobar intracerebral hemorrhage) and diligent neurocritical care can also result in better outcomes than initially expected. Therefore, it is important to treat first and prognosticate later in all but the most catastrophic stroke cases.

Premature withdrawal of life support measures can lead to a "self-fulfilling prophecy." The argument is that delivery of an (unjustified) overly pessimistic prognosis leading to withholding or withdrawing aggressive care could result in an avoidable death. Several studies have found correlations between early limitations of care and greater mortality, particularly in patients with intracerebral hemorrhage. Yet, the benefits of a practice that delivers maximal care for all stroke patients are also uncertain. We think that there is also a "self-fulfilling prophecy in reverse" that takes place when patients with devastating brain injury from stroke receive maximally aggressive treatment that forces them to survive with extreme disability.

The importance of the self-fulfilling prophecy in the practice of neurocritical care has been hotly debated. Unquestionably, observational studies assessing the value of prognostic factors may be biased if these factors were used to discuss prognosis and decide on intensity of care for the patients included in the study. But it is also indisputable that clinicians have a responsibility to estimate prognosis in patients with severe stroke using the best information available and that maximal care is not uniformly the best course of action for every patient with severe destruction of important regions of the brain.

When prognosticating at the bedside, the treating clinician should be forthright, cautious, and thoughtful. Forthrightness is necessary to acknowledge some degree of uncertainty. Caution should be exercised when discussing an unknowable prognosis with families. Thoughtfulness places the estimated chances of recovery in the context of the patient's wishes and values.

A few other observations are important. Patients with profound aphasia *can* recover, and many do. Limb paralysis may be permanent, but increased tone allows standing and sometimes walking. Neglect can be persistent and very disabling, but not infrequently improves over time. Depression is common but can be managed. The speed of improvement is difficult to predict, and the full extent of recovery may not be reached until a year after the ictus. We continue to be surprised by the recovery potential of young stroke patients, particularly when they have the appropriate support from family and friends. There has been a long interest in developing adjunctive treatments to improve poststroke rehabilitation to diminish the impact of long-term sequelae. Electrical devices for neurostimulation are being actively studied and may represent a useful alternative for patients with spastic hemiplegia even after spontaneous recovery has stalled for some time. Brain-computer interfaces may become an option in some patients, but optimal candidates have not been precisely defined.

Our patient experienced slow but consistent improvement in the neuro ICU. She was extubated on day 3 and became progressively more communicative over the course of the following 2 weeks. We repeatedly explained to her family (and then to her as she became more lucid) that meaningful recovery was possible but would be gradual. She required placement of a ventriculoperitoneal shunt. Fortunately, despite her extensive comorbidities, she did not suffer any secondary complications in the hospital. She was discharged to a specialized nursing facility but was able to go home 4 weeks later. Five months after the event, she had regained independence in most activities of daily living, though she still required help with transfers and used a wheeled walker for ambulation. She told us that despite her residual deficits, she considered her quality of life to be acceptably good.

We were uncertain about her outcome. We guess more than a few would have been much more pessimistic. This example highlights the general problem of predicting outcome in patients with fixed deficits (i.e., deficits that are not a result of worsening edema and brain tissue shift). Once there is some clinical stability and the structural damage remains localized, meaningful improvement may start to occur. Wasn't it John Hughlings Jackson—one of the forebears of neurology—who said that neurologic symptoms can change, and sometimes for the better? For example, flaccidity may transition into spasticity with ability to ambulate. He wrote: "Destructive diseases do not directly cause positive symptoms, but rather produce a negative state from which only positive symptoms can arise." In his *Principle of Compensation*, Hughlings Jackson postulated the recruitment of undamaged areas, and we now have imaging that partially corroborate this theory. There are indeed, in his words, "residual representations ready to compensate."

KEY POINTS TO REMEMBER

- Age and severity of the neurological deficits at presentation and premorbid state are crucial prognostic indicators in ischemic or hemorrhagic strokes.
- Chances of improvement with therapy and actual improvement after treatment must always be considered when estimating prognosis.
- Prognostic scores for acute ischemic stroke and intracerebral hemorrhage are helpful to predict outcomes in large groups of patients, but it is not advisable to use them when discussing chances for recovery in individual cases.
- Information from prognosis research should inform discussions on prognosis of patients with severe stroke, but the individual estimation of prognosis cannot be solely guided by this information. Estimation of prognosis and its communication to patients and families must be tailored to each individual case.

Further Reading

Hemphill, J. C., 3rd, D. C. Bonovich, L. Besmertis, et al. "The ICH Score: A Simple, Reliable Grading Scale for Intracerebral Hemorrhage." [In eng]. *Stroke* 32, no. 4 (Apr 2001): 891–97. https://doi.org/10.1161/01.str.32.4.891.

Kremers, F., E. Venema, M. Duvekot, et al. "Outcome Prediction Models for Endovascular Treatment of Ischemic Stroke: Systematic Review and External

Validation." [In eng]. *Stroke* 53, no. 3 (Mar 2022): 825–36. https://doi.org/10.1161/strokeaha.120.033445.

Rabinstein, A., and T. Rundek. "Prediction of Outcome After Ischemic Stroke: The Value of Clinical Scores." [In eng]. *Neurology* 80, no. 1 (Jan 1 2013): 15–16. https://doi.org/10.1212/WNL.0b013e31827b1b5c.

Silva AB, Littlejohn KT, Liu JR, Moses DA, Chang EF. The speech neuroprosthesis. *Nat Rev Neurosci.* 2024 Jul;25(7):473–492. doi: 10.1038/s41583-024-00819-9. Epub 2024 May 14. PMID: 38745103.

Wartenberg, K. E., D. Y. Hwang, K. G. Haeusler, et al. "Gap Analysis Regarding Prognostication in Neurocritical Care: A Joint Statement From the German Neurocritical Care Society and the Neurocritical Care Society." [In eng]. *Neurocrit Care* 31, no. 2 (Oct 2019): 231–44. https://doi.org/10.1007/s12028-019-00769-6.

Zahuranec, D. B., D. L. Brown, L. D. Lisabeth, et al. "Early Care Limitations Independently Predict Mortality After Intracerebral Hemorrhage." [In eng]. *Neurology* 68, no. 20 (May 15 2007): 1651–57. https://doi.org/10.1212/01.wnl.0000261906.93238.72.

54 Prognostication After Cardiopulmonary Resuscitation

A family member found a 60-year-old woman unconscious with gasping breathing. Her daughter performed cardiopulmonary resuscitation (CPR) and called emergency medical services, who documented pulseless ventricular tachycardia. After several shocks restored circulation, she remained unconscious. After arrival to the intensive care unit, she was treated with a cooling device to a targeted temperature of 36°C for 24 hours. She was sedated with propofol and fentanyl. Substantial doses of vasopressors and inotropes were required to treat cardiac shock. Neurological examination, 2 days after rewarming, reveals no eyelid opening to pain, no motor response to pain, normal pupil response to light, intact corneal reflexes, intact grimacing, and nonsustained clonus at both ankles. Her family wants to know what to expect, as does the cardiologist.

What do you do now?

Estimating neurological prognosis for a patient who remains comatose after CPR for cardiac arrest is a very common consultation. Both cardiologists and family members may hope for immediate answers on prognosis. Can we do that confidently? Where did this idea come from? Can we foretell outcome after a major brain insult—perhaps the worst of its kind—when the brain is not perfused or marginally perfused during resuscitation?

But the ball is not entirely in the neurologist's court. Next to neurological assessment, other predictors of poor outcome at the time of resuscitation have been identified. The cardiac rhythm causing circulatory arrest is a major determinant of outcome. Patients with a "nonshockable" rhythm (asystole, pulseless electrical activity) have worse outcomes than patients with ventricular fibrillation or pulseless ventricular tachycardia who receive rapid defibrillation.

The clinical picture of postcardiac resuscitation syndrome is troubling. Patients may have major myocardial (possibly reversible) dysfunction, a systemic ischemic-reperfusion syndrome, intravascular volume depletion, and acute coronary syndrome requiring emergent reperfusion therapy. Hemodynamics are often labile after cardiac arrest due to massive catecholamine release and myocardial stunning, and intravenous vasopressors and inotropes are often necessary. In severe cases of persistent shock or hypoxia, more invasive treatments, such as intra-aortic balloon pump or extracorporeal membrane oxygenation, are life-saving. Acute kidney injury and shocked liver may be present or develop over the following couple of days. Consulting neurologists may not appreciate these confounders, especially when administered sedative drugs cannot be cleared appropriately due to lingering organ dysfunction. The response to treatment of these systemic complications plays an important role in outcome and influences the decision to continue with aggressive care. In other words, how the rest of the body responds to the time of inadequate perfusion is (almost) just as important as how the brain responds to it. Ultimately, even if anything else gets better, the brain—the most vulnerable of all organs—may not.

Once we think we can properly examine the patient, our neurological assessment should focus on motor response to stimuli, presence of spontaneous eye movements, response to certain stimuli, appearance of myoclonus or seizures, and presence of brainstem injury resulting in loss of key brainstem reflexes. The immediate presence of localizing motor responses is the best evidence that the duration of ischemia to the brain has been brief. Long-lasting circulatory arrest results in a more profound insult and may be apparent by the documentation of abnormal extensor or flexor response or no response to a noxious stimulation in the extremities.

Traditionally, incorporating motor response as a prognosticator is considered premature less than 72 hours from the cardiac arrest. We may even need to wait longer because of sedative infusions and altered drug metabolism, which became more of a problem after the wide adoption of therapeutic hypothermia (no longer recommended as elaborated in detail in Chapter 25). Motor response after CPR, however, has never been a very reliable predictor of functional outcome and that was already the case before targeted hypothermia became a common practice. Patients with withdrawal responses to pain may not wake up or may regain only minimal consciousness. Less commonly, patients with transient extensor posturing may get to do well. Meanwhile, discriminating whether absent motor response to pain in patients with renal and liver impairment is caused by structural brain injury or by lingering sedation effects is a virtually impossible task.

The presence of multisegmental myoclonus is always alarming. Myoclonus involves the face, limbs, and axial muscles. These brief jerks are spontaneous and, in the first hours after CPR, may be unrelenting and forceful. The patient may move in the bed—sometimes reducing ventilator synchrony—and cause considerable upset to family members. However, not all patients are the same. Status myoclonus refers to spontaneous multisegmental jerks persisting for hours and most frequently accompanied by malignant patterns on electroencephalography (EEG) (burst suppression or polyspike and wave patterns); prognosis in these cases is very poor. By contrast, a few jerks for a brief time or intermittently, often restricted to the face or a limb alone, may have no prognostic implications.

Brainstem reflexes are mostly normal because the brainstem is more resistant to anoxic-ischemic injury. Yet, absent pupillary and corneal reflexes or loss of all brainstem reflexes may be seen after prolonged periods of resuscitation. Fixed and dilated pupils are more frequently seen with asystole than with ventricular fibrillation, which may simply reflect more prolonged and profound anoxic-ischemic injury. Successful cardiac resuscitation with good neurological recovery more often occurs in patients with persistently reactive pupils from the onset. Abnormal eye movements can be seen, from roving to dipping to ping-pong, but none have prognostic value. The only eye finding that indicates severe injury to the brain is forced upward gaze, and it is commonly seen with myoclonus status.

Are there laboratory tests that can assist with prognostication, and which tests have the best predictive value? Somatosensory evoked potentials (SSEPs) with bilateral median nerve stimulation are key to evaluating patients who remain comatose after CPR. Bilateral absence of N20 (cortical) responses is a reliable indicator of a poor neurological outcome (Figure 54.1). Absence of N20 responses is a useful predictor only in the most severely affected patients. Most patients *do* have N20 responses (>90% in our experience), which limits its utility in predicting outcome. Also, technical difficulties and operator skill may, of course, influence the results. Of note, a single dose of a neuromuscular blocker can overcome muscle artifacts and improve recognition of N20 in some instances. The bilateral absence of N20 (cortical) responses should only be considered real if there is evidence of good conduction before reaching the cortex (P14 in the cervicomedullary junction and N18 in the upper midbrain and thalamus). SSEP, however, remains a test that is not widely available or used.

EEG may provide supplemental information to prognostication but is not conclusive. In many patients, it shows nonspecific increase in slow-wave activity. Generalized suppression less than 20 μV, burst suppression patterns, electrographic seizures on a suppressed or flat background (Figure 54.2), and absence of EEG reactivity are troubling findings, but unfortunately, interrater reliability of these EEG patterns is suboptimal. Moreover, EEG can evolve favorably, and sometimes "malignant" EEG patterns seen early may resolve.

Patients with EEG patterns of generalized periodic epileptiform discharges, burst suppression, or generalized suppression with a nonreactive background usually remain comatose despite aggressive treatment with antiseizure medications. As shown by the TELSTAR trial, aggressively treating these EEG patterns does not improve the chances of awakening with good

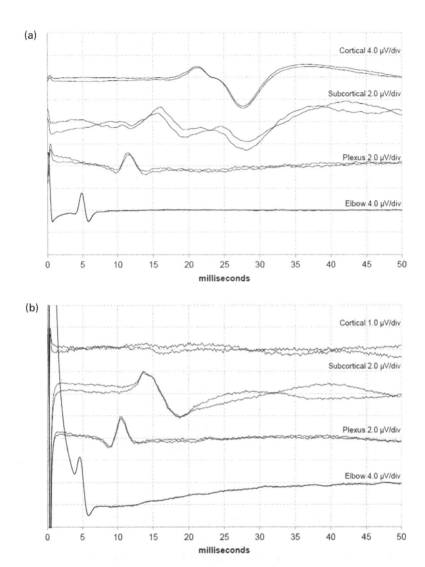

FIGURE 54.1 SSEP showing normal (A) and absent cortical N20 (B) responses.

function. Thus, these EEG patterns may reflect severe anoxic-ischemic injury rather than a treatable condition. Finding actual electrographic seizures is much more uncommon than epileptiform discharges interspersed over a suppressed background.

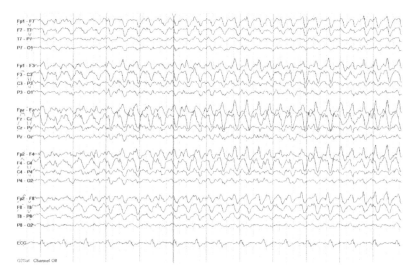

FIGURE 54.2 Electroencephalogram shows generalized epileptiform discharges, typically an ominous finding.

Prior to the introduction of induced hypothermia, physicians relied on the serum biomarker neuron-specific enolase (NSE) to predict poor outcome when it exceeded 33 ng/mL between post-CPR days 1 and 3 (though a more reliable threshold may be closer to 80 ng/mL). Differences in laboratory assays have made comparisons difficult, and not infrequently, hemolysis of the blood sample spuriously increases NSE levels. NSE is a useful biomarker when increased threefold from baseline. Neurofilament light chain (NfL) has better prognosticating value than NSE and may soon replace it. There no absolute cut-off value, but values above 500 to1000 pg/mL are problematic and, when measured serially, may rise just as with NSE. Logistical problems with timely return of these tests remain formidable.

Neuroimaging usually includes a baseline computed tomography scan, which is often normal. Some patients have early effacement of sulci and loss of gray-white matter differentiation. Such findings (when correctly assessed) strongly correlate with a poor neurological examination.

Failure to awaken several days after CPR in the absence of multiple indicators of poor prognosis justifies magnetic resonance imaging (MRI).

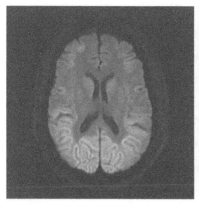 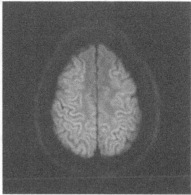

FIGURE 54.3 MRI (DWI sequence) of a comatose patient shows extensive restrictive diffusion affecting the cerebral cortex and basal ganglia.

Imaging parameters associated with poor outcome include widespread cortical diffusion-weighted imaging (DWI) abnormalities, and the combination of cortical and deep gray matter DWI/fluid-attenuated inversion recovery abnormalities (Figure 54.3). However, 20% to 50% of patients with good outcomes have (usually limited) DWI abnormalities on MRI, and conversely, we have seen patients with a repeatedly normal MRI during hospitalization who did very poorly (even progressing to a persistent vegetative state). In those situations, generalized brain atrophy may come much later. MRI is not the ultimate test for prognostication of neurological outcome after cardiac arrest, and studies evaluating its usefulness may have been very selective even when prospective. However, the abnormalities seen in Figure 54.3 are quite definitive.

What is the best approach in our patient? We usually proceed with summarizing clinical signs and laboratory data inarguably linked to poor prognosis in a comatose patient (Table 54.1).

She did not demonstrate myoclonic status epilepticus or absent pupil or corneal reflexes. SSEPs showed preserved cortical responses, and a single early serum NSE level was 45 ng/mL. EEG, however, showed generalized epileptiform discharges. Thus, in this patient, we were unable to prognosticate with certainty and continued support was warranted. She gradually awakened but remained in a severely disabled state, requiring

TABLE 54.1 Poor Outcome Anticipated in Postresuscitation Coma

Time	Findings
0–24 hours	Status myoclonus
24–72 hours	Somatosensory evoked potentials: absent cortical (N20) responses
≥72 hours	Absent pupil reflexes
	Absent corneal reflexes[a]
	Extensor motor responses
	Absent motor responses[a]

[a] Not as reliable if sedatives have recently been administered may linger.

nursing home placement. This case illustrates the current limitations of early prognostication in patients remaining comatose after cardiac resuscitation. The whole notion of being able to predict outcome remains a challenge for the neurologist, although with more time and additional data, the prognosis may become clearer.

Over the years, neurologists have relied on best available scientific facts. In daily practice, however, the outcome cannot be reliability determined in many patients. Indeed, this is the case in more than half of the patients we see post-CPR. We may usually know who will do poorly, but we often cannot predict who will regain independence and recover full use of their intellectual capabilities. Prognostication parameters changed when cooling or targeted temperature management (TTM) became part of care (including in this patient example) but cooling is now rarely practiced as we discussed in Chapter 25. Several pieces of information are needed. The new terminology now is *multimodality prognostication*, but that is what we have been doing all along. No experienced neurologist would put faith in a single laboratory test or a single early examination. We hope there are no physicians who would only observe for 72 hours and then make a major decision on level of care when the outcome appears indeterminate. On the other hand, we have no difficulty in predicting poor outcome in persistently comatose patients with continuous myoclonus and absent cortical (N20) responses on SSEP, early brain edema on CT, diffuse cortical damage on MRI, a markedly suppressed pattern or electrographic status epilepticus, and, most definitively, several absent brainstem reflexes. Overall, a combination of serial neurological exams, SSEP, EEG, and MRI abnormalities may provide the best information needed for prognostication.

KEY POINTS TO REMEMBER

- Certain clinical and laboratory findings are helpful in prognostication. Expect poor prognosis in patients with absent pupillary light responses and corneal reflexes, an extensor or absent motor response, or myoclonus status.
- Sedative medications can abolish corneal reflexes and motor responses to noxious stimulation. Their confounding effects need careful judgment.
- Bilateral absence of cortical (N20) responses is a reliable indicator of poor prognosis but only discriminates the worst cases of anoxic brain injury. Also, many patients with intact N20 responses never regain awareness.
- The prognostic value of serum NSE improves with increase over time, but other biomarkers may be more helpful (e.g., serum NfL).
- Antiseizure medications for generalized epileptiform discharges or burst suppression in anoxic-ischemic brain injury are often used reflexively, but there is no benefit in this condition.

Further Reading

Chakraborty, T., S. Braksick, A. Rabinstein, et al. "Status Myoclonus With Post-Cardiac-Arrest Syndrome: Implications for Prognostication." [In eng]. *Neurocrit Care* 36, no. 2 (2022): 387–94. https://doi.org/10.1007/s12028-021-01344-8.

Chan, W. P., C. Nguyen, N. Kim, et al. "Practical Magnetic-Resonance Imaging Score for Outcome Prediction in Comatose Cardiac Arrest Survivors." [In eng]. *Resuscitation* 202 (Aug 22 2024): 110370. doi:10.1016/j.resuscitation.2024.110370.

Dumas, F., D. Grimaldi, B. Zuber, et al. "Is Hypothermia After Cardiac Arrest Effective in Both Shockable and Nonshockable Patients?: Insights From a Large Registry." [In eng]. *Circulation* 123, no. 8 (2011): 877–86. https://doi.org/10.1161/circulation aha.110.987347.

Hirsch, K. G., M. Mlynash, I. Eyngorn, et al. "Multi-Center Study of Diffusion-Weighted Imaging in Coma After Cardiac Arrest." [In eng]. *Neurocrit Care* 24, no. 1 (2016): 82–89. https://doi.org/10.1007/s12028-015-0179-9.

Perera, K., S. Khan, S. Singh, et al. "EEG Patterns and Outcomes After Hypoxic Brain Injury: A Systematic Review and Meta-Analysis." [In eng]. *Neurocrit Care* 36, no. 1 (2022): 292–301. https://doi.org/10.1007/s12028-021-01322-0.

Rajajee, V., S. Muehlschlegel, K. E. Wartenberg, et al. "Guidelines for Neuroprognostication in Comatose Adult Survivors of Cardiac Arrest." [In eng]. *Neurocrit Care* 38, no. 3 (2023): 533–63. https://doi.org/10.1007/s12028-023-01688-3.

Ruijter, B. J., H. M. Keijzer, M. C. Tjepkema-Cloostermans, et al. "Treating Rhythmic and Periodic EEG Patterns in Comatose Survivors of Cardiac Arrest." [In eng]. *N Engl J Med* 386, no. 8 (2022): 724–34. https://doi.org/10.1056/NEJMoa2115998.

Samaniego, E. A., M. Mlynash, A. F. Caulfield, et al. "Sedation Confounds Outcome Prediction in Cardiac Arrest Survivors Treated With Hypothermia." [In eng]. *Neurocrit Care* 15, no. 1 (2011): 113–19. https://doi.org/10.1007/s12028-010-9412-8.

Sandroni, C., A. Cariou, F. Cavallaro, et al. "Prognostication in Comatose Survivors of Cardiac Arrest: An Advisory Statement From the European Resuscitation Council and the European Society of Intensive Care Medicine." [In eng]. *Intensive Care Med* 40, no. 12 (2014): 1816–31. https://doi.org/10.1007/s00134-014-3470-x.

Stammet, P., O. Collignon, C. Hassager, et al. "Neuron-Specific Enolase as a Predictor of Death or Poor Neurological Outcome After Out-of-Hospital Cardiac Arrest and Targeted Temperature Management at 33°C and 36°C." [In eng]. *J Am Coll Cardiol* 65, no. 19 (2015): 2104–14. https://doi.org/10.1016/j.jacc.2015.03.538.

Wihersaari, L., M. Reinikainen, R. Furlan, et al. "Neurofilament Light Compared to Neuron-Specific Enolase as a Predictor of Unfavourable Outcome After Out-of-Hospital Cardiac Arrest." [In eng]. *Resuscitation* 174 (2022): 1–8. https://doi.org/10.1016/j.resuscitation.2022.02.024.

Wijdicks, E. F., A. Hijdra, G. B. Young, et al. "Practice Parameter: Prediction of Outcome in Comatose Survivors After Cardiopulmonary Resuscitation (an Evidence-Based Review): Report of the Quality Standards Subcommittee of the American Academy of Neurology." [In eng]. *Neurology* 67, no. 2 (2006): 203–10. https://doi.org/10.1212/01.wnl.0000227183.21314.cd.

Wijdicks, E. F. M. "Futility of Suppressing Seizurelike Activity in Postresuscitation Coma." [In eng]. *N Engl J Med* 386, no. 8 (2022): 791–92. https://doi.org/10.1056/NEJMe2118851.

Wurm, R., H. Arfsten, B. Muqaku, et al. "Prediction of Neurological Recovery After Cardiac Arrest Using Neurofilament Light Chain Is Improved by a Proteomics-Based Multimarker Panel." [In eng]. *Neurocrit Care* 36, no. 2 (2022): 434–40. https://doi.org/10.1007/s12028-021-01321-1.

SECTION 5

LONG-TERM SUPPORT, END-OF-LIFE CARE, AND PALLIATION

55 Decisions in Persistent Comatose States

A 43-year-old male remained comatose 2 weeks after a severe traumatic brain injury. He underwent a decompressive craniectomy for a large subdural hematoma. He was treated for increased intracranial pressure associated with multiple frontal and temporal lobe contusions. His clinical course was complicated by seizures, pneumonia, and bacteremia. Resolution of the intracranial hypertension produced no change in his neurological examination, and he remained comatose. He did develop sleep-and-wake cycles. On examination, his eyes were open at times, but he could not track a finger or fixate on family members when they were in the room. A loud handclap produced no reaction. He ground his teeth. There was spontaneous extensor posturing. He would occasionally sweat profusely.

The nursing staff noticed no signs of awareness, but the family was less sure. Long-term support—hoping for a substantial recovery over time—was strongly considered. Family members questioned whether improvement could occur and at what level the patient would be able to function.

What do you do now?

Predicting the outcome of young patients after severe traumatic brain injury (TBI) is a necessary task for neurosurgeons and neurologists (see also Chapter 52), but they recognize the unpredictability in so many cases. When patients show early clinical signs of a persistent vegetative state and neuroimaging reveals severe brain injury, the need for long-term care will arise, and decisions must be made.

The general opinion has always been that recovery of awareness is much less likely if the clinical findings of persistent vegetative state (also called by some unresponsive wakefulness syndrome) are still present after 3 months in nontraumatic coma (i.e., anoxic-ischemic encephalopathy, hypoglycemia, central nervous system infections, status epilepticus) and after 12 months in traumatic brain injury. But we always knew that recovery to a minimally conscious state may still occur beyond this time, particularly after trauma. It is difficult to say with absolute certainty that a patient in a persistent vegetative state will never awaken to a minimally conscious state; however, both conditions imply an extremely poor functional state. Specifically, in comatose young individuals, it is difficult to predict long-term outcome after traumatic brain injury because many recover, some after years. Stories abound of families told there was no chance for recovery . . . and then it happened. Outcome is different with advanced age, and age has remained a strong determinant of outcome.

There has been renewed interest in persistent vegetative state and the accuracy of its clinical diagnosis. But the criteria for the diagnosis of persistent vegetative state have been well defined for decades, and neurologists and neurosurgeons have a particularly good understanding of this condition (Box 55.1).

The reliability of neurological examination in persistent vegetative state has withstood the test of time, although errors by nonneurologists are still considerable. These are the usual questions: Is persistent vegetative state truly permanent? Is our neurological examination reliable? Do we have better ways to assess "consciousness"? Can functional magnetic resonance imaging (MRI) scans predict recovery or provide evidence of awareness not detected clinically? Some of these questions cannot yet be answered with certainty. Brain activation on functional MRI (or electroencephalographic [EEG] changes temporally related to verbal commands) does not necessarily prove consciousness, although some neuroscientists are convinced that

> **BOX 55.1 Clinical Signs of a Vegetative State**
>
> Breathing regular (with tracheostomy in place)
>
> Bronchial hypersecretion
>
> Blood pressure stable
>
> Immobile
>
> Flexion-extension contractures
>
> Eyes closed or open
>
> No evidence of focus or holding attention
>
> No eye movements to examiner (except briefly when suddenly confronting)
>
> Eyes roving, nystagmoid or ballistic, gaze preference changing, no eye contact for >5 seconds
>
> Eyes may move upward or downward or assume lateral gaze for 1–2 minutes
>
> No sound (if not made impossible with tracheostomy)
>
> Spontaneous teeth grinding
>
> Spontaneous clonus or shivering
>
> May show repeated yawning

functional MRI can uncover "willful brain behavior" in patients otherwise unable to show it.

Functional MRI can show thalamic integrity suggestive of recovery potential, but it remains a research tool. It is not a factor in clinical decisions to proceed with prolonged care because it cannot accurately predict outcome or even awakening. There has been a recent recategorization of disorders of consciousness using functional MRI scan or EEG. This includes the category of cognitive motor dissociation (CMD), which applies to a subset of patients (Figure 55.1) who seem to fulfill all the criteria for vegetative state and display no behavioral evidence of language function but demonstrate "command following" response on functional MRI scan or EEG when tested. For instance, they demonstrate activity on functional MRI when asked to move a limb, even if no actual movement is seen. Others propose that another subset may exist, a higher-order cortex-motor dissociation (HMD), which only indicates a response of the associated cortices to auditory stimuli, again in patients who demonstrate no clinical evidence of consciousness. These functional imaging or EEG

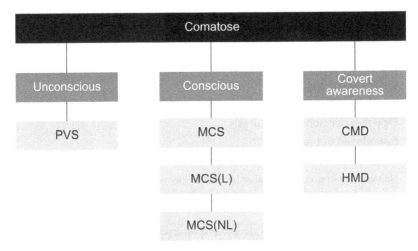

FIGURE 55.1 Categories of persistent disorders of consciousness (see text). CMD, cognitive motor dissociation; HMD, higher-order cortex-motor dissociation; L, language awareness; MCS, minimally conscious state; NL, no language awareness; PVS, persistent vegetative state.

findings suggest that cortical activation to external stimulation may reveal covert consciousness and could predict potential later recovery. Moreover, whether a "diagnosis" of CMD may guide therapy is currently unknown, and despite "recovery," later disability remains substantial. Also, the use of functional MRI or EEG for prognostication is controversial because functional MRI and EEG protocols, paradigms, and interpretation may differ across institutions. Patients who have been diagnosed with CMD using functional MRI and EEG (after making some response to repeated requests to open and close a hand) have focal lesions at the anterior forebrain with preserved thalamocortical projection and preserved functional connectivity. Patients who do not display this responsiveness (the majority) have brainstem injury from a variety of causes. This may suggest the patients with so-called CMD are severely abulic from severe frontal destruction rather than comatose. Nevertheless, growing evidence indicates that patients with these variants may reach states of communication.

Once long-term care has been decided, our main concern is to ensure the best medical support; therefore, a tracheostomy and percutaneous endoscopic gastrostomy (PEG) should be placed, often simultaneously

(Box 55.2). Common contraindications for a PEG are active coagulopathy, inability to perform endoscopy (esophageal obstruction), prior abdominal surgery involving the stomach, and, most importantly, uncertainty about need for long-term care. (It is poor medical practice to place a tracheostomy and PEG if care is withdrawn weeks later.)

Usually, a general surgeon will perform these procedures. Enteral feeding is discontinued 12 hours before surgery. Antibiotic prophylaxis to reduce peristomal infection is administered, and feeding can be restarted a few hours after placement. Complications are infrequent, but some can be anticipated. Pneumoperitoneum is common due to air escaping through the stomach opening and is only worrisome when peritonitis occurs. Air can be obscured by concomitant pulmonary infiltrates, and upright X-ray of the chest can make the diagnosis in these cases.

The advantages of tracheostomy in persistently comatose patients are substantial. These include ease of suctioning, reduced need of sedation, shorter duration of mechanical ventilation, and ability to transfer patients

---

BOX 55.2 **Measures With Gastrostomy and Tracheostomy**

Checks with gastrostomy placement
INR <1.5; platelets >50,000/mm^3
Discontinue intravenous heparin or antiplatelet agents (5 days)
Cefotaxime, 2-gram IV, single dose
Fasting for 4–6 hours
Anticipate use of midazolam (may need airway protection)
Resume tube feeding 1 hour after placement
Monitor for pneumoperitoneum with upright chest X-ray
Monitor white blood cell counts if fever

Checks with tracheostomy placement
Stable cervical spine
No high PEEP (<10 cmH$_2$O) or high FiO$_2$ requirements
INR <1.5; platelets >50,000/mm^3
Discontinue intravenous heparin
Anticipate oxygen desaturation
Anticipate hypotension
Anticipate bleeding at site

FiO$_2$, fraction of inspired oxygen; INR, international normalized ratio; PEEP, positive end-expiratory pressure.

to a long-term care facility. The optimal timing of tracheostomy placement has been a topic of debate. Early performance of tracheostomy (sometimes as early as during the first week of mechanical ventilation) has been proposed in patients expected to require prolonged mechanical ventilation; however, the value of this practice has not been proven. We favor the more conservative approach of proceeding with a percutaneous tracheostomy at least 10 days after the start of mechanical ventilation and when we anticipate the need for more than 3 weeks of mechanical ventilation. Direct tracheostomy (i.e., without previous endotracheal intubation) may be needed in severe neck and facial trauma or when there is inability to secure an airway. Complications of percutaneous tracheostomy are very uncommon (<2%) when done by skilled surgeons, but exclusion criteria include possible cervical neck injury, morbid obesity, and significant coagulopathy. Ongoing need for intravenous heparin may also make management of the bleeding site difficult. Eventually, patients will have the tracheostomy downsized. Uncomplicated plugging ("corking") of the tube for several days indicates that decannulation can be considered.

Long-term care in a nursing home facility is needed, and physicians who follow these patients face a continuous challenge to prevent and treat infections. Superb nursing care and physical therapy are essential to prevent early and late fatal complications. The chronicity of care changes patients' appearance, and they will look worlds away from what they were. It is a life many of us do not want to live. Have we told our loved ones that? (We did!)

KEY POINTS TO REMEMBER

- The prevalence of prolonged disorders of consciousness is not exactly known but likely small because most patients awaken.
- Terminology is changing and expanding, but we have to ensure that we know exactly what we mean and not end up with a Babylonian confusion.
- Disorders of prolonged unconsciousness have been redefined by functional MRI and EEG protocols, and subsets of patients with covert consciousness (or CMD) may exist, but these techniques have not found a clinical application

because they cannot predict outcome or awakening with sufficient certainty.

- Functional MRI and protocolized EEG with command testing may be able to find a small subset of patients who may reach states of communication later, but the imaging technique should not be used outside research protocols.
- Don't start thinking that comatose patients are still "in there".
- Persistent vegetative state will become permanent in most patients, but some patients are still able to improve to a minimally conscious state with full dependence on care and unclear internal life, if any.
- Tracheostomy and PEG tube placement are essentially part of the decision to maintain the best long-term support of the patient and should be considered early.

Further Reading

Bodien, Y. G., J. Allanson, P. Cardone, et al. "Cognitive Motor Dissociation in Disorders of Consciousness." *N Engl J Med* 391, no. 7 (Aug 15 2024): 598–608. doi:10.1056/NEJMoa2400645.

Claassen, J., K. Doyle, A. Matory, et al. "Detection of Brain Activation in Unresponsive Patients With Acute Brain Injury." [In eng]. *N Engl J Med* 380, no. 26 (2019): 2497–505.

Edlow, B. L., J. Claassen, N. D. Schiff, and D. M. Greer. "Recovery From Disorders of Consciousness: Mechanisms, Prognosis and Emerging Therapies." [In eng]. *Nat Rev Neurol* 17, no. 3 (Mar 2021): 135–56. https://doi.org/10.1038/s41582-020-00428-x.

Egbebike, J., Q. Shen, K. Doyle, et al. "Cognitive-Motor Dissociation and Time to Functional Recovery in Patients With Acute Brain Injury in the USA: A Prospective Observational Cohort Study." [In eng]. *Lancet Neurol* 21, no. 8 (Aug 2022): 704–13.

Giacino, J. T., J. J. Fins, S. Laureys, and N. D. Schiff. "Disorders of Consciousness After Acquired Brain Injury: The State of the Science." [In eng]. *Nat Rev Neurol* 10, no. 2 (Feb 2014): 99–114. https://doi.org/10.1038/nrneurol.2013.279.

Goss, A. L., and C. J. Creutzfeldt. "Prognostication, Ethical Issues, and Palliative Care in Disorders of Consciousness." [In eng]. *Neurol Clin* 40, no. 1 (Feb 2022): 59–75. https://doi.org/10.1016/j.ncl.2021.08.005.

Koc, D., A. Gercek, R. Gencosmanoglu, and N. Tozun. "Percutaneous Endoscopic Gastrostomy in the Neurosurgical Intensive Care Unit: Complications and

Outcome." [In eng]. *JPEN J Parenter Enteral Nutr* 31, no. 6 (Nov–Dec 2007): 517–20. https://doi.org/10.1177/0148607107031006517.

Kondziella, D., M. Amiri, M. H. Othman, et al. "Incidence and Prevalence of Coma in the UK and the USA." [In eng]. *Brain Commun* 4, no. 5 (2022): fcac188. https://doi.org/10.1093/braincomms/fcac188.

Kornblith, L. Z., C. C. Burlew, E. E. Moore, et al. "One Thousand Bedside Percutaneous Tracheostomies in the Surgical Intensive Care Unit: Time to Change the Gold Standard." [In eng]. *J Am Coll Surg* 212, no. 2 (Feb 2011): 163–70. https://doi.org/10.1016/j.jamcollsurg.2010.09.024.

Lingsma, H. F., B. Roozenbeek, E. W. Steyerberg, et al. "Early Prognosis in Traumatic Brain Injury: From Prophecies to Predictions." [In eng]. *Lancet Neurol* 9, no. 5 (May 2010): 543–54. https://doi.org/10.1016/s1474-4422(10)70065-x.

Löser, C., G. Aschl, X. Hébuterne, et al. "ESPEN Guidelines on Artificial Enteral Nutrition--Percutaneous Endoscopic Gastrostomy (PEG)." [In eng]. *Clin Nutr* 24, no. 5 (Oct 2005): 848–61. https://doi.org/10.1016/j.clnu.2005.06.013.

Monti, M. M., M. Rosenberg, P. Finoia, et al. "Thalamo-Frontal Connectivity Mediates Top-Down Cognitive Functions in Disorders of Consciousness." [In eng]. *Neurology* 84, no. 2 (Jan 13 2015): 167–73. https://doi.org/10.1212/wnl.0000000000001123.

Monti, M. M., A. Vanhaudenhuyse, M. R. Coleman, et al. "Willful Modulation of Brain Activity in Disorders of Consciousness." *N Engl J Med* 362, no. 7 (2010): 579–89.

Wijdicks, E. F. "Being Comatose: Why Definition Matters." [In eng]. *Lancet Neurol* 11, no. 8 (Aug 2012): 657–58. https://doi.org/10.1016/s1474-4422(12)70161-8.

Wijdicks, E. F. *The Comatose Patient*. 2nd ed. New York: Oxford University Press; 2014.

Wijdicks, E. F. *Guide to the Comatose Patient: Expert Advice for Families and Caregivers*. 1st ed. Rochester, MN: Mayo Clinic Press; 2022.

56 When Withdrawal of Life-Sustaining Treatment Is Considered

A 78-year-old woman is admitted to the neurosciences intensive care unit (ICU) with a destructive (ganglionic hemorrhage involving the diencephalon; Figure 56.1). On examination, she has midsize fixed pupils but with preserved corneal reflexes and a good cough response, and she overbreathes the ventilator. She has flexion withdrawal of both arms with nailbed compression in the fingers and triple-flexion responses of the legs. The family arrives and wants "everything done." The family is clear about her: she is a fighter and, in the past, was able to overcome desperate situations in which physicians had given up any hope for recovery. The family specifically requests that she have all the time she needs to recover and that she be resuscitated if necessary. Three days later, the patient's condition is unchanged.

What do you do now?

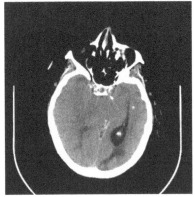 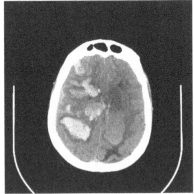

FIGURE 56.1 CT scan showing a massive right intraparenchymal hematoma with intraventricular extension, hydrocephalus, and brain tissue displacement causing complete effacement of the basilar cisterns.

We have discussed prognostication in a ganglionic hemorrhage in Chapter 53. This situation is obviously much different. Not only is there a large clot with shift and trapped ventricles, but also the neurologic examination points to evidence of secondary brainstem injury. We did not expect change, and no change occurred despite optimal medical care. We know intensive care treatment is futile, and even if the patient survives the hospital stay, the only possible outcome is long-term care in a skilled nursing facility. Sad but true. It is thus very reasonable to discuss "goals of care" (a commonly used proxy term that often simply implies limiting care or withdrawal of life sustaining measures) with family members. The goals here are to share what to expect in best-case scenarios, and if the patient had indicated while she was still healthy that she would not want that scenario, comfort care is appropriate.

Over the years, neuropalliative care has developed into an important adjunct but mostly in the setting of chronic neurologic conditions. In the neurocritical care, palliative care services are often sought to resolve conflict situations or to fill in a gap when (neurosurgical) available time is too short for the lengthy discussions often necessary in these cases. It is true that many situations can be approached multidimensionally, but it is much less certain whether routine involvement of palliative care in the neurosciences ICU leads to improved level of support or overall satisfaction. Palliative care services should not be sought if we do not want to take the time to manage ethical issues or conflicts.

End-of-life care in the ICU has become a shared decision-making process in the United States. Intuitively, such an approach must be more satisfactory than decisions based on physicians' authority and experience alone. When catastrophe strikes, families provide insight into the patient's wishes, and physicians estimate the expected degree of disability. When asked in surveys, most families appreciate a physician's openness and directness. Families want to know what to expect and what the limitations of aggressive interventions are. In patients with a poor prognosis, it is important to review the chances of a successful resuscitation effort. Most physicians and many family members recognize that things must come to an end at some point. Yet, as illustrated by our case, things are not always so rational.

Where did a do-not-resuscitate (DNR) order originate? In 1974, the American Medical Association stated in an article devoted to standards that "cardiorespiratory resuscitation was not indicated in certain situations." Other opinions were voiced, including the 1983 President's Commission on "deciding to forego life-sustaining support." This led to a major change in practice, in that doctors now had the opportunity to discuss any intervention before the event. Most major medical organizations supported the view that DNR orders could (and should) be discussed as part of care. How to communicate this to family members or even whether to discuss the actual procedure of cardiopulmonary resuscitation (CPR) has remained an underdeveloped field of medicine, and training of this part of end-of-life care in residencies is not commonplace. How it all pans out in practice is not known, but when studied more closely, the results are troubling. A recent study in the United States found that nearly 25% of ICU patients receive care different than that stipulated in advanced directives at the time of ICU admission. Additionally, more than 15% of patients with DNR orders who died in the ICU did so after receiving CPR.

What do the data say about the success of CPR in the ICU? In most large series of resuscitated critically ill patients with diverse diagnoses, not more than 15% survive to discharge. Advanced age and comorbidity (i.e., cancer) reduce the odds to less than 5%. Patients with acute, deteriorating neurological disease complicated by cardiac arrest and CPR have a very dismal outcome if they survive at all. Some empirical guidelines in patients with acute neurological disease are clearly warranted, but none exist. In an earlier statement, there appeared to be consensus among stroke physicians that DNR orders are appropriate if two of the three following criteria are met: (1) severe deficit, persistent or deteriorating and with impaired consciousness; (2) life-threatening brain damage with brainstem compression involving multiple brainstem levels; or (3) significant comorbidity including pneumonia, pulmonary emboli, sepsis, recent myocardial infarction, and life-threatening arrhythmias. Criteria for other critical neurological conditions have not been developed, but most physicians attending in the neurosciences ICU would discuss DNR orders—if not already made clear by family members—or interpret an advance directive if there is permanent and severe primary brain and brainstem injury.

A DNR order clearly specifies no CPR (no chest compression, no pharmacological or electrical cardioversion). Do-not-intubate orders (no endotracheal intubation or invasive mechanical ventilation) typically accompany the DNR order, but exceptions occur. Orders limiting aggressive care may also discourage use of noninvasive (bilevel positive airway pressure) mechanical ventilation, intravenous drugs, or infusions for cardiac arrhythmias with preserved circulation, cardiac pacemakers, or chest tubes, among other supportive devices—all indicative of aggressive care. However, a DNR order per se should not affect the level of care provided to the patient except obviously in the case of a cardiac arrest. Other restrictions of medical treatment or de-escalation of care should be specified separately from the DNR order.

These distinctions are crucial to avoid unintended problems with a DNR order. Some studies have found that DNR orders negatively influence triage to the ICU. Some patients may feel that a DNR order undermines aggressiveness of care. Multiple studies have found that people from certain cultures perceive a DNR order as equivalent to withholding treatment. It should not. In some situations, a DNR order could be the first step toward de-escalation of care. However, in and of itself, DNR merely defines the limits of care pertaining to a cardiopulmonary arrest.

In the United States, surrogates can make decisions, ideally guided by advance directives. A living will can direct a proxy to withhold or withdraw treatment at the end of life. Unfortunately, living wills are usually formulated in broad terms (often containing sentences such as "if I have terminal disease, I do not want to be resuscitated") and rarely include specifics on acute neurological disease. We would not expect that with documents

> **BOX 56.1 The Family Conference (10 Steps)**
>
> 1. Sit down in a quiet place (separate room).
> 2. Identify yourself.
> 3. Summarize recent developments.
> 4. Proceed with a summary of the clinical course.
> 5. Summarize the big picture and treatment goals.
> 6. Estimate and describe disability.
> 7. Discuss full supportive care, including tracheostomy and gastrostomy.
> 8. Discuss the option of palliative care.
> 9. Answer questions and clarify further if needed.
> 10. Document discussion, code status and level of care.

formulated by attorneys. Decision-makers for the patients therefore will have to interpret such a will. Nonetheless, the mere fact that a living will exists indicates that the patient has anticipated that a difficult medical situation may occur in the future. It expresses a wish by the patient to assist family members in making such decisions. Several states in the US have another option. Called POLST or MOLST, (physician or medical orders for life-sustaining treatment written by a physician) are a means to translate an advance directive into a physician order to be followed by all medical personnel. Physician may use the POLST form to write additional orders.

So, what should we do in this situation? Providing factual information is the first course of action, and this requires a formal family conference (Box 56.1). Sitting down and having a conversation in a separate, private, and quiet room is far more appropriate than a cursory discussion at the bedside. Physicians may need to show computed tomography scans (in this example, showing the large destructive hemorrhage), establish trust under stressful circumstances, and lead multiple conversations, which should include having the family summarize their assessment of the situation as well as what they think the patient would have wanted in such situation. Physicians should respect cultural and religious beliefs, even if these may be an impediment to rational medical care. Many families need considerable time to grasp the finality of the patient's condition. Mutual understanding of family preferences between the ICU team and family; and good medical planning minimizes family distress.

TABLE 56.1	**Information For Family Members When Discussing DNR Order**
Procedure	Chest compression, defibrillation, intubation, mechanical ventilation, invasive catheters, medications; may mean 20–30 minutes with poor brain perfusion (when it works)
Outcome of CPR	Two-thirds survive resuscitation; one-tenth survive to discharge
Consequences of DNR	Care otherwise not different Cardioversion still an option if needed for indications other than cardiac arrest ICU care may continue

Explanations should relay specific information (Table 56.1). If the patient has worsened, the family should understand why the patient has worsened. In some situations, a third party may be helpful in the discussions, and a medical ethics committee may be able to resolve differences if there is an emerging conflict between the patient's family and the treating physician. In fact, withholding or withdrawing treatment is a common reason for consulting the medical ethics committee. Ethics consultants may be able to spend additional time with the family—lack of time is often a limiting factor in ICU communications—explaining the issues at hand with equanimity and compassion. Yet, it remains to be seen whether ethics committees can defuse conflict once a very antagonistic family-physician relationship has developed (see chapter 60).

Families expect an estimate of outcome. what we say as neurologists about prognosis and the way we deliver this message may greatly influence decisions on subsequent level of care. This responsibility must be accepted with full understanding of its weight.

As mentioned earlier in Chapter 53, when communicating a poor prognosis leads to limitations in the level of care or withdrawal of life support, a *self-fulfilling prophecy* may occur. This concept has received considerable attention in the literature over the last decade. Some have even provocatively claimed that the prediction of a poor outcome might be the single factor most strongly associated with mortality in patients with intracerebral hemorrhage. Our prognostic abilities are imperfect, and this should be acknowledged. We should also be mindful of exaggerations or trivialization in the discussion of this important topic. Using this self-fulfilling prophecy concept in medicine can easily lead to ineffective circuitous reasoning, and there is a lot more to the story.

First, the *point of no return*, a condition incompatible with survival or meaningful recovery, is expected with severe brainstem injury, but defining the boundaries of *good, not too bad*, and *poor* outcome has proven far more difficult than it seems. Useful indicators of poor prognosis—often loss of pontomesencephalic reflexes and coma—have been described, but almost invariably the studies supporting their predictive value have not accounted for the potential influence of withdrawal of life support or restriction of aggressive care measures. In other words, an intracerebral hematoma volume exceeding 60 mL has been consistently associated with high mortality and poor recovery, but death in these patients is often preceded by withdrawal of life support, and prognostic studies have rarely accounted for this caveat or provided more neurological detail. Finding a solution to this limitation in studies on prognosis is very difficult because it would require analyzing a population of patients treated aggressively even after clinicians feel that such care has become frankly futile. It also would require a very detailed analysis of the neurological condition. For example, a comatose patient with a destructive hemorrhage causing persistent loss of several brainstem reflexes and extensor posturing is not expected to improve substantially, but a patient with spared brainstem reflexes might, and in such cases, withdrawal of life support may be premature.

Second, the other critical issue to keep in mind is that cognitive and physical incapacity rather than death is the outcome most feared by the vast majority of patients and families. The key question we are asked by families is not whether the patient can survive the acute brain insult but whether survival can be followed by meaningful functional recovery (admittedly the word "meaningful" is subjective and carries a certain arbitrariness). Studies evaluating the possible occurrence of the self-fulfilling prophecy using mortality as the main endpoint fail to address this point. In addition, even the most detailed statistical analysis may be insufficient to account for the effect of the combination of catastrophic brain disease and previous chronic illnesses in an elderly and previously debilitated patient. To sum up, in all honesty, we may not have the answer in all medical conditions, but it would be concerning—and create a truly unworkable environment for physicians—if the concept of self-fulfilling prophesy became a pretext to keep patients alive at whatever effort and cost.

Withdrawal of life support measures consists of extubation and discontinuation of any administered drugs apart from those strictly used to keep the patient comfortable. Central access and arterial catheters are removed, and the monitor is turned off. In our institution, we use the minimum doses of morphine and lorazepam necessary to achieve clear patient comfort. This is achieved by starting a morphine infusion of 0.1 mg/kg/h titrated to resolution of grimacing or labored breathing by increasing the infusion by small increments every 15 minutes. A lorazepam infusion of 0.05 mg/kg/h can be titrated upward slowly until symptoms of agitation or restlessness are controlled. In deeply comatose patients, none of this is indicated unless breathing after extubation becomes markedly labored. Most patients with brainstem injury die within hours after withdrawal of life support. In the event the patient remains stable, transfer to a private room outside of the ICU is best for the family.

How did we approach our quandary? We told the family that it was highly likely the patient would remain comatose. CPR could restore her heartbeat, but she would not recover the capacity to understand her situation. After daily conversations with the family about the patient's condition, it became clear that all of them understood the gravity of the brain injury. In these discussions, long-term care using a tracheostomy and gastrostomy was brought up. The family eventually decided that long-term care was not in her best interest, and a DNR order was placed. Several days later, the family decided to withdraw the ventilator and to provide palliative care only. They requested religious/spiritual practices (prayer, blessing, sacred texts) and sacrament of the sick to reinforce the patient's connection with sacredness. A chaplain conveyed a calming presence to de-escalate the emotionally charged situation.

The case illustrated here may seem an extreme in the spectrum of severity of acute brain damage, but it is a common situation in neurosciences ICUs. It was clear to all of us upon arrival that she could not recover, even with the most aggressive supportive treatment. This was not a quality-of-life discussion but whether to continue aggressive care in a patient likely to remain permanently comatose. We may not seriously harm the patient by continuing care against all odds or limiting care prematurely, but any reasonable person can see that we are already out of options at the onset of a truly catastrophic hemorrhage. To *allow natural death* (now known as AND) appropriately frames this type of situation; "pulling the plug" and "withholding care" are not helpful or adequate terms and they should be avoided. Yet, several family conferences were necessary before the family accepted that their loved one would not regain consciousness. By the time they requested withdrawal of life support measures, they were at peace with their decision and appreciative of the time we had spent with them and the care the patient had received. This may not always be the case and how to manage more demanding situations is discussed in Chapter 60.

KEY POINTS TO REMEMBER

- DNR orders may be warranted in catastrophic neurological injuries.
- The appropriateness of CPR ("full code") depends on the probability of good outcome and absence of life-shortening comorbidity.
- Repeated conversations with family members are extremely important, and quality time should be reserved to do so in an appropriate way.
- Decisions should include a broad picture of validated predictors of outcome, previous functional status, coexistent illnesses, and, most importantly, the patient's preferences.

Further Reading

Becker, K. J., A. B. Baxter, W. A. Cohen, et al. "Withdrawal of Support in Intracerebral Hemorrhage May Lead to Self-Fulfilling Prophecies." [In eng]. *Neurology* 56, no. 6 (Mar 27 2001): 766–72. https://doi.org/10.1212/wnl.56.6.766.

Bryan, A. F., A. J. Reich, A. C. Norton, et al. "Process of Withdrawal of Mechanical Ventilation at End of Life in the ICU: Clinician Perceptions." [In eng]. *CHEST Crit Care* 2, no. 2 (Jun 2024): 100051. doi:10.1016/j.chstcc.2024.100051.

Burns, J. P., J. Edwards, J. Johnson, et al. "Do-Not-Resuscitate Order After 25 Years." [In eng]. *Crit Care Med* 31, no. 5 (May 2003): 1543–50. https://doi.org/10.1097/01.Ccm.0000064743.44696.49.

Curtis, J. R., and M. R. Tonelli. "Shared Decision-Making in the ICU: Value, Challenges, and Limitations." [In eng]. *Am J Respir Crit Care Med* 183, no. 7 (Apr 1 2011): 840–41. https://doi.org/10.1164/rccm.201011-1836ED.

Hart, J. L., M. O. Harhay, N. B. Gabler, et al. "Variability Among US Intensive Care Units in Managing the Care of Patients Admitted With Preexisting Limits on Life-Sustaining Therapies." [In eng]. *JAMA Intern Med* 175, no. 6 (Jun 2015): 1019–26. https://doi.org/10.1001/jamainternmed.2015.0372.

Kluger, B. M., P. Hudson, L. C. Hanson, et al. "Palliative Care to Support the Needs of Adults With Neurological Disease." [In eng]. *Lancet Neurol* 22, no. 7 (Jul 2023): 619–31. https://doi.org/10.1016/s1474-4422(23)00129-1.

Rabinstein, A. A. "Ethical Dilemmas in the Neurologic ICU: Withdrawing Life-Support Measures After Devastating Brain Injury." *Continuum (Minneap Minn)* 15, no. 3 (2009): 13–25. https://doi.org/10.1212/01.CON.0000348807.68685.0b.

Rabinstein, A. A., R. L. McClelland, E. F. Wijdicks, et al. "Cardiopulmonary Resuscitation in Critically Ill Neurologic-Neurosurgical Patients." [In eng]. *Mayo Clin Proc* 79, no. 11 (Nov 2004): 1391–95. https://doi.org/10.4065/79.11.1391.

Rubin, M. A., J. Riecke, and E. Heitman. "Futility and Shared Decision-Making." [In eng]. *Neurol Clin* 41, no. 3 (Aug 2023): 455–67. https://doi.org/10.1016/j.ncl.2023.03.005.

Tian, J., D. A. Kaufman, S. Zarich, et al. "Outcomes of Critically Ill Patients Who Received Cardiopulmonary Resuscitation." [In eng]. *Am J Respir Crit Care Med* 182, no. 4 (Aug 15 2010): 501–6. https://doi.org/10.1164/rccm.200910-1639OC.

White, D. B., C. H. Braddock, 3rd, S. Bereknyei, and J. R. Curtis. "Toward Shared Decision Making at the End of Life in Intensive Care Units: Opportunities for Improvement." [In eng]. *Arch Intern Med* 167, no. 5 (Mar 12 2007): 461–67. https://doi.org/10.1001/archinte.167.5.461.

Wijdicks, E. F. M. *Communicating Prognosis Core Principles of Acute Neurology*. New York: Oxford University Press; 2014.

Wijdicks, E. F. M., and D. Y. Hwang. "Predicting Coma Trajectories: The Impact of Bias and Noise on Shared Decisions." [In eng]. *Neurocrit Care* 35, no. 2 (Oct 2021): 291–96. https://doi.org/10.1007/s12028-021-01324-y.

Wijdicks, E. F. M., and A. A. Rabinstein. "Absolutely No Hope? Some Ambiguity of Futility of Care in Devastating Acute Stroke." [In eng]. *Crit Care Med* 32, no. 11 (Nov 2004): 2332–42.

Wijdicks, E. F. M., and A. A. Rabinstein. "The Family Conference: End-of-Life Guidelines at Work for Comatose Patients." [In eng]. *Neurology 68*, no. 14 (Apr 3 2007): 1092–94. https://doi.org/10.1212/01.wnl.0000259401.36220.1a.

57 Brain Death Determination: Slip-ups and Other Misreadings

A 20-year-old graduate student was sideswiped while driving through an intersection. He was emergently intubated and admitted to the surgical trauma unit. He had multiple frontal and temporal lobe contusions, a pelvic fracture, and pulmonary contusions. He had no motor response to pain, fixed and dilated pupils, and no grimacing to pain. He had no pulse and required cardiopulmonary resuscitation for 30 minutes. He required vasopressors. Responders warmed him because his temperature declined to 35°C.

Neurosurgery placed an intracranial pressure (ICP) monitor that showed normal initial ICP readings, but ICP later increased to 40 to 50 mmHg, not responding to osmotic diuretics. Blood pressure remains unstable, now requiring three vasopressors. He is polyuric and on vasopressin. The trauma surgeon believes the patient is brain dead, as the patient stopped triggering the ventilator. Upon questioning, the intensive care unit (ICU) nurse tells you that the patient is not on any sedative drugs, and the providers discontinued fentanyl infusion 4 hours earlier.

What do you do now?

Severe traumatic brain injury will result in admission to a neurosciences ICU or, alternatively, to a surgical trauma ICU when there are additional multiple injuries. Extreme trauma can rapidly lead to brain death. In most parts of the world, trauma surgeons, neurosurgeons, and neurologists determine whether the patient meets the clinical criteria for brain death. For most of us, we determine brain death in our own patients and in our own ICU. The neurointensivist must carefully assess the situation when consulted to see these patients in other ICUs. Not being the attending physician means you need more time to understand the time course of events and interventions that have taken place. Evaluating a patient with catastrophic brain injury for possible brain death is never straightforward. This is a situation fraught with potential misreadings and slip-ups.

Any physician making the clinical diagnosis of brain death should work through a predetermined set of criteria. It starts with recognizing "red flags," confounders that neurologists recognize as unacceptable, which should make everyone uncomfortable about proceeding to a formal neurological examination (Box 57.1). Equally important is the opposite situation. There may be an unnecessary delay in brain death determination if examiners misinterpret certain clinical findings as incompatible with the diagnosis of brain death (Box 57.2).

First, ask yourself five questions: (1) Have I tried everything to reverse or improve the clinical picture? (2) Is the computed tomography scan compatible with irrecoverable brain injury? (3) Is the temperature normal? (4) Are there any lingering sedatives or illicit drugs? (5) Again and again, what else can deceive me?

BOX 57.1 **Situations Suggesting That the Patient May Not Be Brain Dead**

Insufficient time of observation

Cause of coma not firmly established

Treatable cause of coma

Major systemic instability or organ failure

Evidence of accidental or environmental hypothermia (<32°C)

Unsupported blood pressures, no need for vasopressors

Evidence of alcohol or drug use — or even a reasonable suspicion

> **BOX 57.2 Signs Compatible With Brain Death**
>
> Spinal cord reflexes (neck-arm flexion, arm lifting, head turning, triple-flexion response)
>
> Ventilator auto-triggering (ventilator at fault and auto-triggering due to minor changes in pressure or volume in the circuit)
>
> Preserved intracranial blood flow
>
> Presence of electroencephalographic activity

Another frequently asked question is "How long should one wait to declare a patient brain dead?" The answer must be "as long as it takes to determine a treatment is futile and to exclude confounders." Patients admitted to ICUs who have deteriorated from a major brain injury may "look" imminently agonal, but aggressive treatment—*occasionally*—can lead to substantial improvement. It is absolutely premature to declare brain death before treating an active central nervous system infection, brain edema, undrained hydrocephalus, nondecompressed mass effect, any major uncorrected laboratory abnormality, or marked hypothermia. In these patients, previously absent brainstem reflexes and motor responses can return.

However, when a demonstrably apneic patient has lost all brainstem reflexes—and there is no other explanation—nothing will return, not even after waiting another day. There is a noticeably clear dividing line in neuropathology. The evolutionary, innate resilience of the brainstem explains why so many patients (>90% of all neuro-calamities) never fulfill the criteria of brain death. And furthermore, the number of brain death determinations is declining rapidly, for reasons not well understood. It could be due to rapid withdrawal of support initiated by family members rather than a changing practice of more decompressive surgery. For better or worse, increasing numbers of donors after circulatory death may be another factor; more patients with catastrophic brain injury are now dying after extubation in the operating room (see Chapter 58).

Clearance of sedative drugs requires calculation of time to elimination (the sum of five half-lives is conservative in normal use but inaccurate with large intoxications). The most common drugs are fentanyl ($t_{1/2}$ = 6 hours), lorazepam

($t_{1/2}$ = 15 hours), midazolam ($t_{1/2}$ = 6 hours), phenobarbital ($t_{1/2}$ = 100 hours), and thiopental ($t_{1/2}$ = 20 hours). If there is a massive overdose we should stand back and certainly if the CT scan of the brain is not too abnormal. If patients have been treated by targeted temperature management (rare these days) or if there has been ischemic liver injury after cardiopulmonary resuscitation, it will be exceedingly difficult—if not impossible—to exclude a lingering sedative effect. Most neuromuscular junction blockers dissipate within several hours (the commonly used atracurium $t_{1/2}$ = 30 minutes), but the simplest proof of elimination is the return of deep tendon reflexes. Bedside nerve stimulators are also an option. Other potentially confounding medical conditions are hypothermia (<32°C), severe hyponatremia (<110 mmol/L), hypernatremia (>160 mmol/L), hypoglycemia (<40 mg/dL), or hypercalcemia (>3.4 mmol/L), but these values are not proven cut-offs and only warnings that another process may be present. For example, worsening hypernatremia with frequent use of osmotic agents must not be an impediment to brain death declaration. But it is essential to consider illicit drug and alcohol use and to exclude it quickly with a toxicology screen. It must be said, but when we test brain death determination in our simulation center, learners seldom consider this major confounder.

Box 57.3 summarizes the main decisions and line of action. In any equivocal situation, physicians should simply go back to square one and follow these steps. We often give this simple advice when asked what to do.

The actual neurological evaluation of determining brain death consists of 25 tests and verifications. Brain death determination is complex (more than checking a few brainstem reflexes in an apneic patient), requires expertise (hopefully, a neurologist or neurointensivist), and demands perfect diagnostic accuracy (no room for error). The overriding principle is simple: establish cause, determine futility, exclude confounders, examine brainstem reflexes, and test for apnea. Many physicians have difficulty with the apnea test, but the test—a CO_2 challenge using oxygen diffusion—is simple and safe when the steps are followed carefully. Problems typically arise when physicians proceed without carefully checking all prerequisites. You cannot just remove the patient from the ventilator and provide extra oxygen insufflation without adequate preparation; there are too many patients with a high alveolar-arterial gradient from early neurogenic pulmonary edema or aspiration. For sure, the apnea test remains problematic in any patient with a traumatic pneumothorax.

PROCEDURES AND TESTS TO DECLARE BRAIN DEATH

PREREQUISITES (ALL MUST BE CHECKED)
- ☐ Coma, irreversible and cause known
- ☐ Neuroimaging explains coma *(review CT close to time of examination)*
- ☐ Sedative drug effect absent *(if indicated, order a toxicology screen)*
- ☐ No residual effect or paralytic drug *(if indicated, use peripheral nerve stimulator)*
- ☐ Absence of severe acid-base, electrolyte, or endocrine abnormality *(no cut off values known)*
- ☐ Normal or near normal temperature *(core temperature ≥36°C)*
- ☐ Systolic blood pressure ≥100 mm Hg
- ☐ No spontaneous respirations

EXAMINATION (ALL MUST BE CHECKED)
- ☐ Pupils non-reactive to bright light *(mid-position at 5-7 mm)*
- ☐ Corneal reflexes absent *(saline jet and tissue paper touch)*
- ☐ Eyes immobile, oculocephalic reflexes absent *(tested only if C-spine integrity ensured)*
- ☐ No facial movement to noxious stimuli at supraorbital nerve or temporomandibular joint compression
- ☐ Gag reflex absent *(gloved index finger to posterior pharynx)*
- ☐ Cough reflex absent to tracheal suctioning *(2 passes)*
- ☐ No motor response to noxious stimuli in all 4 limbs *(triple flexion response is spinal-medicated reflex)*

APNEA TESTING (ALL MUST BE CHECKED)
- ☐ Patient is hemodynamically stable *(systolic blood pressure ≥100 mm Hg)*
- ☐ Ventilator adjusted to normocapnia *($PaCO_2$ 35-45 mm Hg)*
- ☐ Patient pre-oxygenated with 100% oxygen for 10 minutes *($PaO2$ ≥200 mm Hg)*
- ☐ Patient maintains oxygenation with a PEEP of 5 cm H_2O *(if not, consider recruitment maneuver)*
- ☐ Disconnect ventilator
- ☐ Provide oxygen via an insufflation catheter to the level of the carina at 6 liters/min or attach T-piece with CPAP valve @ 10-20 cm H_2O and resuscitation bag
- ☐ Spontaneous respirations absent
- ☐ Arterial blood gas drawn at 8-10 minutes, patient reconnected to ventilator
- ☐ $PaCO_2$ ≥60 mm Hg and arterial pH <7.3, or 20 mm Hg rise of $PaCO_2$ from normal baseline value or apnea test aborted and confirmatory ancillary test *(cerebral blood flow study)*

DOCUMENTATION OF BRAIN DEATH
- ☐ Time of death *(use time of final blood gas result or time of completion of confirmatory ancillary test)*

BOX 57.3 The complete procedure of brain death determination shown as one step at a time. There are other things everyone should know: 1) a guideline from a professional organization is an educational tool not a mandate, 2) US state laws may have additional modifications such as type of specialty and a requirement to repeat the examination by a separate examiner, 3) throughout the world major differences exist in examination specifications, and 4) religious and cultural objections should be recognized.

One examination should suffice for adults, but some U.S. states require two physicians to examine the patient. There is enough evidence in adults that a second examination does not change the initial findings when executed appropriately. A second examination also may delay the final determination, and it may take over 12 hours to find a suitable second examiner and we remain a little puzzled why. However, in infants and children (30 days to 18 years), professional organizations continue to recommend repeat examinations and having two examinations performed by two separate examiners and we remain a little puzzled why. The clinical examination always concludes with an apnea test, and the time of completion of this test is the time of death (if the patient meets criteria).

Ancillary tests may have far less specificity than appreciated. Nonetheless, ancillary tests are mandatory in some European, Latin American, and Asian countries. Sometimes it seems to us that the focus in brain death determination has unfortunately shifted to finding an ideal technical test rather than improving clinical competence.

These ancillary tests may not fit the clinical examination. In fact, (partially) preserved blood flow is just a reflection of the ICP, which may not be high enough to stop blood entry through the dura into the skull (i.e., extremely high ICP, no flow; high but not extremely high ICP, preserved flow). The same applies to electrodiagnostic tests; they are just a reflection of cortical function and not brainstem function. To use these tests in patients with confounding drug effects or even intoxication to shorten observation time or to declare brain death—assuming no flow or no electrical brain activity—will lead to errors. No physician wants to declare a patient brain dead using a confirmatory test to override a confounder and later learn from the nursing staff that motor movement are repeated seen or spontaneous breathing has resumed.

So, what should you do? The patient suffered anoxic-ischemic injury in addition to traumatic diffuse axonal and contusional brain injury, and reversal of this condition is not likely. In this patient, it is prudent to wait another day (five half-lives of fentanyl is 30 hours – 4 hours of discontinuation = 26 hours). Obtaining a drug screen to exclude drugs the patient may have co-ingested (alcohol level, serum toxicological screen) is also necessary.

Brain death determination is complex and best performed by an experienced examiner. How to define "experienced" and judge competency is an ongoing discussion. This also relates to training and how to measure proficiency. We can assume that nonneurologists feel reluctant and even non-hospital-based neurologists (the majority) feel challenged by the complex critical care environment. It is not simply reading a guideline and placing the check marks. It is complex work. We think it is more reliable to leave this procedure in the hands of a neurointensivist, but we cannot know for sure. All neurointensivists should actively perform brain death determinations in their respective hospitals; that is the way we learned— embarrassed by our mistakes, oversights, and misreadings that we fortunately caught in time. This should be the neurointensivists' "rite of passage."

Brain death determination allows closure and options for organ donation. The uniform determination of death act (UDDA) is the legal underpinning of such determination and simple in its approach. The UDDA sets forth two standards for determining death (circulatory death and brain death) and leaves to the medical community to elaborate criteria by which physicians can determine when those standards have been met. In the USA, the UDDA has been of paramount importance to families of comatose patients, and the health care professionals who care for them. There is no medical rationale for continuing care if there is no consent for organ donation. No ICU has the obligation to care for a legally deceased person, and in the extreme, it is unethical to hold the bed if it results in refusal of necessary transfers of other patients. (For more information about the quandaries see Chapter 60.)

KEY POINTS TO REMEMBER

- Brain death determination is time consuming and demands strict adherence to a protocol including a detailed neurological examination. No shortcuts can be allowed.
- Most of the time should be spent in finding confounding factors.
- Remember that patients with traumatic brain injury may have taken illicit drugs or alcohol.
- The diagnosis is based on a clinical neurological examination and not on cerebral blood flow or an electrodiagnostic study.
- Brain death determination for infants and children requires two examinations by two separate physicians.
- In the United States, one examination is usually sufficient for adults (>18 years), but hospital protocols may be different. Some states and hospitals require that two physicians examine the patient and document their findings.

- Several countries around the world require brain death confirmation by a second or third (and sometimes even fourth) physician. We strongly disagree.
- Ancillary tests are legally necessary in some countries. We also disagree—again, strongly.

Further Reading

Greer, D. M., M. P. Kirschen, A. Lewis, et al. "Pediatric and Adult Brain Death/Death by Neurologic Criteria Consensus Guideline: Report of the AAN Guidelines Subcommittee, AAP, CNS, and SCCM." [In eng]. *Neurology* (Oct 11 2023): 10.1212/WNL.0000000000207740. https://doi.org/10.1212/WNL.0000000000207740. Epub ahead of print. PMID: 37821233

Jain, S., and M. DeGeorgia. "Brain Death-Associated Reflexes and Automatisms." [In eng]. *Neurocrit Care* 3, no. 2 (2005): 122–26. https://doi.org/10.1385/ncc:3:2:122.

Lustbader, D., D. O'Hara, E. F. Wijdicks, et al. "Second Brain Death Examination May Negatively Affect Organ Donation." [In eng]. *Neurology* 76, no. 2 (Jan 11 2011): 119–24. https://doi.org/10.1212/WNL.0b013e3182061b0c.

Wijdicks, E. F. M. "Brain Death Guidelines Explained." [In eng]. *Semin Neurol* 35, no. 2 (Apr 2015): 105–15. https://doi.org/10.1055/s-0035-1547532.

Wijdicks, E. F. M. "The Clinical Determination of Brain Death: Rational and Reliable." [In eng]. *Semin Neurol* 35, no. 2 (Apr 2015): 103–4. https://doi.org/10.1055/s-0035-1547531.

Wijdicks, E. F. M. "How I Do a Brain Death Examination: The Tools of the Trade." [In eng]. *Crit Care* 24, no. 1 (Nov 18 2020): 648. https://doi.org/10.1186/s13054-020-03376-6.

Wijdicks, E. F. M., and C. Burkle. "The Language of the UDDA is Sufficiently Precise and Pragmatic." [In eng]. *Neurocrit Care* (Jun 11 2024). doi:10.1007/s12028-024-02004-3. Epub ahead of print.

58 When to Mention Organ Donation

A 51-year-old man was admitted with a devastating ganglionic hemorrhage. Soon after arrival, he was intubated in the emergency department. About 2 hours after the ictus, the patient's eyes remained closed without opening to temporomandibular pressure and he had fixed midsize pupils, absent corneal reflexes, and minimal oculovestibular responses but a strong cough response after tracheal suctioning. He also had spontaneous extensor posturing and triple flexion responses with Babinski signs. The computed tomography scan showed a large, destructive ganglionic hemorrhage starting in the putamen and extending into the frontal lobe and diencephalon. There was trapping of the third ventricle and acute hydrocephalus. In a desperate (and likely ineffective) attempt to improve the neurological condition, a ventriculostomy was placed. Over the next hours, more brainstem reflexes disappeared, and only a faint cough reflex and a breathing drive remained, as evidenced by triggering of the ventilator.

The family understood very well that nothing more could be done. The family brought up his previously expressed strong wish for organ donation if something terminal happened to him. The family hoped to donate his organs after withdrawal of support.

What do you do now?

Catastrophic neurological injury may be obvious even within hours after presentation. In extreme cases, acute neurosurgical intervention, or other measures to reduce increased intracranial pressure are futile. In these acute circumstances with rapid onset of coma, neurologists and neurosurgeons try to identify "a point of no return," defined by the degree of destruction, the involvement of crucial structures maintaining awareness (i.e., thalamocortical connections), and persistent upper brainstem dysfunction. Clinically, the injury translates into no pupillary light responses, no corneal responses, and no oculocephalic responses. The lower part of the brainstem (lower pons and medulla oblongata) often still functions, as evidenced by the presence of (abnormal) motor response to a noxious stimulus, a cough response to tracheal suctioning, and the preserved ability to trigger a ventilator.

When it is a foregone conclusion that there will be no recovery, de-escalation or full withdrawal of intensive care support will rapidly come up during a family conference. Both families and physicians may mention organ donation *after* the decision is made to withdraw support. This timepoint in decision-making is crucially important because suggesting organ donation before there is consensus to withdraw support may be misinterpreted by distrustful family members (but also ethicists) as a veiled attempt to obtain donor organs. If feasible, and after a firm decision to withdraw support, organ donation should be explored and discussed in a separate meeting with organ donation procurement officers—at least this is how we like to do it. Organ donation is possible through a donation after cardiac/circulatory death (DCD) protocol or through donation after brain death (DBD).

Two clinical scenarios are possible. First, a proportion of candidates for a DCD protocol may still eventually progress to loss of all brainstem function and be officially declared brain dead. The procedures of DBD are well established. But if patients do not meet the clinical criteria for brain death, they could potentially become candidates for donation after withdrawal of life support through a DCD protocol. Again, it requires two important decisions: to establish with certainty the presence of a hopeless situation and to decide when to withdraw life support measures. Proponents of a DCD protocol have claimed a significant increase in donation rates, but the increase has still been less pronounced than originally hoped.

A DCD procurement protocol is more complicated and restricted than a DBD protocol. Crucial differences between the two protocols are shown in Table 58.1.

To maintain accreditation, many hospitals in the United States must have a DCD protocol in place; however, few physicians fully understand their responsibilities within these protocols. Utilization of DCD protocols worldwide is more variable, with marked differences in utilization between Asian and European countries. (Most notable is the continuous absence of DCD protocols in Germany and is not permitted by the German Medical Association.) DCD protocols are far from uniform, and differences exist in determinations of permanent circulatory arrest, type of consent required, and even definition of circulatory arrest. DCD involves retrieval of abdominal organs, and a few centers have developed protocols that include lung and heart retrieval; the early results are similar to outcomes in brain death donors. In some countries (Belgium, the

TABLE 58.1 **Differences Between DCD and DBD Protocols**

Variables	DCD	DBD
Age	There is an upper limit[a]	All ages (in principle)
Preconditions	No confounders and irremediable cause	No confounders and irremediable cause
Clinical findings	Devastating neurological injury and often loss of upper brainstem function	Coma, absent brainstem reflexes, no motor response and apnea
Eligibility determination	Attending physician and transplant surgeon through organ donation agency	Attending physician (may need confirmation by another physician)
Organ recovery	2–5 minutes circulatory arrest after patient extubation in the operating room	Immediately after arrival to operating room
Organ/tissue	All those consented (heart and lungs rarely procured)	All those consented
Triage	May return to ICU for palliative care if patient breathes after extubation	Morgue

[a] Cut-off is variable depending on the protocol of the individual organ procurement organization (much lower for heart procurement). Often it is age of 60 years.

Netherlands, Canada, and Spain), euthanasia is combined with organ donation. Other situations, which seemingly disregard the "dead donor rule," raise serious ethical concerns, but the transplantation community is moving ahead fast.

In brief, the DCD protocol is based on organ retrieval after circulatory arrest. After a consensus to withdraw life support, the patient may become a candidate for a DCD protocol. Eligibility is decided by an organ procurement coordinator who is in contact with the transplant surgeon, requires a detailed conversation with the family and a signed informed consent, a determination of organ suitability, and a match with a recipient. A detailed medical and social history is obtained from the family. Contraindications to organ donation may include older age, infectious diseases (notably HIV and hepatitis C), potentially transmissible malignancies (including primary brain tumors manipulated by biopsy or ventriculostomy), and, most commonly, unsuitable organs. Blood (or tissue) samples are sent to a laboratory designated by the organ procurement organization for serological testing and tissue typing.

The family needs to understand that the entire DCD procedure may take about 24 to 36 hours to complete. During this time, the patient is examined regularly because progression to brain death may still occur. This later transition to brain death is dependent on the time from the injury but is not expected if no neurological deterioration has been observed for 2 days. The family should also be informed that the patient goes intubated to an operating room. Extubation takes place in the operating room, but after extubation the patient may breathe, pressure may not fall precipitously, and the heart may not stop. Guidelines indicate this maximum period of 60 to 90 minutes between withdrawal of life support and death, after which patients become ineligible for DCD. But some recommend that the liver only be retrieved if death ensues within 30 minutes after withdrawal of life support, while the kidney and pancreas may be still retrieved if death occurs within 60 minutes. Other surgeons link age to the time it takes to circulatory arrest; in other words, older age no longer than 60 minutes wait until circulatory arrest.

If circulatory arrest does not happen within a predefined time interval (~60–90 minutes), the DCD procedure is aborted, and the patient will return to the ICU for further palliative care. Usual palliative care orders will be started, and the arterial catheter will be removed (bleeding may occur and sometimes be profuse due to the high dose of heparin administered during the pre-DCD preparation). We expect the patient to succumb several hours after return to the ICU.

What can the family expect if they decide to go ahead? Organ procurement coordinators work closely with families to ensure that all the details and timing work for the family and for the surgeons. The organs are recovered by a trained transplant surgeon anonymous to the donor's family. All conversations go through the trained organ procurement representative. After all appropriate preparations, the patient is transferred to the operating room and prepared for organ retrieval. In the operating room, the patient is fully draped with the thorax and abdomen sterilized. Instruments are prepared and placed on a tray. For family members, coming to the operating room is a major event and a new, likely difficult experience despite the best intentions and preparation of the surgical staff. (Some of our neuroscience staff have had a visceral response after witnessing the procedure and many prefer not to participate.) In the dimly lit, serene operating room, the family sits close to the patient's head, behind a sterile drape. Usually, only the attending physician, an anesthesiologist, a surgical nurse, and the organ procurement coordinator are present. The surgical team is out of the operating room and out of sight.

The team present is a designated physician who can declare the patient and has written orders for possible comfort medication. Morphine 2 mg intravenously is administered if major discomfort is noted with breathing and this medication has been brought to the operating room. (The organ donation agency is not involved in directing medication administration.)

The patient is extubated. After extubation, the patient may gasp for several minutes, becoming deeply cyanotic until breathing stops. It may take several minutes for circulatory arrest to occur. (Asystole is not a criterion, although both asystole and circulatory arrest often occur simultaneously.) This circulatory arrest is noted when the arterial line is consistently unable to measure pressures (shown by the monitor with the appearance of a question mark sign where numbers used to be). The determination of circulatory arrest requires absent pulse in the carotid artery and zero reading of the invasive arterial pressure tracing. At that point, the family is told that the patient has died and they are escorted out of the operating room. After circulatory arrest is determined and documented, a "death watch" begins with monitoring for any change. This is to ensure that the circulatory arrest is permanent. The timeframe may vary according to institution but ranges between 2 and 5 minutes. After that interval has passed, the surgical team enters the operating room and proceeds quickly with a large, thoracoabdominal-splitting incision followed by rapid cooling, cannulation of major arteries, infusion of preservation fluids, and mobilization of transplantable organs. The transplant surgeon may determine on inspection that certain organs are unsuitable for organ donation. The deceased patient then goes to the morgue.

There is growing interest in heart procurement from DCD donors. Centers allowing donation of the heart after a clinical trial showed feasibility and safety of transplantation of hearts from circulatory-death donors. There are two main approaches. One is where the surgically retrieved donor heart enters a perfusion system (recent technology such as the TransMedics Organ Care System™ [OCS™], nicknamed "Heart in a Box"). The other (more problematic) method requires the use of normothermic regional perfusion of the donor following circulatory death by means of central extracorporeal life support. In other words, after spontaneous circulation has stopped, it is then restarted through a pump connected to cannulae inserted into the ascending aorta and the right atrium. Restoration of brain perfusion is excluded by clamping of the aortic arch arteries (the problematic part). The initial qualms about the ethical standing of DCD may have subsided, but heart procurement brings up a much more challenging set of issues: Circulatory arrest happened but was then reversed after 5 minutes of "death watch." The brain could be perfused if it weren't for the intentional (and rather crude) closure of the feeding arteries. If we can resuscitate patients after being down for some time with some as alert as if nothing had happened, it is no wonder that some of our colleagues are strongly opposed to playing any part in these procedures. (This concern is immaterial in patients who have remained comatose with loss of several brainstem reflexes but never fully progressed to brain death.)

Again, if circulatory arrest does not occur within the prespecified time (usually 60–90 minutes), the patient is transported back to the ICU (or to a regular room) to receive palliative measures. These failed DCD attempts can be distressing to families and discouraging to the medical team. They also use considerable resources.

The time to respiratory and circulatory arrest in the operating room after extubation is difficult to predict; most studies show a 50/50 chance of respiratory/circulatory arrest within the allotted observation time. The organ procurement coordinator often will try to do a "mini apnea test" in the ICU, basically placing the patient on a continuous positive airway pressure of 5 cmH$_2$O and watching for respiratory deterioration. In the absence of respiratory deterioration, the chance that the patient will develop a respiratory arrest after extubation in the operating room later is smaller. Some organ procurement officers will call the procedure off and have the patient not go to the operating room. However, most available predictive scores are not specifically adapted for neurological patients. In a multicenter study, we devised and tested a new score (DCD-N) and attached 1 point to absent corneal reflexes, 2 points to absent cough reflex, 1 point to extensor or absent motor response, and 1 point for oxygenation index greater than 3. The sum score provides a probability of survival beyond 60 minutes (Figure 58.1).

The original study on DCD-N found that a score of 3 or more translated into a 74% chance of death within 60 minutes (positive predictive value), and a score of 0 to 2 translated into a 77% chance of survival beyond

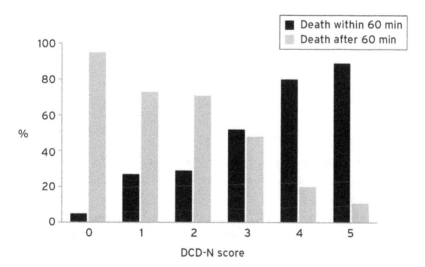

FIGURE 58.1 Percentage of patients with survival or death within 60 minutes. High predictability with highest scores.

60 minutes (negative predictive value). A recent validation study showed the DCD-N score had a lower positive predictive value of 36.4% and a negative predictive value of 91.7% to predict death within 60 minutes after withdrawal of support. Because brainstem reflexes may change during the waiting period, prediction may change. No other currently available model has better predictive values, but high odds of no circulatory arrest within 60 minutes should not necessarily discourage teams from moving forward—in other words, it may be still worth trying. Nonetheless, we can estimate the number of non-utilizations to be possibly still at 30-50%. Obviously, this must exclude patients who transitioned to brain death while waiting for transport to the operating room and who obviously will not breathe. But failed donations could put additional psychological strain on procurement teams and families. It should be emphasized that Families must be forewarned that their loved one may return to the ICU if circulatory arrest does not occur.

DCD protocols create an important opportunity to donate tissue and organs, but the decisions—starting with the determination to withdraw support—are far more complicated and ethically challenging than in cases of DBD. With an expected increase in DCD donors—still only about 20% to 30% of all donors but growing—physicians should be aware of these procedures.

Organ donation is for the lucky ones, and in the United States approximately 6000 patients die yearly on the growing organ donation waiting list with over 100,000 patients. The other sad fact is that there are not enough organs available for everyone who needs one.

KEY POINTS TO REMEMBER

- Catastrophically injured patients may be candidates for a DCD protocol after the decision is made to proceed with comfort care measures.
- Some patients in a DCD protocol become brain dead. It therefore remains important to repeatedly examine the patient's neurological status until it is time to go to the operating room.

- The DCD procedure involves many steps and requires close communication with an organ procurement coordinator.
- Patients return to the ICU for palliative care if respiratory and circulatory arrest does not occur after extubation in the operating room.

Further Reading

Blondeel, J., M. Blondeel, N. Gilbo, et al. "Simultaneous Lung-Abdominal Organ Procurement From Donation After Circulatory Death Donors Reduces Donor Hepatectomy Time." [In eng]. *Transplantation* 108, no. 1 (Jan 1 2024): 192–7. https://doi.org/10.1097/tp.0000000000004669.

Cannon, R. M. "Prediction of Organ Donation After Circulatory Death: In Search of a Better Crystal Ball." [In eng]. *Transplantation* 105, no. 6 (Jun 1 2021): 1165–66. https://doi.org/10.1097/tp.0000000000003431.

Citerio, G., M. Cypel, G. J. Dobb, et al. "Organ Donation in Adults: A Critical Care Perspective." [In eng]. *Intensive Care Med* 42, no. 3 (Mar 2016): 305–15. https://doi.org/10.1007/s00134-015-4191-5.

Domínguez-Gil, B., B. Haase-Kromwijk, H. Van Leiden, et al. "Current Situation of Donation After Circulatory Death in European Countries." [In eng]. *Transpl Int* 24, no. 7 (Jul 2011): 676–86. https://doi.org/10.1111/j.1432-2277.2011.01257.x.

Emanuel, E. J., B. D. Onwuteaka-Philipsen, J. W. Urwin, and J. Cohen. "Attitudes and Practices of Euthanasia and Physician-Assisted Suicide in the United States, Canada, and Europe." [In eng]. *Jama* 316, no. 1 (Jul 5 2016): 79–90. https://doi.org/10.1001/jama.2016.8499.

Fugate, J. E., M. Stadtler, A. A. Rabinstein, and E. F. Wijdicks. "Variability in Donation After Cardiac Death Protocols: A National Survey." [In eng]. *Transplantation* 91, no. 4 (Feb 27 2011): 386–89. https://doi.org/10.1097/TP.0b013e318204ee96.

Morrissey, P. E., and A. P. Monaco. "Donation After Circulatory Death: Current Practices, Ongoing Challenges, and Potential Improvements." [In eng]. *Transplantation* 97, no. 3 (Feb 15 2014): 258–64. https://doi.org/10.1097/01.TP.0000437178.48174.db.

Murphy, N. B., M. Slessarev, J. Basmaji, et al. "Ethical Issues in Normothermic Regional Perfusion in Controlled Organ Donation After Determination of Death by Circulatory Criteria: A Scoping Review." [In eng]. *Transplantation* (Aug 28 2024). doi:10.1097/TP.0000000000005161.

Nijhoff, M. F., R. A. Pol, M. Volbeda, et al. "External Validation of the DCD-N Score and a Linear Prediction Model to Identify Potential Candidates for Organ Donation After Circulatory Death: A Nationwide Multicenter Cohort Study." [In eng].

Transplantation 105, no. 6 (Jun 1 2021): 1311–16. https://doi.org/10.1097/tp.00000 00000003430.

Rabinstein, A. A., A. H. Yee, J. Mandrekar, et al. "Prediction of Potential for Organ Donation After Cardiac Death in Patients in Neurocritical State: A Prospective Observational Study." [In eng]. *Lancet Neurol* 11, no. 5 (May 2012): 414–19. https:// doi.org/10.1016/s1474-4422(12)70060-1.

Schroder, J. N., C. B. Patel, A. D. DeVore, et al. "Transplantation Outcomes With Donor Hearts After Circulatory Death." [In eng]. *N Engl J Med* 388, no. 23 (Jun 8 2023): 2121–31. https://doi.org/10.1056/NEJMoa2212438.

Smith, M., B. Dominguez-Gil, D. M. Greer, et al. "Organ Donation After Circulatory Death: Current Status and Future Potential." [In eng]. *Intensive Care Med* 45, no. 3 (Mar 2019): 310–21. https://doi.org/10.1007/s00134-019-05533-0.

Wijdicks, E. F. M. *Brain Death*. 3rd ed. New York: Oxford University Press; 2017.

SECTION 6

THE OTHER SIDE OF NEUROCRITICAL CARE: COMMUNICATION CONUNDRUMS

59 Patients Coming In and Going Out

Triage nurse: I have a call from an outside physician about a possible transfer. I will connect the two of you.

MD: Hi. I am an emergency physician in a small hospital, and I have a 67-year-old man here who was found down, was intubated in the field, and has a cerebellar bleed, and I want to send him over.

YOU: Tell me more.

MD: He is now sedated, but his pupils were anisocoric and responsive to light. Corneal reflexes were both absent, he had a spontaneous vertical nystagmus, and his eyes looked skewed. He had bilateral extensor posturing. He is not triggering the ventilator and may be apneic. His platelets are normal, but his international normalized ratio is 4. So we immediately gave him four-factor prothrombin complex. The computed tomography (CT) scan shows a large cerebellar hematoma with acute hydrocephalus. I gave him a bolus of 23% hypertonic saline through his femoral artery. We will fly him.

YOU: Thank you, and we will give a heads up to our neurosurgeons because he may need decompression and evacuation of the hematoma; we will expect him soon.

What do you do now?

Do you remember having a conversation like this? Probably not. We wish all transfer requests had this level of detail. But we often hear "brain bleed, GCS [Glasgow Coma Scale] of 3, intubated, and on its way." In a fast-moving medical world, we want to save time, but ironically, we often end up wasting time just sorting through useless information. There are problems in our current ways of communication, even with more digital communication platforms at hand.

Ideally, communicating with each other must be disease specific. We cannot expect or demand superior knowledge of the neurologic examination and full understanding of the clinical patterns from those less experienced in assessing acutely ill neurologic patients, but still an abbreviated summary of clinical course, diagnosis (or differential diagnosis) and neuroimaging results is needed.

Also, once we start texting each other with fragments of information, which are often not shared with others, situations become chaotic, and nobody seems fully knowledgeable and "in charge." Some people may have more information than others, the full picture gets lost, and that is confusing to the attending neurointensivist.

What can we do about it? When it comes to communication about a triage over the phone, we think that following a mnemonic called TELL ME (Figure 59.1) may help physicians (or any other referring health care professional) standardize and focus their communication. These are knowing the time course (new and unexpected or ongoing for some time), extracting essential information from less essential particulars, communicating which tests are pending (CT and laboratory), relaying how much support will be needed (e.g., secretion burden, intubation), knowing which emergency drugs have been administered (e.g., mannitol, antiepileptics, anticoagulation reversal agents), and planning for worst-case scenarios. With this information, the receiving staff knows what to expect and can be well prepared to intervene quickly. The mnemonic invites a back-and-forth discussion because it queries why crucial support is needed, what is already provided, and how the patient has been managed. But if our questions continuously lead to new information (the proverbial "the plot thickens"), we have a communication issue. Once we end the interaction, we must summarize what we understood.

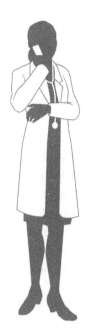
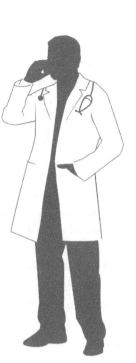

Time Course
Essence
Laboratory
Life-Sustaining Interventions

Management
Expectation

FIGURE 59.1 TELL ME mnemonic.

We can all agree that a busy environment affects structure and processes. Information sharing must "check a few boxes" before we can confidently understand the full picture, and this must include the basic chronology of events. Incorporating a checklist into the electronic health record allows data to autopopulate and eliminates reliance on the provider's memory for specific details of, for instance, medication dosages or administration times.

Starting a conversation with a final working diagnosis and then discussing how you arrived there is a good approach when the diagnosis seems sufficiently certain. The listener's mind is better primed to hear the key findings rather than waiting for the presenting puzzling story to unravel. A few options can be mentioned, but going over a long differential diagnosis just takes too long and comes later. When the diagnosis is uncertain, however, jumping to one from the start may bias the receiving physician ("anchoring" in the wrong diagnosis is always a major risk).

Cut to the very essence of the problem. Some information, while significant, may also not be immediately essential; for example, the symmetry or absence of reflexes is not essential information (unless the patient has Guillain-Barré syndrome), and the same with tone (unless the patient has a serotonin syndrome or exhibits dysautonomic storming). Communicating these essential findings is a learned skill that requires knowledge and remains the crux of all communication problems. Physicians should lean toward simple diagnoses and simple solutions but remain able to recognize something unusual. Scale and score numbers help but may also confuse; we seldom know how the person arrived at the numbers, particularly when the scores and scales are summed up—a GCS of 7 may mean different things depending on the scoring of its individual components. Using simple scales and sum scores may adversely affect how we communicate the results of the neurologic examination and neuroimaging. "The CT scan shows no bleed" is not an appropriate description. Instead, "the CT scan shows no hyperdense middle cerebral artery (MCA) or basilar sign, the basal cisterns are open, the ventricles are normal in size, there are normal cortical sulci, and gray and white matter structures can be distinguished" provides a ton of useful information. Becoming articulate takes time and training.

So, which patients are the best candidates for the neurosciences intensive care unit (neuro-ICU) and, indeed, should not be admitted anywhere else? By its nature, the neuro-ICU is for the medical and neurosurgical management of critical neurologic disorders and for the postoperative care of neurosurgical patients. An unstable acute neurological disease belongs in the neuro-ICU as well as severe physiologic derangements or any other progression of a prior medical illness in neurological or neurosurgical patients. Admission to the neuro-ICU must be free of bias and requires excellent rapport among the physician, nurse manager, and charge nurse. Criteria for neuro-ICU admission should be flexible. Neurocritical illness is rarely defined by systemic criteria but by the high likelihood the patient may deteriorate quickly from consequences of the initial brain injury. We need to consider carefully causes of deterioration in a specific acute brain injury. Also, sedation for marked agitation or monitoring of airway patency alone may justify admission for some patients. Patients with unsalvageable acute brain injury may be admitted to the neuro-ICU simply because transition to comfort care rarely takes place in the emergency department. These patients are, therefore, appropriately, or not, admitted to the neuro-ICU to await the arrival of their families or to allow time for the families to say their goodbyes. We also have encountered situations in which families have not understood the gravity of the patient's condition and need additional clarification. Palliation may also involve the activation of an organ procurement protocol, and these complex logistics are better managed in the neuro-ICU.

Triage out of the neuro-ICU is equally complex. Valuable information is needed on medications and recent changes or discontinuation. Patients with an inability to clear secretions require close attention, and we cannot expect the same level of attention on the ward. Patients with fluctuating blood pressure despite oral medication will likely return to the ICU ("bounce back"). On the other hand, patients with previously stable blood pressures may develop a blood pressure surge refractory to medication soon after transfer. We must accept that nothing is perfect, and a justified return to the ICU is not a failure. Unfortunately, however, administrators now use ICU and hospital readmissions as a quality measure. Moreover, excessively restrictive criteria for ICU discharge may jeopardize admission of more needy patients. A machine learning algorithm has identified patients that are not readmitted to the ICU and will not die within 48 h after discharge. Will this also work for neurological patients? Is that too much to hope for?

KEY POINTS TO REMEMBER

- Discussing a multifaceted neurocritical disease requires practice—and lots of it. It is a fundamental skill.
- Many patients with neurological conditions are admitted elsewhere under the care of general care physicians, and the receiving neurointensivist must be patient and cordial when getting the sign-out from these colleagues.
- Checklists may assist in triage but are never sufficiently individualized.
- Only a few "bounce-backs" are avoidable.
- Patients who are agitated, require hourly attention to blood pressure, or need close secretion management are at high risk to return to the ICU, sometimes only hours after they have arrived on the ward.

Further Reading

Cohen, M. D., and P. B. Hilligoss. "The Published Literature on Handoffs in Hospitals: Deficiencies Identified in an Extensive Review." [In eng]. *Qual Saf Health Care* 19, no. 6 (Dec 2010): 493–97. https://doi.org/10.1136/qshc.2009.033480.

Coon, E. A., N. M. Kramer, R. R. Fabris, et al. "Structured Handoff Checklists Improve Clinical Measures in Patients Discharged from the Neurointensive Care Unit." [In eng]. *Neurol Clin Pract* 5, no. 1 (Feb 2015): 42–49. https://doi.org/10.1212/cpj.0000000000000094.

Coughlin DG, Kumar MA, Patel NN, Hoffman RL, Kasner SE. Preventing Early Bouncebacks to the Neurointensive Care Unit: A Retrospective Analysis and Quality Improvement Pilot. *Neurocrit Care.* 2018 Apr;28(2):175–183. doi: 10.1007/s12028-017-0446-z.

Fakhry, S. M., S. Leon, C. Derderian, et al. "Intensive Care Unit Bounce Back in Trauma Patients: An Analysis of Unplanned Returns to the Intensive Care Unit." [In eng]. *J Trauma Acute Care Surg* 74, no. 6 (Jun 2013): 1528–33. https://doi.org/10.1097/TA.0b013e31829247e7.

Gandhi, T. K. "Fumbled Handoffs: One Dropped Ball After Another." [In eng]. *Ann Intern Med* 142, no. 5 (Mar 1 2005): 352–58. https://doi.org/10.7326/0003-4819-142-5-200503010-00010.

Nathan, C. L., L. Stein, L. J. George, et al. "Standardized Transfer Process for a Neurointensive Care Unit and Assessment of Patient Bounceback." [In eng]. *Neurocrit Care* 36, no. 3 (Jun 2022): 831–39. https://doi.org/10.1007/s12028-021-01385-z.

Riesenberg, L. A., J. Leitzsch, and B. W. Little. "Systematic Review of Handoff Mnemonics Literature." [In eng]. *Am J Med Qual* 24, no. 3 (May–Jun 2009): 196–204. https://doi.org/10.1177/1062860609332512.

Riesenberg, L. A., J. Leitzsch, J. L. Massucci, et al. "Residents' and Attending Physicians' Handoffs: A Systematic Review of the Literature." [In eng]. *Acad Med* 84, no. 12 (Dec 2009): 1775–87. https://doi.org/10.1097/ACM.0b013e3181bf51a6.

Rojas, J. C., P. G. Lyons, T. Jiang, et al. "Accuracy of Clinicians' Ability to Predict the Need for Intensive Care Unit Readmission." [In eng]. *Ann Am Thorac Soc* 17, no. 7 (Jul 2020): 847–53. https://doi.org/10.1513/AnnalsATS.201911-828OC.

Ropper, A. H. "How to Determine If You Have Succeeded at Neurology Residency." [In eng]. *Ann Neurol* 79, no. 3 (Mar 2016): 339–41. https://doi.org/10.1002/ana.24592.

Tangonan R, Alvarado-Dyer R, Loggini A, Ammar FE, Kumbhani R, Lazaridis C, Kramer C, Goldenberg FD, Mansour A. Frequency, Risk Factors, and Outcomes of Unplanned Readmission to the Neurological Intensive Care Unit after Spontaneous Intracerebral Hemorrhage. *Neurocrit Care.* 2022 Oct;37(2):390–398. doi: 10.1007/s12028-021-01415-w. Epub 2022 Jan 24.

Tschoellitsch T, Maletzky A, Moser P, Seidl P, Böck C, Tomic Mahečić T, Thumfart S, Giretzlehner M, Hochreiter S, Meier J. Machine learning prediction of unexpected readmission or death after discharge from intensive care: A retrospective cohort study. *J Clin Anesth.* 2024 Oct 14;99:111654. doi: 10.1016/j.jclinane.2024.111654. Epub ahead of print.

Wang, J., M. Ren, H. Wang, et al. "Analysis of Urgent Inpatient Neurologic Consultations in a Large Tertiary Hospital Center: Follow-up on the Effect of Standardized Training of Residents." [In eng]. *Brain Behav* 13, no. 5 (May 2023): e2983. https://doi.org/10.1002/brb3.2983.

Wijdicks, E. F. M. "Communicating Neurocritical Illness: The Anatomy of Misunderstanding." [In eng]. *Neurocrit Care* 34, no. 2 (Apr 2021): 359–64. https://doi.org/10.1007/s12028-020-01131-x.

60 When Families Do Not Agree With Our Approach and Care

A 50-year-old man is admitted with a large pontine hemorrhage extending into the thalamus. He has remained comatose since onset with extensor motor posturing, pinpoint pupils, and ocular bobbing. When our expectations of his (poor) outcome are discussed, the conversation with the family members immediately turns sour. Members of the family accuse each other using rude language, and conversations with the health care staff are not productive. Other family members turn up drunk. Nursing staff is accused of disinterest and neglect. The situation rapidly gets out of hand with nobody daring to speak for fear of abuse and even physical altercations. Care continues with full resuscitative measures, but the health care team considers it very inappropriate. The current medical situation and care plan is at variance with reasonable practice.

What do you do now?

Once a patient is admitted with a catastrophic acute brain injury, family members wish for detailed information about the patient's clinical status. Certainly, they need and want to know, and we must be available to inform them with considerable detail. Our immediate task is explaining and planning. We not only strive for a good-natured relationship with the patient's family but we also try quickly to build rapport. With our good effort, this is virtually always achieved. Patients' families value our professional opinion, and we value their insight into the person they have lived with and known so well. Family members can only infer how their loved one would experience permanent disability, and many are quick to say, "He/she does not want to live like this." Cultural beliefs comes into play when families deviate from what many of us would consider a reasonable judgment. Do we have the competence to understand that?

But at times, we find ourselves in a most unfair dispute, and our patience and our solicitousness are stretched to a breaking point. We can expect that to occur in any acute major stressful situation because strong personal emotions often drive irrational thinking. Regrettably, when dealing with verbal aggression, anger, and hostility, trust evaporates quickly, and an eerie silence may prevail. We quickly realize that the slightest gesture or word can change the course of communication. Bad feelings may also result when we explain that severe irreversible brain injury cannot be treated and that all interventions are ineffectual. Why do some families deny the reality of the situation and refuse to come to terms? Why do families dispute physicians' ability to assess the situation correctly? What are the main mechanisms sustaining this failure to reach a satisfactory and reasonable conclusion? Why does the atmosphere become antagonistic and belligerent? Intensive care unit (ICU) teams are highly familiar with these situations and how they take up all the attention. They represent the other, less rigorously studied management side of our specialty.

We realize that acute brain injury is wholly unexpected (unlike a known, prior illness reaching its end) and immediately disabling. Most patients' core goals of independence, vigor, and joy are gone forever. Even with such a devastating outlook, families do not always accept the inevitable. Physicians may be guilty of this as well. Continuation of care may also be demanded by neurosurgeons, who are hesitant to withdraw support from patients following complex, hours-long surgeries or following surgery complicated by some mishap.

How these troublesome interactions occur is not entirely known, but some feel that giving families too much autonomy may limit physicians' freedom to implement what they feel to be in the patient's best interest. Being forced to provide aggressive, futile care may violate their sense of moral integrity. For some physicians, it represents a deplorable affront; others simply shrug it off as "the difficult family (or patient)." None of these sentiments are particularly helpful in a major crisis, and our primary goal is to ensure that our patients receive appropriate care, whether in our hands or others.

Some families will always hope for a miraculously good outcome in a futile situation. There is no satisfactory, all-encompassing, psychologic or sociologic explanation. It is not simple denial; most families emphatically know the reality. The potential for subsequent guilt for "doing something you may have to live with the rest of your life" may play a role. Previous conversations with their loved one on limiting care (i.e., ""Don't forget, I am a fighter; don't let them give up on me!") may drive the conversation. Combat metaphors of a fighting spirit and battles to win are common. Moreover, in an increasingly diverse care environment, ethnic minorities may hold a different view of how best to cope with major adversity. In many cultures, a keen sense of obligation to their loved one compels family members to do everything possible even if they fully realize the unlikely chance of recovery. Moreover, in Asian cultures, nondisclosure is quite common. Discussing the details of serious illness is considered confrontational, disrespectful, and a cause of too much anxiety to the patient. Collusion is often justified by the mistaken assumptions that it causes their loved one to lose hope and motivation to get better and increase the risk of depression and later suicide. The elderly are highly respected and revered, and speaking positively and offering hope are standard social norms. Other religions emphasize that life always has value. Expense does not deter these families from continuing futile care if costs are carried by health care insurance. There may be multiple other reasons. Families might be unhappy with the treatment the patients have received and may have a lingering feeling that "not everything has been done." These obstacles to a rational discussion cannot be overcome even by an independent ethics committee.

These conflicts can lead to appalling circumstances and honestly a mess. We, as neurointensivists, are not specifically trained (or lack sufficient experience) to manage them appropriately, and some conflicts cannot be solved by anyone. Once we are in the thick of a conflict, we need to find a workable solution. The main elements of resolution are shown in Figure 60.1, and it is often pure common sense.

In large teaching centers, we deal with many opinions. Disagreements should be recognized, but before meeting with the family, the lead physician and nursing staff must develop a similar understanding of what

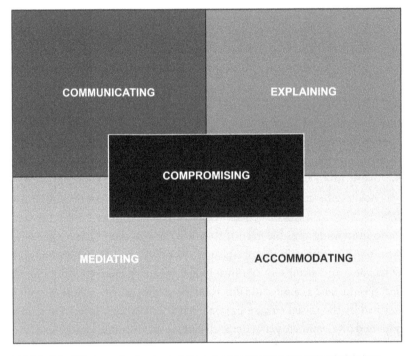

FIGURE 60.1 Diffusing a situation (and what solutions to consider). The main principle is to keep the lines of communication open. We must avoid any remarks that might be perceived as patronizing. The neurointensivist's role is fivefold: first, to explain what is known and not known about the neurologic condition and to acknowledge flexibility and that the situation may change; second, to clarify the family's tolerance for an open discussion about these matters; third, to respect their opinions and to seek patient or family consent before you do anything; fourth, to continue to explain the unchanged condition and lack of improvement; and fifth, to compromise where needed and to try, in some way, to accommodate the patient and family's position. This is a very time-intensive process and should take place in a quiet setting with everyone sitting down.

is happening to the patient and a consensus about the appropriate level of care. A conversation with the family cannot proceed if the health care providers are not "on the same page." Physicians should also recognize that with staff rotations or "changing of the guard," the new attending physician may change the overall approach. We have seen new physicians starting their rotation armed with good intentions to "solve this problem" suddenly confronting family members and confusing (or antagonizing) them even more.

In those situations, we can legitimately ask ourselves whether involvement of an ethics or palliative care committee might be helpful. Tried approaches are mediation and accommodation or the so-called "structured, time-limited trial approach" (with a timeline we can all agree upon). When there is the threat of a major conflict, mediation may be possible through another senior neurologist, a social worker, clergy, or elders. For some families, the best compromise is simply to allow them time to come to grips with the situation and to discuss the new reality with other family members. But if families will not back down, we must tolerate their choice, proceed with gastrostomy and tracheostomy placement, and facilitate admission to a skilled care facility. It may start an endless cycle of return to the ICU with serious infections and other complications.

Clinicians have duties of care to patients, even the odious ones or the ones with unpleasant relatives. Physicians' expectations of their role as well-meaning carers must remain. However, unilaterally refusing life-sustaining treatment risks liability under not only malpractice but also intentional infliction of emotional distress. Contacting the hospital legal department may escalate the problem even more. It is better to keep the law out of it.

And then there is another major conundrum that we unfortunately cannot ignore. Catastrophic brain injury may lead to brain death and requires a formal examination. Suddenly, we are now facing unprecedented new questions on whether we can declare a patient brain dead. Its origin may be manifold and include greater acceptance of the family's personal viewpoint (and morality) rather than a universal position, but theirs cannot be an absolute right. There is now some debate whether physicians should ask for consent to perform the apnea test. We have not come across that specific objection too often. However, it is a strong indication that the family does not accept that a patient is dead despite the lack of brain function and necessity of machine-supported breathing and life-sustaining medication, and they do not want us to make that declaration.

These personal family positions are also supported by some bioethicists whose positions are easily found on the internet. Bioethicists may argue that the apnea test can harm the brain through hypercapnia or hypoxemia, a seriously flawed if not ridiculous argument (how can we harm a dead brain?).

If families fail to accept brain death as death, there are two options. First, the physician can consider maintaining full support for 2 to 3 days. During this hiatus, the physician could seek assistance from a hospital ethics committee to meet with the family and reassure them that brain death is, in fact, the death of a person. Spiritual counsel may be sought. It is very unclear if any of this will make any difference. Physicians should appreciate these sensitivities and try to help family members come to a sense of closure. Continuing support should be full support; it is poor practice to maintain mechanical ventilation but stop vasopressors, effectively hastening cardiac arrest. However, cardiopulmonary resuscitation is not warranted under any circumstances.

If the family refuses to come to an agreement, legal advice must be obtained. We cannot support brain-dead patients indefinitely. A local judge will then decide and can be expected to declare the patient dead, which would then allow withdrawal of support. However, judges may grant families temporary injunctions to keep the patient supported while evidence is gathered.

Guilt (or remorse) is a powerful, anxiety-laden emotion. It may quickly follow the decision to withdraw support. Most of these early emotions subside, but we have seen family members revisit their actions years later, even when the decisions were made in the setting of overwhelming futility. Guilt in this context is also partly related to questioning the physician's medical knowledge ("Were his/her recommendations sound?") and revisiting their own decisions ("Did I fully understand what I was told?"). Guilt may become pathological and excessive. Bereavement support should be sought, and ideally, health care professionals should find ways to follow up if problems are anticipated.

Many newly qualified intensivists recognize that they are skating on thin ice. Because we are all essentially eternal novices in comprehending communication patterns, conundrums remain and present in unexpected ways. Knowledge from research studies and opinion papers do not necessarily help in real practice, and the sheer number of surprise encounters are not easily simulated in training sessions. Using hired actors to play patients and families and to give us feedback on our bedside manner, emotional control, and eye contact only goes so far. We must remain civil towards each other and have the patient's best interest at heart. Some guidance is provided here, but we stop short in saying it leads to a definitive solution. Years of attending complex family conferences will allow us to develop several workable approaches. Human interaction under these trying circumstances does not always work the way the bioethical and philosophy books tell us.

KEY POINTS TO REMEMBER

- When a discussion gets heated, take a "timeout."
- One staff person should act as the liaison who provides updates to the family. (Avoid "multiple captains on a ship" phenomenon.)
- Simplify topics to discuss.
- Make a sincere effort to persuade without coercion.
- Stay the course and provide a consistent message.
- If conflict remains, step back and consider consulting a hospital medical ethics committee.
- Only involve the legal department as a very last resort.

Further Reading

Cohen, M. S., and D. S. Prough. "Reducing the Angst Associated With Withdrawal of Life-Sustaining Therapy." [In eng]. *Crit Care Med* 44, no. 6 (Jun 2016): 1241–42. https://doi.org/10.1097/ccm.0000000000001810.

Fiester, A. "The 'Difficult' Patient Reconceived: An Expanded Moral Mandate for Clinical Ethics." [In eng]. *Am J Bioeth* 12, no. 5 (2012): 2–7. https://doi.org/10.1080/15265161.2012.665135.

Kim, S., H. Mills, T. Brender, et al. " 'My Mom is a Fighter': A Qualitative Analysis of the Use of Combat Metaphors in Intensive Care Unit Clinician Notes." [In eng]. *Chest* (Aug 26 2024): S0012-3692(24)05052-9. doi:10.1016/j.chest.2024.07.178.

Kopar, P. K., A. Visani, K. Squirrell, and D. E. Brown. "Addressing Futility: A Practical Approach." [In eng]. *Crit Care Explor* 4, no. 7 (Jul 2022): e0706. https://doi.org/10.1097/cce.0000000000000706.

Krebs, E. E., J. M. Garrett, and T. R. Konrad. "The Difficult Doctor? Characteristics of Physicians Who Report Frustration With Patients: An Analysis of Survey Data." [In eng]. *BMC Health Serv Res* 6 (Oct 6 2006): 128. https://doi.org/10.1186/1472-6963-6-128.

Luce, J. M. "A History of Resolving Conflicts Over End-of-Life Care in Intensive Care Units in the United States." [In eng]. *Crit Care Med* 38, no. 8 (Aug 2010): 1623–29. https://doi.org/10.1097/CCM.0b013e3181e71530.

Misak, C. J., D. B. White, and R. D. Truog. "Medical Futility: A New Look at an Old Problem." [In eng]. *Chest* 146, no. 6 (Dec 2014): 1667–72. https://doi.org/10.1378/chest.14-0513.

Pope, T. M. "Counterpoint: Whether Informed Consent Should Be Obtained for Apnea Testing in the Determination of Death by Neurologic Criteria? No." [In eng]. *Chest* 161, no. 5 (May 2022): 1145–47. https://doi.org/10.1016/j.chest.2021.11.029.

Rich, B. A. "Distinguishing Difficult Patients From Difficult Maladies." [In eng]. *Am J Bioeth* 13, no. 4 (2013): 24–26. https://doi.org/10.1080/15265161.2013.767957.

Rivera, S., D. Kim, S. Garone, et al. "Motivating Factors in Futile Clinical Interventions." [In eng]. *Chest* 119, no. 6 (Jun 2001): 1944–47. https://doi.org/10.1378/chest.119.6.1944.

Shewmon, D. A. "Point: Whether Informed Consent Should Be Obtained for Apnea Testing in the Determination of Death by Neurologic Criteria? Yes." [In eng]. *Chest* 161, no. 5 (May 2022): 1143–45. https://doi.org/10.1016/j.chest.2021.11.026.

Stienen, M. N., F. Scholtes, R. Samuel, et al. "Different but Similar: Personality Traits of Surgeons and Internists—Results of a Cross-Sectional Observational Study." [In eng]. *BMJ Open* 8, no. 7 (Jul 7 2018): e021310. https://doi.org/10.1136/bmjopen-2017-021310.

Udwadia, F. R., J. Zhu, H. M. Khan, and S. Das. "Futility Considerations in Surgical Ethics." [In eng]. *Ann Med Surg (Lond)* 85, no. 1 (Jan 2023): 1–5. https://doi.org/10.1097/ms9.0000000000000114.

Ward, M., and S. Cook. "When Communication Breaks Down: Handling Hostile Patients." [In eng]. *Med Clin North Am* 106, no. 4 (Jul 2022): 689–703. https://doi.org/10.1016/j.mcna.2022.01.009.

Index

For the benefit of digital users, indexed terms that span two pages (e.g., 52–53) may, on occasion, appear on only one of those pages.

Tables, figures, and boxes are indicated by an italic *t*, *f*, and *b* following the page/paragraph number.

abscess, 243*t*
acid maltase deficiency, 87
action myoclonus
  case of 62-year-old man, 227*b*, 228, 231
  differences between postarrest myoclonus
    and posthypoxic, 229*t*
  See also myoclonus
acute autonomic failure, Guillain-Barré
    syndrome (GBS), 396–97, 400
acute bacterial meningitis, need for
    intracranial pressure (ICP) monitor,
    307*b*, 311
acute disseminated encephalomyelitis, 243*t*
  causes and neuroimaging, 63*t*
acute embolus
  occluded basilar artery, 120*f*, 120–21,
    123–24
  predictors in patients treated with
    endovascular clot retrieval, 121*b*
acute encephalitis
  bacterial infections, 65*t*
  case of 60-year-old woman, 61*b*, 62*f*,
    69–70
  causes of, 63*t*, 65*t*
  computed tomography (CT) scan of
    patient with acute HSV-1, 61*b*, 62*f*,
    62–64
  diagnosis of, 64
  diagnostic tests, 65*t*
  electroencephalography (EEG), 67–68
  fungal infections, 65*t*
  intracranial pressure (ICP) monitoring
    for brain swelling, 69
  issues requiring admission to intensive
    care unit (ICU), 69

  key points to remember, 70
  neuroimaging and, 62–64, 63*t*
  principle aspects of management, 65*t*
  protozoal infections, 65*t*
  role of brain biopsy and, 68
  testing for autoimmune, 68
  treatment for presumed, 68–69
  treatment in emergency department,
    69–70
  viral infections, 64–67, 65*t*
acute ischemic stroke
  factors associated with worse prognosis,
    446–47, 446*t*
  patients presenting with severely
    disabling, 446–47
  predicting outcome of patients, 444–45,
    445*t*
  prognosis of, 444
  prognostic scores for, 449
  See also prognostication after acute
    ischemic stroke and cerebral
    hemorrhage
acute neuromuscular disease
  bedside respiratory tests predicting need
    for mechanical ventilation in GBS, 87*t*
  bedside spirometry gauges, 85, 86–87
  case of 21-year-old woman, 83*b*, 88
  clinical findings predicting worsening of
    respiratory weakness, 83*b*
  decision-making in respiratory failure,
    88*f*, 88–89
  diagnosis of respiratory failure, 85–86
  failure of breathing mechanics, 84–85
  Guillain-Barré syndrome (GBS), 84,
    86–87, 87*t*

acute neuromuscular disease (*cont.*)
  intubation of patients, 83*b*
  key points to remember, 89
  mechanical ventilation, 83*b*, 85–86
  myasthenia gravis, 84, 86–87, 87*t*
  procrastination, 84
  respiratory failure, 84, 85–86, 88
  restlessness, 84
acute respiratory distress syndrome
    (ARDS), 222, 372–73
  aspiration pneumonitis evolving into,
    375–76
  definition of, 373–74
  sepsis management, 355*b*
acute stroke
  algorithm for control of hypertension,
    363*f*
  bouncing back from, 101–2
  candidates for endovascular
    recanalization therapy for, 101*b*
  case of 62-year-old man, 99*b*, 105
  computed tomography (CT) angiogram
    for occlusion site, 103
  CT angiogram showing a flow
    gap, 100*f*
  CT scan without contrast showing no
    ischemic changes, 99*b*, 100*f*
  endovascular reperfusion therapy, 105*f*,
    105
  follow-up CT scan showing hypodensity
    in left basal ganglia, 105, 106*f*
  indicators of worse prognosis after
    therapy for, 102*b*
  IV recombinant tissue plasminogen
    activator (rt-PA), 103–4
  key points to remember, 106–7
  managing blood pressure after
    reperfusion, 104–5
  mechanical thrombectomy, 100–1, 104
  perfusion injury, 104
  recanalization and reperfusion, 100–1
  risks of asymptomatic intracranial
    hemorrhage, 104
  See also stroke(s)

acute subdural hematoma
  case of 21-year-old accident victim, 35*b*,
    40–41
  computed tomography (CT) scan of
    initial, 35*b*, 36*f*
  craniotomy and decompressive
    craniectomy, 38
  delayed epidural hematoma, 37
  electroencephalography (EEG) studies
    of, 40
  extra-axial hematomas, 38
  extradural hematoma as complication, 40
  head injury, 37
  key points to remember, 41–42
  magnetic resonance imaging (MRI),
    36–37
  multiple CT scans for evolving, 37
  neurologic examination guides, 37
  neurosurgeons approach to, 38–40
  postoperative CT after evacuation, 36*f*
  postoperative CT scans, 40
  rapid reoccurrence postoperatively, 41*f*
  RASH score, 39–40, 39*t*
  surgery for, 38
  traumatic brain injury, 37
acyclovir
  acute encephalitis, 68–69
  emergency room for encephalitis, 69–70
  suspected encephalitis, 70
Addison disease, 209
adrenal bleeding, IV thrombolysis, 93
adrenal hemorrhage, major complication of
    IV thrombolysis, 96*b*
adrenocorticotropic hormone deficiency, 210
adynamic ileus
  Guillain-Barré syndrome (GBS), 398–99
  treatment of, 399
agitation, extreme
  delirium tremens, 341
  pharmacological options for, 341–42,
    342*t*
AIDS patients, 242–44
Alberta Stroke Program Early CT score
    (ASPECTS), 99*b*, 101–3

bouncing back from stroke, 101–2
major stroke, 109*b*, 111–12
mechanical thrombectomy, 103
standardizing assessments, 103
See also acute stroke
alcohol intoxication, traumatic brain injury
(TBI), 26
alcohol use disorder
case of 43-year-old male, 345*b*
malnutrition and alcoholism, 347
mental confusion triggering
hospitalization, 350
See also central pontine myelinolysis
(CPM); Wernicke-Korsakoff syndrome
alcohol withdrawal
benzodiazepines, 341, 342*t*, 343
brain chemistry, 340
case of 52-year-old man, 339*b*, 343
delirium, 341
dexmedetomidine, 341–42, 342*t*
diazepam, 342*t*
differential diagnosis of paroxysmal
sympathetic hyperactivity, 383*t*
"front-loading" therapy, 341, 343
ICU patients with encephalopathy, 327*t*
key points to remember, 343
lorazepam, 342*t*
medical emergency, 340
patients in emergency room after
traumatic brain injury, 340–41
pharmacological options for treatment of
delirium tremens, 341–42, 342*t*
phenobarbital, 341–42, 342*t*
propofol, 341–42, 342*t*
seizures, 341
supportive care, 343
treatment of, 353*b*
altered mental status
five Ss (sedatives, stroke, seizures, sudden
metabolic derangement, and slow drug
clearance), 270
term, 266
amebiasis, cause, diagnostic test and
management, 65*t*

American Clinical Neurophysiology Society,
301
American College of Obstetricians and
Gynecologists, 217
American Heart Association, 20, 131
American Medical Association, 473
American Society for Transplantation and
Cellular Therapy, 259
amiodarone, atrial fibrillation, 391–92,
393, 393*t*
ampicillin
bacterial meningitis, 55*b*
Listeria monocytogenes, 54
meningitis patient, 53*b*
amyloid angiopathy, 7–8
amyotrophic lateral sclerosis (ALS),
respiratory failure, 87
anaphylactoid reaction, major complication
of IV thrombolysis, 96*b*
ancillary tests, brain death determination,
486, 488
andexanet alfa, reversal of Xa inhibitors,
17*t*, 21
aneurysmal rebleeding in subarachnoid
hemorrhage, differential diagnosis of
paroxysmal sympathetic hyperactivity,
383*t*
aneurysmal subarachnoid hemorrhage
(aSAH)
case of 44-year-old woman, 147*b*, 148,
150
cerebral vasospasm, 148, 150–52, 153
computed tomography (CT) scan of
head, 147*b*, 148*f*
CT angiogram and CT perfusion in
patients, 151–52
delayed cerebral ischemia, 175–78
delayed cerebral vasospasm, 150–51
diabetes insipidus (DI) in neurosciences
ICU, 421*b*
"good grade" patients becoming "poor
grade", 152
hydrocephalus and, 148–49, 152–53
hypertension, 367

aneurysmal subarachnoid hemorrhage
  (aSAH) (*cont.*)
  key points to remember, 152–53
  major risks to patient, 148
  middle cerebral artery versus cervical
    internal carotid artery (MCA/ICA
    ratio or Lindegaard ratio), 151
  modalities for diagnosis and monitoring
    cerebral vasospasm and delayed
    ischemic damage, 151*t*
  patient stability, 148
  rebleeding and, 148, 149–50, 152
  risk factors for development of delayed
    cerebral ischemia after, 150*b*
  transcranial Doppler (TCD), 150,
    151–52
  treatment of hypertension, 366
  Ultra-early transexamic acid after
    subarachnoid hemorrhage (ULTRA)
    trial, 149–50
  See also delayed cerebral ischemia in
    aneurysmal subarachnoid hemorrhage
    (aSaH); subarachnoid hemorrhage
    (SAH)
angioedema
  lip swelling, 92
  treatment, 96
angiotensin-converting enzyme (ACE)
    inhibitor(s)
  angioedema risk, 96
  ischemic stroke patient, 364
  stroke risk and, 92
anoxic-ischemic brain injury, 26, 243*t*
antibiotic-associated encephalopathy,
    334–35
  case of 65-year-old woman, 333*b*,
    336–37
  cefepime neurotoxicity, 334–37
  key points to remember, 337
  See also cefepime
antibiotics
  bacterial meningitis, 54–56, 55*b*, 58
  septic shock, 356*b*

septic shock treatment with broad-
    spectrum, 357, 358
  toxicity from, 334
antibodies, encephalitis link with or
    without malignancies, 77*t*
anticholinergic toxicity, ICU patients with
    encephalopathy, 327*t*
anticoagulation
  cerebral venous sinus thrombosis
    (CVST), 141–43, 144
  need to resume, 289–90
  restarting, 292
  timing for resumption of, 289–90
  traumatic brain injury (TBI), 26
anticoagulation in cerebral hemorrhage
  anticoagulation reversal in ICH, 15*b*
  case of 70-year-old man, 13*b*
  costs for reversal treatment, 17–18
  direct oral anticoagulants (DOACs),
    14, 17
  key points to remember, 20–21
  patients with thrombocytopenia, 16
  resuming anticoagulation, 19–20
  reversal of antiplatelet agents, 18–19
  reversal of DOACs, 17–18, 17*t*
  reversal of IV thrombolysis, 16–17
  warfarin reversal, 15*b*, 15–16
antidepressants, 392
antidopaminergics, alcohol withdrawal,
    341–42
antiepileptic drugs, postresuscitation status
    myoclonus, 230–31
antihistamines, angioedema
    treatment, 96
anti-N-methyl D-aspartate receptor
    (NMDAR) encephalitis, 75, 76–77,
    78–79
antipsychotics, 392
antiseizure medication
  barbiturates, 284
  brivaracetam, 280–83, 281*t*
  case of 72-year-old man, 279*b*, 284
  drug-drug interactions, 284

drug rash with eosinophilia and systemic
symptoms (DRESS) syndrome,
283–84
fosphenytoin, 281*t*, 283–84
key points to remember, 285
lacosamide, 279*b*, 280, 281*t*, 284
levetiracetam, 280–83, 281*t*
liver and renal failure, 284
main side effects and interactions, 280,
281*t*
phenobarbital, 284
phenytoin, 281*t*, 283–84
side effect profile, 280
valproic acid, 281*t*, 283
aortic repair
case of 58-year-old man, 181*b*, 186
hypothermia during procedures, 184
lumbar drain placement and adverse
events, 184–85, 186
risk factors for spinal cord infarction
(SCI), 183
spinal cord infarction (SCI) or ischemia,
182
See also spinal cord infarction (SCI)
apixaban, 26
anti-factor Xa levels, 17–18
reversal of DOACs, 17, 17*t*
Apixaban after Anticoagulation-associated
Intracerebral Hemorrhage in Patients
with Atrial Fibrillation (APACHE-AF)
trial, 19–20
apnea test, consent for performing, 513–14
apnea testing, brain death determination,
485*f*
apoplexia, Greek word, 208
arboviruses, cause, diagnostic test and
management, 65*t*
areflexia, 182
arginine vasopressin (AVP), deficiency of,
420
arrhythmia(s)
drug-induced, 392
treatment for, 393*t*

aSAH. *See* aneurysmal subarachnoid
hemorrhage (aSAH)
aspergillosis, cause, diagnostic test and
management, 65*t*
aspiration, after acute brain injury, 375*t*
aspiration pneumonitis, 372–73
aspirin, duration of action, 18–19
astrocyte dysfunction, thiamine deficiency,
349
astrocytoma, 243*t*
ATACH-2 trial, 446–47
blood pressure, 365
atracurium, TBI treatment, 27–28
atrial fibrillation, 390–91
amiodarone, 391–92, 393*t*
diltiazem, 391–92, 393*t*
metoprolol, 391–92, 393*t*
treatment for, 391–92, 393*t*
atrioventricular block, treatment for, 393*t*
autoimmune depression, 79
autoimmune disorders, immunosuppressive
drugs and, 79
autoimmune encephalitis
antibodies linked to, with or without
malignancies, 77*t*
anti-N-methyl D-aspartate receptor
(NMDAR) encephalitis, 75
cancer risk factors and, 76
case of 27-year-old woman, 73*b*, 78–79
characterization of, 74
clinical spectrum of, 75
computed tomography (CT) scans, 76–77
diagnosis of, 74, 79
elderly patients, 76
electroencephalogram (EEG) showing
extreme delta brush, 73*b*, 74*f*
herpes simplex encephalitis (HSE) and,
75
ICU admission, 78–79
incorrect diagnosis of, 79
key points to remember, 80
neuro-intensive care unit (ICU) for cases
of, 74, 78

autoimmune encephalitis (*cont.*)
noninfectious, 64
presenting with rapidly progressive
encephalopathy, 75
seizures, 78–79, 80
seizures and, 80
supportive clinical features, 76
testing, 68
treatment objectives disabling antibodies,
77–78
when to consider, 75*b*
autoimmune epilepsy, 79
autoimmune limbic encephalitis, causes and
neuroimaging, 63*t*
autoimmune movement disorders, 79
autoimmune psychiatry, 74
autoimmune psychosis, 79
autoimmune thyroiditis, 243*t*
autonomic dysreflexia from spinal cord
injury, differential diagnosis of
paroxysmal sympathetic hyperactivity,
383*t*
azathioprine, myasthenia gravis, 406

baclofen
paroxysmal sympathetic hyperactivity
(PSH), 384, 385*t*, 386
bacterial infections, cause, diagnostic test
and management, 65*t*
bacterial meningitis
acute hydrocephalus, 58
antibiotics, 58
antibiotic treatments, 54–56, 55*b*
brain as innocent bystander, 54–55
case of 50-year-old woman, 53*b*,
57–58
cerebral edema, 58
corticosteroids, 54–55, 58
deterioration causes that are
untreatable, 58
deterioration of patient, 56–57, 56*t*
hydrocephalus, 57–58
key points to remember, 59
Listeria monocytogenes, 54

lumbar drainage, 57–58
magnetic resonance imaging (MRI), 46*f*,
53*b*, 57*f*
outcome in forms of, 58–59
outcome of acute, 58–59
Streptococcus pneumoniae, 46, 53*b*,
54–55
balloon angioplasty, 160*f*
cerebral vasospasm, 158, 161
barbiturates, 284
aborting status epilepticus (SE), 193
basal ganglia, MRI in rapid progressive
brain disease, 243*t*
basal ganglia injury, movement disorders,
229–30
basilar artery
acute embolus occluding, 120–21
Basilar Artery Occlusion Chinese
Endovascular Trial (BAOCHE), 124
case of 71-year-old man, 119*b*, 121
clinical trajectory and manifestations of
acute embolus, 121, 123*f*
clot retrieval, 122–23, 123*f*
computed tomography (CT) angiogram
of head and neck, 119*b*, 120*f*
critical area perfusion score (CAPS),
124–25
diagnosis of occlusion, 125
Endovascular Treatment for Acute Basilar
Artery Occlusion (ATTENTION),
124
Endovascular Treatment versus Standard
Medical Treatment for Vertebrobasilar
Artery Occlusion (BEST), 124
European guidelines for patients with
occlusion, 124–25
hyperdense, reflecting embolus, 119*b*
hyperdense sign, 119*b*, 120*f*, 125, 126
key points to remember, 126
magnetic resonance imaging of brain,
121, 122*f*
mechanical embolectomy for restoration
of flow, 120*f*, 121
neuro-ophthalmologic signs, 122–23

predictors in patients treated with endovascular clot retrieval, 121*b*

randomized trials, 124

signs and symptoms by obstructing distal embolus, 123–24

Basilar Artery Occlusion Chinese Endovascular Trial (BAOCHE), 124

batoclimab, myasthenia gravis treatment, 406

B-cell lymphoma, CAR T-cell infusion, 257*b*

bedside spirometry gauges, 85

bentracimab, ticagrelor reversal, 18–19

benzodiazepines

alcohol withdrawal, 343, 353*b*

delirium and, 324–26, 331

paroxysmal sympathetic hyperactivity (PSH), 384, 385*t*

seizures with multiple doses of, 380

status epilepticus (SE), 190–91, 192*t*

traumatic brain injury (TBI), 26

Berkowitz, Aaron, 245–46

beta-lactams, antibiotic-associated encephalopathy, 334–35

bilevel positive airway pressure (BiPAP), myasthenia gravis, 403*b*, 407

biomarkers, prognostication tools, 440

bipolar disorder, autoimmune encephalitis and, 74

bivalirudin, anticoagulation, 289–90

blastomycosis, cause, diagnostic test and management, 65*t*

bleeding, traumatic brain injury (TBI), 26

bleeding at arterial and venous puncture sites, minor complication of IV thrombolysis, 96*b*

blood pressure, 238

control of, 19

eclampsia and management of, 217–18, 219

Guillain-Barré syndrome (GBS), 398*b*, 400

management after reperfusion, 104–5

posterior reversible encephalopathy syndrome (PRES), 237–38

See also hypertension

brain biopsy

rapidly progressive brain disease, 241*b*, 244–45

role in encephalitis, 68

brain death determination

actual neurological evaluation, 484

allowing closure and options for organ donation, 487

ancillary tests, 486, 488

brain injury, 486

brainstem reflexes, 483

case of 20-year-old male student, 481*b*

clearance of sedative drugs and, 483–84

clinical diagnosis of, 482

decisions and line of action, 484, 485*f*

diabetes insipidus (DI), 421*b*

donation after brain death (DBD), 490

experienced examiner for, 486–87

how long to declare, 483

key points to remember, 487–88

procedures and tests for declaring, 485*f*

questions to ask, 482

second examination for, 485–86

signs compatible with, 483*b*

situations suggesting that patient may not be brain dead, 482*b*

tests not fitting clinical examination, 486

uniform determination of death act (UDDA), 487

See also organ donation

brain disease

drug neurotoxicity, 334

toxic encephalopathy, 335*f*

See also rapidly progressive brain disease

brain edema

case of 48-year-old woman, 233*b*, 237–38

head computed tomography (CT) scan showing cerebral and cerebellar edema, 233*b*, 234*f*

See also posterior reversible encephalopathy syndrome (PRES)

brain injury
case of 17-year-old boy, 371*b*, 375
catastrophic, 513–14
computed tomography (CT) scan of brain, 371*b*, 372*f*
deterioration from major, 483
fever, 358–59
glucose management, 357–58
increased ammonia as damaging neurotoxin, 429–30
septic shock, 359
systemic complications, 359
See also traumatic brain injury (TBI)
BrainPath (NICO Corporation), 6–7
brain "sagging", mechanical shift postoperatively, 275
brainstem injury
displacement-associated, 14
Sequential Organ Failure Assessment (SOFA), 358–59
brainstem reflexes
after cardiac resuscitation, 453–54
brain death determination, 483
brain surgery. *See* stupor after brain surgery
brain swelling, treatment of, 69
Brain Trauma Foundation, 26–27
brain tumors
brain metastasis as serious, 203
case of 64-year-old man, 199*b*, 202
causes of neurological deterioration in patients with, 200*b*
decline of brain metastasis or malignant, 204
diabetes insipidus (DI) in neurosciences ICU, 421*b*
emergency department treatment, 202
head CT scan showing cerebral mass, 202, 203*f*
key points to remember, 204
patients with primary malignant, 200
precipitating causes, 200, 204
surgery, 204
surgery as complex decision, 202–3
surgical resection, 202–3

surgical resection of brain metastasis, 202–3
treatment options, 200–2
vasospasm after surgery, 276
breast cancer, spinal cord compression, 174
breathing mechanics, clinical manifestations of failure of, 84–85
brivaracetam
adverse effects and drug interactions, 281*t*
levetiracetam and, 280–83
broad-spectrum antibiotics, treatment of, 376
bromocriptine, paroxysmal sympathetic hyperactivity (PSH), 384

calcium channel blockers, intra-arterial therapy, 158–61, 159*t*
cancer
antibodies and, 76
radiation, 178
risk of radiation myelopathy, 178
spinal cord compression, 174*f*, 174
surgical resection of brain metastasis, 202–3
Tokuhashi revised scoring system, 174–75, 176*t*
treatment of acute spinal cord compression, 177*b*
types, 174
See also spinal cord compression
CAR (CD19 chimeric antigen receptor) T-cell therapy
American Society and Transplantation and Cellular Therapy, 259, 260*t*
case of 58-year-old woman, 257*b*, 262–63
cerebrospinal fluid (CSF) analysis, 262–63
computed tomography (CT) scan, 261*f*
consensus grading for cytokine release syndrome (CRS) and neurologic toxicity associated with immune effector cells, 260*t*

cytokine release syndrome (CRS) as
complication, 258
description, 258
immune effector cell-associated
neurotoxicity syndrome (ICANS),
258–59
infectious disease human herpesvirus
type 6 (HHV-6) encephalitis in, 262
key points to remember, 263
magnetic resonance imaging (MRI),
261f, 262
neurotoxicity from, 258–59
oncologic approach, 258
pathophysiology of cerebral edema
following, 259–62
profound white matter (vasogenic
edema) in patient treated with, 261f
RocKet trial, 259
carbamazepine, postresuscitation status
myoclonus, 230–31
carbon monoxide, 243t
cardiac arrest
hypothermia after, 223–24
in-hospital (IHCA), 225
out-of-hospital (OHCA), 225
recommendations for targeted
temperature management, 225b
See also action myoclonus; Lance-Adams
syndrome; myoclonus; targeted
temperature management
cardiac arrhythmias
after acute ischemic stroke, 390–91
atrial fibrillation, 390–92
case of 86-year-old woman, 389b
drug-induced, 392
electrocardiogram (ECG) showing
repolarization changes, 389b, 390f,
390
guideline for treatment of, 393t
Guillain-Barré syndrome
(GBS), 398b
key points to remember, 393
morphological ECG changes, 392–93
onset of new, 392

prevalence of, 392
cardiac dysfunction, postarrest, 230
cardioembolism, 267
cardiopulmonary resuscitation
(CPR), 119b
appropriateness of, 479
case of 60-year-old woman, 451b,
457–58
chest compressions, 221b
do-not-resuscitate (DNR) order and,
473–74
electroencephalopathy (EEG), 453,
454–55, 457–59
motor response as prognosticator after
cardiac arrest, 453
myoclonus and, 453
neurological assessment, 452–53
postcardiac resuscitation syndrome, 452
procedure, 473
success in ICU, 473–74
See also prognostication after
cardiopulmonary resuscitation;
targeted temperature management
cavernous sinus, localization of the lesion,
319t
cefepime, 333b
administration, 334
empirical dosing of, 334–35
encephalopathy, 337
hypothesis for brain function
suppression, 336
neurotoxicity, 334–37
patients with neurotoxicity, 336
risk of encephalopathy, 334–35
septic shock treatment, 356b
switching patient to piperacillin-
taxobactam, 336–37
ceftriaxone
bacterial meningitis, 55b
meningitis patient, 53b
central nervous system necrotic vasculitis,
differential diagnoses of posterior
reversible encephalopathy syndrome
(PRES), 236b

central pontine myelinolysis
(CPM), 345*b*
alcoholism with malnutrition, 347
key points to remember, 350
MRI facilitating diagnosis, 347–48
MRI showing restricted diffusion, 345*b*,
346*f*
osmotic endothelial injury, 347–48
progression to locked-in syndrome,
347–48
sodium correction, 347–48
centronuclear myopathies, 87
cephalosporin, *Listeria monocytogenes*, 54
cerebellum, MRI in rapid progressive brain
disease, 243*t*
cerebral amyloid angiopathy, 19–20
cerebral amyloid angiopathy-related
inflammation, 244
cerebral and cerebellar edema
head computed tomography (CT) scan
of, 233*b*, 234*f*
See also posterior reversible
encephalopathy syndrome (PRES)
cerebral angiogram, posterior communicating
artery aneurysm, 315*b*, 316*f*
cerebral angiography, 155*b*, 161–62
acute subarachnoid hemorrhage, 155*b*,
161–62
cerebral disease, Sequential Organ Failure
Assessment (SOFA), 358–59
cerebral edema
bacterial meningitis, 58
coma and, 237
cerebral hemorrhage
hemostatic therapy, 6
mechanical valve and, 19–20
neurosurgical evacuation of, 4
neurosurgical options, 4–5
theories of expansion, 5
tirofiban therapy, 291*f*
ventriculostomy placement, 4–5, 8
See also anticoagulation in cerebral
hemorrhage; lobar cerebral

hemorrhage; prognostication after
acute ischemic stroke and cerebral
hemorrhage
cerebral infarction, craniotomy, 275
cerebral ischemia, mean arterial pressure
(MAP), 354–55
cerebral perfusion pressure (CPP),
intracranial pressure (ICP) and,
26–27, 29
cerebral salt wasting (CSW)
evaluation and management of
hyponatremia, 414*f*
fludrocortisone, 415
hyponatremia in subarachnoid
hemorrhage (SAH), 412
syndrome of inappropriate secretion of
antidiuretic hormone (SIADH) and,
413*f*
cerebral spasm
after aneurysmal subarachnoid
hemorrhage (aSaH), 156
ischemia and, 156–57
randomized trial, 156–57
treatment options, 159*t*
cerebral vasospasm, 148
after brain surgery, 277
after craniotomy, 277
aneurysm rupture and, 148, 153
case of 23-year-old man, 273*b*, 277
cause of postsurgical, 276
cerebral angiogram identifying, 276
cerebral angiogram showing diffuse,
273*b*, 274*f*
delayed cerebral ischemia from,
150–51
digital subtraction catheter angiography,
160*f*
by endothelial dysfunction,
151–52
monitoring and documenting, 153
pathophysiology of, 276
supraclinoid internal carotid
artery, 160*f*

cerebral venous sinus thrombosis (CVST)
ACTION-CVT trial, 142
anticoagulation, 141–43
case of 46-year-old woman, 139*b*,
143–44
causes of deterioration in, 143*b*
cerebral edema, 142
clinical trials, 142
diagnosis of, 140–42
evaluation of, 141*b*
key points to remember, 145
magnetic resonance (MR) venogram,
139*b*
mechanical thrombectomy, 143–44,
144*f*
outcomes of anticoagulation, 144
perspective on, 145
RESPECT-CVT trial, 142
screening patients, 141–42
seizures, 142
cerebritis, 58
cerebrospinal fluid (CSF)
acute encephalitis, 62–64
autoimmune encephalitis patient, 73*b*
draining after aortic surgery, 184
dynamics, 47
extra-axial CSF accretion, 47, 48
Guillain-Barré syndrome (GBS), 254
hydrodynamics, 48
lumbar drain placement and adverse
events, 184–85, 186
polymerase chain reaction (PCR) for
patients with presumed encephalitis,
62–64, 70
posterior reversible encephalopathy
syndrome (PRES), 235–36, 237
preventive treatment for leakage, 49
rapidly progressive brain disease, 241*b*,
242–44, 246
resolving leaks, 50
skin leaks, 46–47
subarachnoid hemorrhage (SAH), 165*b*,
166–68

chemoprophylaxis with heparin, 29
chemotherapy, 243*t*, 245
chest X-ray
case of 17-year-old boy, 371*b*, 375
clinical suspicion of acute pulmonary
emboli, 376
myasthenia gravis, 403*b*–4, 405*f*, 407*t*,
408
pulmonary conditions after acute brain
injury, 375*t*
white-out lungs, 371*b*, 372*f*
Cheyne-Stokes breathing pattern, 3*b*,
13*b*
chlordiazepoxide, detoxification
with, 341
chlorpropamide, diabetes insipidus (DI),
423
chronic inflammatory demyelinating
polyneuropathy, 253
chronic kidney disease, 230
chronic myopathies, 87
ciprofloxacin, *Listeria monocytogenes*, 54
circulatory arrest
organ donation and, 494, 497
respiratory and, 495
Clazosentan to Overcome Neurological
Ischemia and Infarction Occurring
After Subarachnoid Hemorrhage
(CONSCIOUS) trials, 156–57
clevidipine
blood pressure control, 19
Guillain-Barré syndrome (GBS), 397–98,
400
hypertension treatment, 366–67, 367*t*
clinical diagnosis, brain death, 482*b*, 482,
483*b*
Clinical Feature Scale (CFS), paroxysmal
sympathetic hyperactivity (PSH), 381*t*
Clinical Institute Withdrawal Assessment of
Alcohol (CIWA), 341
Clinical Institute Withdrawal Assessment
of Alcohol revised version (CIWA-Ar),
341

Clinical Research Study With Clazosentan to Evaluate Its Effects on Preventing Complications Due to the Narrowing of the Blood Vessels (Vasospasm) in the Brain, Caused by Bleeding Onto the Surface of the Brain (REACT) trial, 156–57

clonazepam
  posthypoxic myoclonus, 229–30
  postresuscitation status myoclonus, 230–31

clonidine, 366–67
  Guillain-Barré syndrome (GBS), 397–98, 398*b*, 400
  paroxysmal sympathetic hyperactivity (PSH), 384, 385*t*, 386

clopidogrel, duration of action, 18–19

clot. *See* acute stroke

Clot Lysis Evaluation of Accelerated Resolution of Intraventrical Hemorrhage (CLEAR) III trial, 8

coccidioidomycosis, cause, diagnostic test and management, 65*t*

cognitive motor dissociation (CMD), 465–66, 466*f*, 468–69

Collaborative European Neurotrauma Effectiveness Research in Traumatic Brain Injury (CENTER-TBI), 38

collusion, 511

coma
  cerebral edema, 237
  postoperative examination, 269
  situations suggesting patient may not be brain dead, 482*b*
  See also persistent comatose states

communication. *See* triage communication

computed tomography (CT) angiography, 3*b*
  helical, of chest, 372–73

computed tomography (CT) perfusion, black-and-white drawing of results for major stroke, 113*f*, 113

computed tomography (CT) scan(s)
  acute encephalitis, 61*b*, 62*f*
  acute stroke, 99*b*, 100*f*
  acute subarachnoid hemorrhage (aSaH), 155*b*
  acute subdural hematoma, 36*f*, 41*f*
  antibody and cancer, 76–77
  bilateral cerebellar strokes with acute obstructive hydrocephalus, 265*b*, 266*f*
  brain with cerebral mass, 202, 203*f*
  brain with heterogenous sellar and suprasellar mass, 207*b*, 208*f*
  brain with progressive cortical hypodensities, 427*b*, 428*f*
  brain with unusual bilateral deep brain infarctions, 139*b*
  central pontine myelinolysis (CPM) abnormalities, 347–48
  cerebellar hematoma, 501*b*
  characteristics predicting unstable hematoma, 6
  head, showing diffuse cerebral and cerebellar edema, 234*f*, 236*b*
  head CT of thalamic hemorrhage, 443*b*, 444*f*
  hematoma, 290
  hemorrhagic infarcts involving bilateral thalami and basal ganglia, 139*b*, 140*f*
  hyperdense basilar artery sign, 119*b*, 120*f*
  hypertension, 361*b*
  intracerebral hematoma, 287*b*, 288*f*
  intraparenchymal hematoma, 471*b*, 472*f*
  multiple, for evolving contusion, 37
  rapidly progressive brain disease, 244–45
  spine tumors, 173*b*
  subarachnoid hemorrhage (SAH), 165*b*, 166*f*
  subarachnoid hemorrhage (SAH) with aneurysmal pattern, 147*b*, 148*f*
  subdural hygroma, 45*b*, 46*f*
  thalamic hematoma, 13*b*, 14*f*

traumatic brain injury (TBI) showing
subdural hematoma, 305*b*, 306*f*
traumatic subarachnoid hemorrhage,
435*b*–36, 437*f*
conflicts
accommodation, 512*f*, 513
communicating, 512*f*, 512–13
compromise, 512*f*, 513
explaining, 512*f*, 512–13
mediation, 512*f*, 513
resolutions and, 512*f*, 512–13
Confusion Assessment Method for the
Intensive Care Unit score (CAM-ICU),
331
congenital myopathies, respiratory failure, 87
corneal reflexes, postresuscitation coma,
458*t*
cortex, MRI in rapid progressive brain
disease, 243*t*
cortical (N20) responses, postresuscitation
coma, 48, 458*t*, 459
corticosteroid(s)
angioedema treatment, 96
bacterial meningitis, 54–55, 58, 59
brain tumor, 199*b*, 200–1
cerebral edema, 59
immune checkpoint inhibitor-associated
myopathy, 253, 255
immune effector cell-associated
neurotoxicity syndrome (ICANS), 262
immune therapy, 80
injections for rheumatoid arthritis, 61*b*
posterior reversible encephalopathy
syndrome (PRES), 236–37
septic shock treatment, 357
short-term side effects and preventive
measures, 201*t*
spinal cord ischemia, 185
viral encephalitis and, 69
Corticosteroid Randomization After
Significant Head Injury (CRASH)
model, 438
cortisol, pituitary apoplexy, 210

CPR. *See* cardiopulmonary resuscitation
(CPR); prognostication after
cardiopulmonary resuscitation
craniectomy
case of 40-year-old roofer, 45*b*, 49
cerebrospinal fluid (CSF) leaks, 45*b*, 48, 49
decompressive, 4–5
extradural hygroma, 47
hydrocephalus, 46*f*, 46
key points to remember, 49–50
major complications after, 46*f*
neurosurgeon on CSF leaks, 46–47
open, 5
post-traumatic hydrocephalus (PTH),
47–48
sinking skin flap syndrome, 48–49
subdural hygroma, 46*f*, 46, 47
syndrome of the trephined, 46*f*, 46
treatment of intracranial pressure (ICP),
28*f*, 28–29
ventriculostomy placement, 48
See also hemispheric stroke
craniectomy-associated progressive
extra-axial collections with treated
hydrocephalus (CAPECTH), 48
craniopharyngioma, causes of central
diabetes insipidus (DI), 421*b*
cranioplasty, 47–48
bone-flap placement, 48
craniotomy
acute subdural hematoma, 38
causes of deterioration after, 274, 275*b*
cerebral infarction after, 275
trial of patients with lobar hematoma, 6
Creutzfeldt-Jakob disease, 243*t*, 244
critical care trials, 222
cryoprecipitate, IV thrombolysis, 95
cryptococcosis, cause, diagnostic test and
management, 65*t*
cryptogenic epilepsy, 75
crystalloids
diabetes insipidus (DI) treatment, 424
resuscitation, 354–55, 355*b*

INDEX   529

cultures, family members and, 511

Cushing response, differential diagnosis of paroxysmal sympathetic hyperactivity, 383t

CVST. *See* cerebral venous sinus thrombosis (CVST)

cyclophosphamide, immunosuppression, 77–78

cytokine release syndrome (CRS)
complication of CAR T-cell therapy, 258
consensus grading for, 260t
tocilizumab, 262
treatment of, 258

cytomegalovirus
cause, diagnostic test and management, 65t
causes and neuroimaging, 63t

cytomegalovirus infection, ganciclovir and foscarnet, 68–69

dabigatran, 17
idarucizumab and, 26
idarucizumab reversing, 17t, 21
reversal of DOACs, 17, 17t

DAWN trial, major stroke, 110–11

death. *See* brain death determination

death watch, circulatory arrest and, 493–94

decision makers
do-not-resuscitate (DNR) order and, 474–75
family conference, 475b, 475–76, 479
See also withdrawal of life-sustaining treatment

decompressive craniectomy
acute subdural hematoma, 38, 40
case of 48-year-old man undergoing, 129b, 130f, 134
criteria for, in large hemispheric stroke, 132b
critical questions for best candidates, 132b, 132
elderly patients, 131–32, 135
gunshot injury, 25

intracranial pressure (ICP), 28–29, 31
neurosurgical option, 4–5
outcome of patients, 131
patients younger than 60 years of age, 132, 135
swollen hemispheric stroke, 130–31
treatment of intracranial pressure (ICP), 28f, 28
See also hemispheric stroke; ischemic stroke

decompressive craniotomy, treatment of intracranial pressure (ICP), 28f, 28–29

decompressive hemicraniectomy, encephalitis and, 69

deep-seated hematomas, stereotactic surgery with needle aspiration, 6–7

deep venous thrombosis, TBI treatment, 29, 30, 31

delayed cerebral ischemia in aneurysmal subarachnoid hemorrhage (aSAH), 156
balloon angioplasty, 157, 158, 161
case of 66-year-old woman, 155b, 161–62
cerebral angiography, 161–62
cerebral vasospasm, 158
Clazosentan to Overcome Neurological Ischemia and Infarction Occurring After Subarachnoid Hemorrhage (CONSCIOUS-1) trial, 156–57
Clinical Research Study With Clazosentan to Evaluate Its Effects on Preventing Complications Due to the Narrowing of the Blood Vessels (Vasospasm) in the Brain, Caused by Bleeding Onto the Surface of the Brain (REACT) trial, 156–57
computed tomography (CT) scan showing aSaH, 155b
CONSCIOUS-2 trial, 156–57
CONSCIOUS-3 trial, 156–57
digital subtraction catheter angiography for vasospasm of internal carotid artery, 158, 160f

EARLY DRAIN trial, 157–58
hemodynamic augmentation therapy, 158
intra-arterial medication options treating cerebral vasospasm, 158–61, 159*t*
key points to remember, 162
Magnesium for aneurysmal subarachnoid hemorrhage (MASH)-2 trial, 156–57
Simvastatin in aneurysmal subarachnoid hemorrhage (STASH) trial, 156–57
transluminal balloon angioplasty, 158, 160*f*, 161
triple H (hypervolemia, hypertension, hemodilution), 158
See also aneurysmal subarachnoid hemorrhage (aSaH)
delirium
alcohol withdrawal, 341
approach to evaluating patients with ICU delirium, 329, 330*t*
assessment of sedation and, in ICU, 325*f*
case of 72-year-old man, 323*b*, 329–30
causes and mechanisms of, 324–26
common complication in ICU, 324
description of, 329
differential diagnoses in ICU patients with encephalopathy, 327*t*
evaluation of, 330, 330*t*
key points to remember, 331
monitoring tools for nursing staff, 324
quiet delirium, 324
Richmond Agitation Sedation Scale (RASS), 324–26, 326*b*
risk with opiates, 324–26
word, 324
delirium by fabulation, 349
dementia, 7–8
depression, autoimmune encephalitis and, 74
depressive craniectomy, cerebral hemorrhage, 4–5
desaturation, 88*f*, 88–89
desmopressin, 18–19

administration for diabetes insipidus (DI), 423–24, 424*b*, 425
before surgery, 18–19
desmopressin acetate (DDAVP), managing diabetes insipidus (DI), 419*b*, 420–21
dexamethasone
angioedema, 92–93
bacterial meningitis, 55*b*
brain tumors in emergency department, 199*b*, 202
immune effector cell-associated neurotoxicity syndrome (ICANS), 262
meningitis patient, 53*b*
tumor swelling, 419*b*
dexmedetomidine
alcohol withdrawal, 341–42, 353*b*
delirium and, 324–26
dysautonomia, 78
paroxysmal sympathetic hyperactivity (PSH), 384, 385*t*
treatment of delirium tremens, 342*t*
diabetes insipidus (DI)
arginine vasopressin (AVP) secretion and, 420
calculating free water deficit, 422
case of 40-year-old woman, 419*b*, 424
causes of central, in neurosciences ICU, 421*b*
desmopressin acetate (DDAVP) for managing, 419*b*, 420–21
desmopressin administration, 423–24, 424*b*, 425
desmopressin when polyuria is severe, 423
diagnosis of, 420–21
hypernatremia, 420–22, 423, 424*b*
key points to remember, 425
management of, 421–22
patients with aneurysmal subarachnoid hemorrhage, 423
pituitary gland, 420
protocol for treating, 424*b*
serum sodium concentration, 422–23
treatment in intensive care unit (ICU), 424

diabetes mellitus, third-nerve palsies and, 318

diagnosis
  anchoring in wrong, 503
  essential information for, 504
  seeking working, 503
  See also triage communication

diazepam
  paroxysmal sympathetic hyperactivity (PSH), 384, 385*t*, 386
  refractory status epilepticus (SE), 192*t*
  treatment of delirium tremens, 342*t*

diffusion-weighted imaging (DWI), failure to awaken after CPR, 456–57

diffusion-weighted imaging-fluid-attenuated inversion recovery (FLAIR), mild to moderate strokes, 112–13, 115*f*, 116

diltiazem, atrial fibrillation, 391–92, 393, 393*t*

diphenhydramine, angioedema, 92–93

direct oral anticoagulants (DOACs)
  anticoagulation-associated cerebral hemorrhages, 14
  resumption of, 19–20
  reversal of DOACs, 17–18

Direct oral anticoagulant versus warfarin in the treatment of cerebral venous thrombosis (ACTION-CVT), 142

dobutamine, septic shock, 354–55

documentation, brain death determination, 485*f*

donation of organs
  differences between DCD and DBD protocols, 491*t*
  donation after brain death (DBD), 490
  donation after cardiac/circulatory death (DCD), 490–93
  heart procurement from DCD donors, 494
  morphine, 493

United States hospitals with DCD protocol, 491–92
  See also organ donation

do-not-resuscitate (DNR) order
  catastrophic neurological injuries, 479
  cognitive and physical incapacity vs. death, 477–78
  communicating with family, 476–77, 476*t*
  criteria, 473–74
  decision makers, 474–75
  discussion of, 473–74
  family conference, 475*b*, 475
  good, not too bad, and poor outcomes, 477
  information to convey to family when discussing, 476–77, 476*t*
  origination of, 473
  point of no return, 477
  self-fulfilling prophecy, 476–77
  unintended problems, 474
  See also withdrawal of life-sustaining treatment

dopamine, 354–55

DRESS (drug rash with eosinophilia and systemic symptoms) syndrome, 283–84

drug-induced leukoencephalopathy, differential diagnoses of posterior reversible encephalopathy syndrome (PRES), 236*b*

Duchenne dystrophy, 87

dural venous sinus thrombosis, ICU patients with encephalopathy, 327*t*

dysarthria, stroke, 91*b*

dysautonomia, 88*f*, 88–89
  Guillain-Barré syndrome (GBS), 396–99
  IV dexmedetomidine for, 78

dysphagia, 88*f*, 88–89

dysphonia, 88*f*, 88–89

dyssynchronous breathing, 88*f*, 88–89

EARLY DRAIN trial, 157–58
Early Minimally Invasive Removal of
  Intracerebral Hemorrhage (ENRICH)
  trial, 6–7
eclampsia
  blood pressure management, 217–18,
    219
  case of 25-year-old female, 215*b*
  head computed tomography (CT), 215*b*
  intrapartum, 217
  key points to remember, 219
  magnesium sulfate treatment, 217–18,
    219
  magnetic resonance imaging (MRI),
    215*b*, 216*f*
  nicardipine, 218
  nifedipine, 219
  postpartum, 216–17
  pregnancy, 219
  pregnancy and, 216–17, 219
eculizumab, myasthenia gravis treatment,
  406
e-Delphi survey, 307–8
edema. *See* posterior reversible
  encephalopathy syndrome (PRES)
edoxaban, anti-factor Xa levels, 17–18
efalizumab, 61*b*
Efficacy and Safety of MRI-Based
  Thrombolysis in Wake-Up Stroke
  (WAKE-UP) trial, 112–13
efgartigimod, myasthenia gravis treatment,
  406
electroencephalographic (EEG)
  monitoring, treatment of increased
  ICP, 27–28
electroencephalography (EEG)
  bitemporal seizures, 73*b*, 74*f*
  brain death and, 483*b*
  case of 64-year-old man, 297*b*, 301–2
  continuous EEG, 302, 303
  convulsive seizures, 298–99
  epileptologists and intensivists
    interpreting, 301

generalized, anterior-predominant theta-
  to-delta-range rhythmic activity, 297*b*,
  298*f*
generalized epileptiform discharges,
  454–55, 456*f*
indications and rationale for EEG
  monitoring in ICU, 300*t*
key points to remember, 302–3
myoclonus after cardiopulmonary
  resuscitation (CPR), 453, 454–55,
  457–59
myoclonus status patterns, 229
nonconvulsive seizures (NCSs),
  298–301
nonconvulsive status epilepticus (NCSE),
  298–99, 301–2
persistent vegetative state, 464–66, 469
posterior reversible encephalopathy
  syndrome (PRES), 237–38
showing extreme delta brush, 73*b*, 74*f*
electroencephalography (EEG) studies
  acute encephalitis, 67–68, 70
  acute subdural hematoma, 40
electromyography (EMG), 249*b*
  Guillain-Barré syndrome (GBS), 254
embolectomy
  selectin of candidates for, 107
  stroke, 106
embolus. *See* basilar artery
emergency department, posterior reversible
  encephalopathy syndrome (PRES),
  238
emergency noncardiac surgery, risk of stroke
  after, 266–67
emergency room, treatment for encephalitis,
  69–70
empyema, magnetic resonance imaging
  (MRI), 57*f*
encephalitis, 243*t*
  diagnosis of, 70
  differential diagnoses of posterior
    reversible encephalopathy syndrome
    (PRES), 236*b*

encephalitis (*cont.*)
  differential diagnosis of paroxysmal
    sympathetic hyperactivity, 383*t*
  ICU patients with encephalopathy, 327*t*
  nivolumab/pembrolizumab, 252
  See also acute encephalitis; autoimmune
    encephalitis
encephalopathy
  cefepime and risk of, 334–35
  differential diagnoses in ICU patients
    with, 327*t*
  drug toxicity as cause, 334
  hepatic, 428–29
  hypothermia in post anoxic, 222–23
  multifactorial, 334
  prolonged hyperammonemic, 430
  term, 326–29
  toxic, 337
  toxic, in sepsis, 335*f*
  See also antibiotic-associated
    encephalopathy
encephalopathy/delirium, nivolumab/
  pembrolizumab, 251*f*
end-of-life care, intensive care unit (ICU),
  473
endotracheal intubation, traumatic brain
  injury (TBI), 26
endovascular aneurysms, treatment of,
  319–20
endovascular reperfusion therapy
  patient as ideal candidate for, 105
  patient selection, 107
endovascular stroke therapy, 100–1
  eligibility of patients, 106
  indicators of worse prognosis after, 102*b*
  recanalization, 100–1, 101*b*
endovascular therapy, cerebral venous sinus
  thrombosis (CVST), 145
Endovascular Therapy Following Imaging
  Evaluation for Ischemic Stroke
  (DEFUSE-3) trial, 110–11
endovascular thoracoabdominal aortic
  surgery, 183

Endovascular Treatment for Acute Basilar
  Artery Occlusion (ATTENTION),
  124
Endovascular Treatment versus Standard
  Medical Treatment for Vertebrobasilar
  Artery Occlusion (BEST), 124
Enterobacteriaceae, 334
epidural empyema, 56–57
epidural hematoma, traumatic brain injury
  (TBI), 37
epilepsy, 189*b*
  See also status epilepticus (SE)
epinephrine, 354–55
Erasmus University, SAH Study Group,
  166–67
erythromycin, gastroparesis, 399
esmolol, atrial fibrillation, 393
Established Status Epilepticus Treatment
  Trial (ESETT) trial, 190–91
European Cooperative Acute Stroke Study
  (ECASS-2) trial, 93
experienced examiner, brain death
  determination, 486–87
external ventricular drain (EVD),
  intracranial pressure (ICP) monitor,
  307–8
extubation, myasthenia gravis, 406–7, 407*t*,
  408
eye. *See* pupil, fixed and dilated

failure to awaken after surgery
  "altered mental status", 266
  anesthetics and, 270
  case of 56-year-old woman, 265*b*, 268
  causes to consider in patients with, 267*b*
  computed tomography (CT) scan of
    bilateral cerebellar strokes, 265*b*, 266*f*
  five Ss (sedatives, stroke, seizures, sudden
    metabolic derangement, and slow drug
    clearance), 270
  hypoglycemia, 135, 269
  hyponatremia, 135, 269
  ischemic stroke, 268

key points to remember, 270
perioperative stroke, 267
postoperative coma, 269
postoperative stupor, 269, 270
risk of perioperative stroke, 266–67
risk of stroke after emergency noncardiac
    surgery, 266–67
status epilepticus, 269
VISION (Vascular Events in Noncardiac
    Surgery Patients Cohort Evaluation)
    study, 266–67
family members, dealing with
    accepting brain death as death, 514
    case of 50-year-old man with pontine
        hemorrhage, 509*b*
    communication, 514–15
    conflicts and resolution, 512*f*, 512–13
    consent for apnea test, 513–14
    continuation of care, 510–11
    cultures and, 511
    dispute with ICU teams, 510
    hoping for miraculous outcome in futile
        situation, 511
    key points to remember, 515
    legal advice, 514
    professional opinion and, 510
    qualified intensivists with, 514–15
    troublesome interactions with physicians,
        511
famotidine, 392
fascicles, localization of the lesion, 319*t*
fat embolism syndrome
    ICU patients with encephalopathy,
        327*t*
    patient presentation of, 371*b*, 374
fat embolization syndrome
    after acute brain injury, 375*t*
    Gurd's criteria for, 374, 374*t*
    key points to remember, 376
    long bone fracture and, 376
    magnetic resonance imaging (MRI)
        abnormalities, 374–75
    treatment of, 374

fenestrated-branched endovascular aortic
    repair (F-BEVAR), 183–84
fentanyl
    brain death determination and, 483–84,
        486
    TBI treatment, 27–28
fever, brain injury, 358–59
fibrinogen, IV thrombolysis, 95
Fisher, C. Miller, 334
fixed and dilated pupil. *See* pupil, fixed and
    dilated
fludrocortisone, hyponatremia, 415, 416
fluid-attenuated inversion recovery
    (FLAIR), magnetic resonance imaging
    (MRI), 101–2
fluorodeoxyglucose positron emission
    tomography (FDG PET)
    hypermetabolism, 76
    screening of antibody and tumor,
        76–77
fluoxetine, postresuscitation status
    myoclonus, 230–31
fondaparinux, 16
fosphenytoin, 392
    administration of, 283–84
    adverse effects and drug interactions,
        281*t*
    intravenous, 297*b*
    management of status epilepticus (SE),
        195*f*
    posterior reversible encephalopathy
        syndrome (PRES), 237–38
    refractory status epilepticus (SE), 192*t*
    seizure therapy, 190–91
four-factor prothrombin complex
    concentration, 288–89, 290
    patient with hematoma, 290
Foville syndrome, 123
free water deficit, calculation of, 422
fresh frozen plasma (FFP), 13*b*, 288–89
    reversing antagonistic effect of warfarin,
        15*b*, 15–16
frontotemporoparietal craniectomy, 310

INDEX   535

fulminant hepatic failure
  clinical manifestations of, 430–31
  intracranial pressure (ICP) monitors,
    308–9, 311
  need for ICP monitor, 307*b*
fulminant meningitis, 58–59
fulminant multiple sclerosis, 243*t*
fulminant myositis, 254
funduscopy, 317
fungal infections, 243*t*
  cause, diagnostic test and management,
    65*t*
  causes and neuroimaging, 63*t*

gabapentin
  alcohol withdrawal, 341–42
  paroxysmal sympathetic hyperactivity
    (PSH), 384, 385*t*
  PSH, 384–86
gamma-aminobutyric acid (GABA),
  cefepime and, 336
ganglionic hemorrhage, case of 51-year-old
  man with, 489*b*
gastrointestinal hemorrhage, major
  complication of IV thrombolysis, 96*b*
gastrointestinal prophylaxis, TBI treatment,
  30
Glasgow Coma Scale (GCS), 445*t*, 502,
  504
Glasgow Modified Alcohol Withdrawal
  Scale, 341
glial fibrillary acidic protein (GFAP),
  biomarker for prognostication, 440
gliomatosis, differential diagnoses of
  posterior reversible encephalopathy
  syndrome (PRES), 236*b*
gliomatosis cerebri, 243*t*
glucose management, patients with brain
  injury, 357–58
glycocorticoids, 210
goals of care, 472
  See also withdrawal of life-sustaining
    treatment

grade IV hepatic encephalopathy,
  intracranial pressure (ICP) monitor,
    308–9
gram-negative bacilli (GNB), infections, 49
granulomatosis with polyangiitis, diabetes
  insipidus (DI) in neurosciences ICU,
    421*b*
granulomatous inflammation of central
  nervous system, nivolumab/
  pembrolizumab, 252
grey matter, MRI in rapid progressive brain
  disease, 243*t*
Guillain-Barré syndrome (GBS), 238
  acute autonomic failure in, 399
  acute neuromuscular disorder, 84
  administration of intravenous morphine,
    399
  axonal type of, 88
  bedside respiratory tests, 87*t*
  blood pressure fluctuations, 397
  bronchial function, 398
  case of 73-year-old man, 395*b*, 399
  diagnosis of, 254
  drug sensitivity, 397–98
  dysautonomia, 396–99
  early management of, 396*b*
  EMG and NCSs determining, 254
  essential information, 504
  hypertension treatment, 397–98, 398*b*
  intubation of patients, 89
  key points to remember, 400
  marked dilated colonic loops on
    abdominal X-ray, 397*f*
  mechanical ventilation, 87*t*, 396, 399
  myasthenia gravis and, 86–87
  neurologic complication, 251*f*, 253
  patients with adynamic ileus, 398–99
  patient with severe, 396
  pembrolizumab/nivolumab, 253
  respiratory failure, 84, 86, 88–89
  spirometry, 85, 86
  treatment of acute autonomic failure,
    396–97

536 INDEX

gunshot injury, traumatic brain injury (TBI) and, 25–26
Gurd's criteria, fat embolization syndrome, 374, 374t

H1N1, outbreaks of encephalitis, 64
haloperidol, 384
heart failure, end-stage, 288, 289
heart transplant, 289
hematoma(s)
    computed tomography (CT) scan of expansion of, 14f
    deep ganglionic, 8–9
    enlargements, 5
    gunshot injury, 25–26
    neurosurgical evacuation, 21
    speed of growth, 6
    surgery for deep-seated, 6–7
    traumatic brain injury (TBI) and, 25
    ultra-early evacuation, 6–7
    See also acute subdural hematoma
hematoma mass effect, hematoma expansion, 5
hematuria, minor complication of IV thrombolysis, 96b
hemicraniectomy
    critical questions for, 132
    hemispheric stroke and, 130–31, 133
hemispheres, MRI in rapid progressive brain disease, 243t
hemispheric stroke
    computed tomography (CT) angiography, 129b, 130f
    craniectomy, 133
    criteria for decompressive craniectomy in, 132b, 132
    elderly patients, 131–32, 135
    hemicraniectomy, 130–31, 133
    magnetic resonance imaging (MRI) for monitoring, 132b, 132
    medical management of large swollen, 130–31, 133–34, 135
    neurocritical management avoiding brain injury, 133
    neurosurgical treatment for swollen, 130–31, 133
    See also decompressive craniectomy
hemorrhage. See aneurysmal subarachnoid hemorrhage (aSAH)
hemostatic therapy, hematoma expansion, 6
hemostatic therapy (SPOTLIGHT/ STOP-IT) trial, 446–47
heparin, anticoagulation reversal in ICH, 15b
heparin infusion, testing the waters, 289–90
hepatic encephalopathy, 428–29
    ICU patients with encephalopathy, 327t
hepatitis C, infectious disease, 492
herpes simplex encephalitis (HSE), 243t
    autoimmune encephalitis and, 75
herpes simplex virus (HSV), polymerase chain reaction (PCR), 73b
herpes simplex virus type 1 (HSV-1), IV acyclovir treating, 68–69
herpes simplex virus type 1 (HSV-1) encephalitis
    brain imaging of patient, 62f
    cause, diagnostic test and management, 65t
    causes and neuroimaging, 63t
    electroencephalography (EEG), 70
    magnetic resonance imaging (MRI), 62–64
herpes simplex virus type 2 (HSV-2), IV acyclovir treating, 68–69
higher-order cortex-motor dissociation (HMD), 465–66, 466f
high-flow nasal oxygen (HFNO), acute respiratory distress syndrome (ARDS), 373–74
hippocampi, MRI in rapid progressive brain disease, 243t
histoplasmosis, cause, diagnostic test and management, 65t

HIV. *See* human immunodeficiency virus
(HIV)
human herpesvirus type 6 (HHV-6)
encephalitis, CAR T-cell recipients, 262
human immunodeficiency virus (HIV)
cause, diagnostic test and management,
65*t*
highly active antiretroviral therapy
(HAART) for infected patients, 68–69
infectious disease, 492
hydralazine
blood pressure control, 19
hypertension treatment, 366–67, 367*t*
hydrocephalus
aneurysmal rupture, 148–49
bacterial meningitis, 57–58
complication after craniectomy, 46*f*, 46
symptomatic, demanding immediate
CSF diversion, 149
hydrocortisone, 210
septic shock treatment, 356*b*, 357
5-hydroxytryptophan, postresuscitation
status myoclonus, 230–31
hyperammonemia, 269
correction of, 428–29
key points to remember, 431
lactulose with or without rifaximin to
treating, 427*b*, 430
liver cirrhosis case, 427*b*
MRI findings in acute, 430
hyperglycemia, 222
hypernatremia, 420–22
brain death determination and, 483–84
diabetes insipidus (DI) treatment, 424*b*
lowering serum sodium, 425
protocol for treating diabetes insipidus
(DI), 424*b*
stupor after brain surgery, 275*b*, 275–76
See also diabetes insipidus (DI)
hyperosmolar therapy
mannitol or hypertonic saline, 309–10
posterior reversible encephalopathy
syndrome (PRES), 237–38

hypertension, 158
aneurysmal subarachnoid hemorrhage,
366
blood pressure targets, 362
case of 56-year-old man, 361*b*, 364
definition, 217
drugs for use in, 366–68, 367*t*
head computed tomography (CT) scan,
361*b*
intracerebral hemorrhage (after first 24
hours), 366
intracerebral hemorrhage (first 24 hours),
365
ischemic stroke after first 24 hours, 365
ischemic stroke as candidate for
thrombosis (first 24 hours), 362–64
ischemic stroke not candidate for
reperfusion therapy (first 24 hours),
364–65
ischemic stroke treated with mechanical
thrombectomy, 364
key points to remember, 367
options for treatment of acute stroke
patients, 367*t*
paroxysmal sympathetic hyperactivity
(PSH), 386
permissive, 364–65
recommended algorithm for control of,
363*f*
hypertonic saline
hyperosmolar therapy, 309–10
treatment of intracranial pressure (ICP),
28*f*, 28
hyperventilation
intracranial pressure (ICP) monitor,
309–10
treatment of intracranial pressure (ICP),
28*f*, 28
hypervolemia, 158
hypocalcemia, 392
hypoglycemia
brain death determination and, 483–84
failure to waken after surgery, 269, 270

hypogonadism, 210
hypokalemia, 347–48, 392
  temperature management, 224
hypomagnesemia, 392
hyponatremia, 347–48
  algorithm for evaluation and
    management of, 414f
  brain death determination and, 483–84
  correction of, 482–84
  definition, 412
  failure to waken after surgery, 269, 270
  fludrocortisone, 415, 416
  hypotonic intravenous fluids, 415–16, 415t
  key points to remember, 416
  serum osmolality, 414f
  sodium correction of, 347–48
  stupor after brain surgery, 275b, 275–76
hypophysitis, anti-CTLA-4 therapy, 252
hypopituitarism, 209, 210, 252
hypotension and fever spike
  case of 50-year-old man, 353b, 358
  initial treatment of septic shock, 356b
  key points to remember, 359
  recommendations from Surviving Sepsis
    Campaign, 355b
hypothalamic hamartoma, causes of central
    diabetes insipidus (DI), 421b
hypothermia
  adoption of therapeutic, 222
  after cardiac arrest, 223
  brain death determination and, 483–84
  induction of, 224
  targeted temperature management,
    222–24
Hypothermia for Brain Enhancement
    Recovery by Neuroprotective
    and Anticonvulsivant Action for
    Convulsive Status Epilepticus
    (HYBERNATUS), 194
hypothyroidism, 210, 419b
hypotonic intravenous fluids, sodium
    content, 415–16, 415t
hypovolemia, 158, 309–10, 421–22

ICI. See immune checkpoint inhibitors (ICI)
idarucizumab, reversal of dabigatran, 17t, 21
immune checkpoint inhibitors (ICI)
  case of 78-year-old man, 249b, 253
  electromyography (EMG), 249b, 254
  key points to remember, 255
  myopathy, 252–53
  neurologic complications with anti-PD-1
    therapy, 250–51, 251f
  programmed death 1 (PD-1), 251–52
  reintroduction of, 253–54
  severe cases, 250f, 250
immune effector cell-associated
    neurotoxicity syndrome (ICANS),
    258–59
  brain imaging and
    electroencephalography (EEG), 262
  diagnosis of, 259, 263
  fulminant fatal cerebral edema and, 263
  neurotoxicity from CAR T-cell therapy,
    258–59
  posterior reversible encephalopathy
    syndrome (PRES) and, 259, 261f
  progress of, 259
  risk factors for, 258–59
  treatment, 263
  treatment of, 262–63
  See also CAR (CD19 chimeric antigen
    receptor) T-cell therapy
immunosuppression toxicity, 243t
immunosuppressive drugs, autoimmune
    disorders and, 79
immunotherapy
  management of status epilepticus (SE),
    195f
  myasthenia gravis treatment, 406, 409
infections, rapidly progressive brain disease,
    242, 244
Influence of Cooling during on Efficacy
    in Cardiac Arrest Patients (ICECAP)
    trial, 223–24
influenza, cause, diagnostic test and
    management, 65t

insulin therapy, glucose level, 355*b*, 357–58

Intensive Ambulance-delivered Blood Pressure Reduction in Hyper-Acute Stroke Trial (INTERACT-4), 362, 365

intensive care unit (ICU)
  acute encephalitis and, 69
  alcohol withdrawal, 339*b*, 340
  approach to patient with ICU delirium, 329, 330*t*
  brain death determination, 481*b*
  cooling devices for targeted temperature management, 222
  delirium as complication in, 324
  diagnosis of ICU delirium, 327*t*, 331
  differential diagnoses in ICU patients with encephalopathy, 327*t*
  drug toxicity as cause of encephalopathy, 334
  end-of-life care in, 473
  families and physicians, 510
  immunotherapy complications, 254
  indications and rationale for EEG monitoring in, 300*t*
  neuropalliative care, 472
  neurotoxicity of CAR T-cell therapy, 257*b*
  severe traumatic brain injury (TBI), 482
  stroke patient, 105
  See also delirium; neuroscience intensive care unit (neuro-ICU)

INTERACT-2 trial, 446–47

International Mission for Prognosis and Analysis of Clinical Trials in Traumatic Brain Injury (IMPACT), 437, 440

intra-arterial therapy, calcium channel antagonists, 159–61, 159*t*

intracerebral hematoma (ICH)
  case of 72-year-old man with LVAD, 287*b*, 288
  head computed tomography (CT) scan of, 287*b*, 288*f*
  importance of site for prognostication, 445
  key points to remember, 292

neurologic complications with LVADs, 290–91
patients with LVADs, 288–90
See also left ventricular assist device (LVAD)

intracerebral hemorrhage (ICH)
  after first 24 hours, 366
  algorithm for control of hypertension, 363*f*
  anticoagulation reversal in, 15*b*
  consequences of, 5
  factors associated with worse prognosis, 446–47, 446*t*
  factors favoring surgery for, 3*b*–5*b*
  first 24 hours, 365
  hypertension, 367
  intracranial pressure (ICP) monitor, 307–8
  IV heparin, 16
  key points to remember, 9
  low-molecular-weight heparin (LMWH), 16
  need for intracranial pressure (ICP) monitor, 307*b*
  neurosurgical evacuation of hematomas, 7–8
  predicting outcome of patients, 444–45, 445*t*
  prognosis of, 437
  prognostic scores for, 449
  reversal of IV thrombolysis, 16–17
  surgery for, 6–7
  thrombocytopenia, 16
  trials evaluating surgical evacuation for spontaneous ICH, 6

intracranial abscesses, magnetic resonance imaging (MRI), 57*f*

intracranial hemorrhage (ICH)
  anticoagulation, 289–90
  ICU patients with encephalopathy, 327*t*
  IV thrombolysis complication, 93

intracranial internal carotid artery (ICA)
  computed tomography (CT) angiogram showing clot in, 99*b*, 100*f*

CT scan showing hyperdensity in, 99*b*, 100*f*

intracranial pressure (ICP)
rapid release of, 47
traumatic brain injury, 30*b*, 31
traumatic brain injury (TBI) and, 26–27

intracranial pressure (ICP) monitor
brain swelling and, 69
case of 53-year-old man, 305*b*, 310–11
clinical scenarios indicating need for, 307*b*
considerations, 306–8
fulminant hepatic failure, 308–9, 311
hyperosmolar therapy, 309–10
hypertonic saline, 310
intracranial hypertension, 309
key points to remember, 311
neurosurgery, 481*b*
noncontrast head CT in TBI showing subdural hematoma, 305*b*, 306*f*
patients with traumatic brain injury (TBI), 306–7, 311
placement of, 308
rescue surgery, 310
traumatic brain injury (TBI), 435*b*–36, 439–40

intraparenchymal probe, intracranial pressure (ICP) and, 26–27

intravenous (IV) dexamethasone, *Streptococcus pneumoniae*, 54–55

intravenous fluid solutions, sodium content, 415–16, 415*t*

intravenous immunoglobulin (IVIG), myasthenia gravis, 403*b*, 406

intravenous thrombolysis
adrenal bleeding into hemodynamic collapse, 93
case of 82-year-old woman, 91*b*
computed tomography (CT) scans of asymptomatic ICH in left frontal lobe, 95*f*
emergency evaluation and management of wake-up stroke, 115*f*

hemorrhage in opposite hemisphere after IV recombinant tissue plasminogen activator (rt-PA), 91*b*, 94*f*, 94

intracranial hemorrhage (ICH), 93
key points to remember, 96–97
major and minor complications of, 96*b*
outcome of ischemic strokes, 95–96
reversing the thrombolytic effect, 94, 95*f*
stroke patients, 116
swollen tongue after, 93
symptomatic intracranial hemorrhage (sICH), 93–94, 94*f*
treatment algorithms, 95

intravenous vitamin K, 13*b*
reversing antagonistic effect of warfarin, 15–16

ischemic stroke
after first 24 hours, 365
algorithm for control of hypertension, 363*f*
best candidates for decompressive hemicraniectomy, 132
candidate for thrombosis (first 24 hours), 362–64
case of 48-year-old man, 129*b*, 134
complication of vascular surgery, 268
computed tomography (CT) scan series showing evolving infarct, 129*b*, 130*f*
criteria for decompressive craniectomy in large hemispheric stroke, 132*b*, 132
decompressive craniectomy and, 134–35
decompressive hemicraniectomy for patients (60 years old and younger), 132, 135
elderly patients and, 131–32, 135
hemicraniectomy for some patients, 130–31
ICU patients with encephalopathy, 327*t*
key points to remember, 135
low to normal blood pressure after, 390–91
mechanical thrombectomy, 364
medical management of swollen hemispheric, 130–31, 133–34, 135

ischemic stroke (*cont.*)
neurocritical management, 133
neurosurgical intervention, 134–35
not candidate for reperfusion therapy
(first 24 hours), 364–65, 367
outcome of hemicraniectomy, 131
seizures and, 133
timing of surgery, 133
See also hemicraniectomy; hypertension;
prognostication after acute ischemic
stroke and cerebral hemorrhage;
stroke(s)
isoflurane
management of status epilepticus
(SE), 195*f*
rescue therapy, 193–94
IV immunoglobulin (IVIG)
immune therapy, 80
immunosuppression, 77–78
IV thrombolysis, anticoagulation reversal in
ICH, 15*b*, 16–17

JC virus, 242–44
See also progressive multifocal
leukoencephalopathy (JC virus)

ketamine
addition to midazolam or propofol, 193
failure to awaken postoperatively, 270
management of status epilepticus
(SE), 195*f*
refractory status epilepticus (SE), 192*t*
ketogenic diet, management of status
epilepticus (SE), 195*f*
kidney injury
drug neurotoxicity, 334–35
hypertonic saline, 309–10
Korsakoff, Sergei, 349
Korsakoff syndrome, 349
Krebs cycle, 350

labetalol
blood pressure control, 19, 219

Guillain-Barré syndrome (GBS), 398*b*
hypertension treatment, 366–67, 367*t*
lacosamide
adverse effects and drug interactions,
281*t*
antiseizure medication, 279*b*, 280, 281*t*,
284
management of status epilepticus (SE),
195*f*
prescribing after electrocardiogram
review, 280
refractory status epilepticus (SE), 192*t*
stabilizing neuronal membranes, 284
lactulose and rifaximin, hyperammonemia
treatment, 427*b*, 430
lamotrigine, postresuscitation status
myoclonus, 230–31
Lance-Adams syndrome
case of 62-year-old man, 227*b*, 228, 231
treatment of, 230–31
See also myoclonus
Langerhans cell histiocytosis, diabetes
insipidus (DI) in neurosciences ICU,
421*b*
left ventricular assist device (LVAD)
case of 72-year-old man, 287*b*, 288
as destination therapy, 288
intracranial hemorrhage (ICH) in
patients with, 289–90
key points to remember, 292
neurologic complications with, 290–91
patients with, 288–89
saving lives with risk and consuming
resources, 291–92
See also intracerebral hematoma (ICH)
leptomeningeal carcinomatosis, 254
levetiracetam
adverse effects and drug interactions,
281*t*
brain tumors in emergency department,
202
disabling myoclonus, 231
head trauma and, 341

management of status epilepticus (SE),
195*f*

medication for acute seizures, 280–83

posthypoxic myoclonus, 229–30

postresuscitation status myoclonus,
230–31

refractory status epilepticus (SE), 192*t*

seizure control, 290

seizure therapy, 190–91

levofloxacin, urinary infection, 61*b*

levothyroxine, hypothyroidism, 419*b*

life support, premature withdrawal of, 447

limb-girdle dystrophy, 87

limbic encephalitis, 243*t*

lingual hematoma, 96

lip swelling, angioedema, 92

Listeria monocytogenes

infection with, 54

meningitis, 58–59

liver cirrhosis

case of 38-year-old female, 427*b*, 429, 431

computed tomography (CT) scan of
cortical hypodensities, 427*b*, 428*f*

hyperammonemia, 427*b*, 428–29, 430,
431

key points to remember, 431

magnetic resonance imaging (MRI),
428*f*, 429

serum ammonia, 427*b*, 428, 431

liver failure

drug neurotoxicity, 334

opiates, 358

lobal hematoma, clot removal, 8–9

lobar cerebral hemorrhage

case of 78-year-old woman, 3*b*, 8

computed tomography (CT) angiogram
of hyperdensity in hematoma, 4*f*

computed tomography (CT)
angiography, 3*b*

CT scan of temporal lobe hematoma, 4*f*

evacuation through open craniotomy, 5

factors favoring surgery for ICH
(intracerebral hemorrhage), 3*b*–5*b*

factors when considering surgery for, 8–9

hematoma evacuation, 4–5

neurosurgical evacuation, 7–8

placement of ventriculostomy, 8

points to remember, 9

postoperative CT showing hematoma
evacuation, 4*f*

lobar hematomas, CT scan showing
temporal, 4*f*

lobar intracerebral hemorrhage, key points
to remember, 9

long-term care

neuropalliative care, 472

persistent comatose states, 468, 469

lorazepam

brain death determination and, 483–84

intravenous, at emergency room, 194–96

management of status epilepticus (SE),
195*f*

refractory status epilepticus (SE), 192*t*

seizure therapy, 190–91

treatment of delirium tremens, 342*t*

waking up slowly, 265*b*

withdrawal of life support, 478

low-molecular weight heparin (LMWH), 29

anticoagulation reversal in ICH, 15*b*, 16

protamine and, 16, 20

lumbar drain, placement, 184

lumbar drainage

bacterial meningitis, 57–58

perioperative, 184–85

lung cancer, spinal cord compression, 174

Lyme, cause, diagnostic test and
management, 65*t*

lymphohistiocytic myocarditis, 250

lymphoma, 243*t*

causes of central diabetes insipidus (DI),
421*b*

lymphomatosis cerebri, 243*t*

macrolides, 392

Magnesium for aneurysmal subarachnoid
hemorrhage (MASH)-2 trial, 156–57

magnesium sulfate, eclampsia and, 217–18, 219
magnetic resonance angiogram (MRA), cerebral vasospasm, 276
magnetic resonance imaging (MRI)
acute subdural hematoma, 36–37
bacterial meningitis, 53*b*, 54*f*, 56–57, 57*f*
Bilsky grading scale for tumors, 175, 177*t*
brain, 73*b*
brain biopsy guided by, 68
brain MRI of stroke patient with frontal infarction, 113, 114*f*
diffusion-weighted imaging (DWI), 103
diffusion-weighted, for major stroke, 110
empyema, 57*f*
failure to awaken after CPR, 456–57, 457*f*
functional MRI of persistent vegetative state, 464–66, 469
herpes simplex virus type 1 (HSV-1) encephalitis, 62–64
hyperintensities in thalamus, brainstem, and occipital lobe, 121, 122*f*
liver cirrhosis patient, 428*f*, 429
multiple intracranial abscesses, 57*f*
neuroimaging for suspected encephalitis, 70
patient in stupor and lesions, 268
pituitary adenomas with hemorrhage, 208
posterior reversible encephalopathy syndrome (PRES), 234–35
preoperative and postoperative, for tumor resection, 419*b*, 420*f*
prognostic models on usefulness of, 438
progressive parenchymal loss, 245
rapidly progressive brain disease, 241*b*, 242*f*, 242–45, 243*t*
restricted diffusion on bilateral dorsal medial thalami, mamillary bodies, periaqueductal gray matter and the pons, 345*b*, 346*f*
spinal cord infarction (SCI), 182*f*, 182

spinal tumors, 173*b*, 175, 177*t*
strokes by diffusion-weighted imaging-fluid-attenuated inversion recovery (DWI-FLAIR), 112–13, 115*f*, 116
subarachnoid hemorrhage (SAH), 165*b*, 167, 168*f*, 170
traumatic brain injury (TBI) and, 25
treatment for encephalitis, 69–70
maintenance immunosuppression, treatments, 78
malaria, cause, diagnostic test and management, 65*t*
malignancies, antibodies linked to encephalitis with or without, 77*t*
malignant hyperthermia, ICU patients with encephalopathy, 327*t*
malnutrition, 345*b*
alcoholism and, 347
Mancall, Elliott Lee, 347–48
mannitol
acute brain edema, 55*b*
hyperosmolar therapy, 309–10
treatment of intracranial pressure (ICP), 28*f*, 28
Marchiafava-Bignami disease, 347
Mayo Clinic, 210, 253, 347–48
mean arterial pressure (MAP), spinal cord perfusion, 184–85
measles, cause, diagnostic test and management, 65*t*
mechanical embolectomy, recanalization of basilar artery, 120*f*, 121
mechanical thrombectomy
best imaging selection for, 103
catheter cerebral angiogram with complete recanalization, 113, 114*f*
emergency evaluation and management of wake-up stroke, 115*f*
indications for, 104, 107
ischemic stroke treatment, 364
major acute ischemic stroke, 110
recanalization and reperfusion, 100–1
mechanical valves, cerebral hemorrhage, 19–20

medical staff. *See* family members, dealing with; triage communication

meningioma, causes of central diabetes insipidus (DI), 421*b*

meningitis
ICU patients with encephalopathy, 327*t*
nivolumab/pembrolizumab, 251*f*, 252
See also bacterial meningitis

metabolic leukodystrophies, 243*t*

metastasis, 243*t*
causes of central diabetes insipidus (DI), 421*b*

metastatic melanoma, pembrolizumab for, 249*b*

methanol, 243*t*

methotrexate, 61*b*

methylnaltrexone, treating adynamic ileus, 399

methylprednisolone
immune checkpoint inhibitor-associated myopathy, 253
immune effector cell-associated neurotoxicity syndrome (ICANS), 262–63

methylprednisolone, high-dose IV, immunosuppression, 77–78

metoprolol, atrial fibrillation, 391–92, 393*t*

midazolam
antiepileptic agent, 191–93
brain death determination and, 483–84
intravenous, in neuro-intensive care unit (ICU), 78
ketamine and, 193
management of status epilepticus (SE), 195*f*
refractory status epilepticus (SE), 192*t*
treatment in intensive care unit, 194–96

milrinone
cerebral vasospasm treatment option, 159*t*
inducing cerebral vasodilation, 158

mineralocorticoids, subarachnoid hemorrhage (SAH), 415

mini apnea test, organ donation, 495

minimally invasive instruments, neurosurgical, 4

mitochondrial encephalomyopathy (MELAS), 243*t*

modified Thrombolysis in Cerebral Infarction (mTICI) score, 100–1

monoclonal antibodies, programmed death 1 (PD-1), 251–52

monoclonal antibody therapy, rituximab, 253–54

mononeuritis multiplex, 253

morphine, 384–86
comfort medication, 493
intravenous, for Guillain-Barré syndrome (GBS), 397–98, 398*b*, 399, 400
withdrawal of life support, 478

morphine sulfate, paroxysmal sympathetic hyperactivity (PSH), 385*t*, 386

motor responses, postresuscitation coma, 458*t*

multifactorial encephalopathy, 334

multifocal atrial tachycardia, treatment for, 393*t*

multifocal myoclonus, 297*b*

multimodality prognostication, term, 458–59

mumps, cause, diagnostic test and management, 65*t*

myalgia, nivolumab/pembrolizumab, 251*f*

myasthenia gravis (MG)
acute neuromuscular disorder, 84
anti-muscle-specific kinase (MuSK) variant, 408
bilevel positive airway pressure (BiPAP), 403*b*, 407
case of 60-year-old man, 403*b*–4*b*, 408
cerebrospinal fluid (CSF), 254
checkpoint inhibitor-induced, 253
chest X-ray showing atelectasis of left lung, 403*b*–4, 405*f*
electromyography (EMG), 254
extubation, 406–7, 407*t*, 408
Guillain-Barré syndrome (GBS), 86–87
key points to remember, 409
management of, 405

INDEX 545

myasthenia gravis (MG) (*cont.*)
  nerve conduction studies (NCSs), 254
  nivolumab-induced, 253
  nivolumab/pembrolizumab treatment, 251*f*, 252–53
  postextubation stridor, 408
  pyridostigmine assisting weaning of patient, 406, 409
  respiratory failure, 84, 86, 88–89
  treatment of, 408
  triple M syndrome, 252–53
  weaning patients from ventilator, 405–6
mycobacterium tuberculosis, cause, diagnostic test and management, 65*t*
mycophenolate mofetil, myasthenia gravis, 406
myelitis, nivolumab/pembrolizumab, 251*f*, 252
myeloma, spinal cord compression, 174
myocarditis
  lymphohistiocytic, 250
  treatment for steroid-refractory, 255
  triple M syndrome, 252–53
myoclonic status epilepticus, postresuscitation coma, 458*t*
myoclonus
  action, 228, 229, 230–31
  basal ganglia injury, 229–30
  brainstem, 228–29
  cardiac arrest and, 230
  cefepime and acute encephalopathy, 337
  classification, 228
  clinical and EEG differences between postarrest, and posthypoxic action, 229*t*
  cortical, 228–29
  cortical polymyoclonus, 228
  definition, 228
  electroencephalographic (EEG) recordings, 229, 229*t*
  generalized, 228–29
  key points to remember, 231
  Lance-Adams syndrome, 228, 229, 230–31

  movements, 229
  multifocal, 228–29
  multisegmental, after cardiopulmonary resuscitation (CPR), 453
  patients with cefepime neurotoxicity, 336
  postresuscitation status, 230–31
  segmental, 228–29
  status, 230, 231
  subcortical, 228
  treatment of posthypoxic, 229–30
  treatments, 230–31
  See also action myoclonus; Lance-Adams syndrome
myopathy
  immune checkpoint inhibitor (ICI)-associated, 253
  immune-mediated, 250
  immune-mediated necrotizing, 253
myositis
  necrotic, 250
  nivolumab/pembrolizumab, 251*f*, 252–53
  oculobulbar variant of, 254
  triple M syndrome, 252–53
Myriad device (NICO Corporation), 6–7
mysoline, postresuscitation status myoclonus, 230–31

naloxegol, treating adynamic ileus, 399
naloxone, postoperative stupor, 269
National Inpatient Sample database, 134–35
National Institute of Neurological Disorders and Stroke (NINDS) trial, 93
National Institutes of Health Stroke Scale (NIHSS), 91*b*, 93, 99*b*, 104, 122–23, 361*b*
  ceiling effect of the score, 104
  major stroke, 109*b*, 110
  neurosciences ICU, 364
  See also acute stroke
natural death, withdrawal of life support for, 478–79
necrotic myositis, 250

neocritical care, self-fulfilling prophecy of, 447

neostigmine, treating adynamic ileus, 399

nerve conduction studies (NCSs)
    Guillain-Barré syndrome (GBS), 254
    myasthenia gravis, 254

Neurocritical Care Society, 131

neurofilament light chain (NfL), prognosticating value, 456

neurogenic pulmonary edema, 372–73, 375–76
    after acute brain injury, 375t

neuroimaging, posterior reversible encephalopathy syndrome (PRES), 235–36, 237

neuroleptic malignant syndrome
    differential diagnosis of paroxysmal sympathetic hyperactivity, 383t
    ICU patients with encephalopathy, 327t

neurological deterioration, malignant brain tumors, 200b

neurological evaluation, brain death determination and, 484

neuromuscular respiratory failure, myasthenia gravis, 405–6

neuron-specific enolase (NSE), serum biomarker, 456

neuropalliative care, intensive care unit (ICU), 472

neuroscience intensive care unit (neuro-ICU)
    brain tumors, 199b, 202
    cardiac arrhythmias, 389b, 391–92
    case of 78-year-old woman with acute brain damage, 471b, 478–79
    causes of central diabetes insipidus (DI), 421b
    ischemic stroke patient, 364
    neuropalliative care, 472
    patients as best candidates for, 504–5
    patient with thalamic hemorrhage, 443b, 444f, 448
    stroke patient, 91b

See also intensive care unit (ICU)

neurosurgical evacuation, hematomas, 4–5, 6, 7–8

neurosurgical intervention, traumatic brain injury (TBI) and, 24–26

neurosurgical management, cerebral hemorrhage, 4

neurosyphilis, 245–46

neurotoxicity, cefepime, 334–37

New England Journal of Medicine (journal), 222

nicardipine, 392
    blood pressure control, 19
    cerebral vasospasm treatment option, 159t
    eclampsia and, 218
    Guillain-Barré syndrome (GBS), 397–98, 398b, 400
    hypertension treatment, 366–67, 367t
    intra-arterial therapy, 159–61
    ischemic stroke patient, 364

nifedipine, 366–67
    eclampsia and, 219

nimodipine, 155b, 366
    cerebral vasospasm treatment option, 159t
    intra-arterial therapy, 159–61

nivolumab, treatment, 252

nonaneurysmal subarachnoid hemorrhage
    case of 44-year-old female, 165b
    See also subarachnoid hemorrhage (SAH)

nonconvulsive seizures (NCSs), electroencephalography (EEG), 298–301

nonconvulsive status epilepticus, patients with cefepime neurotoxicity, 336

non-Hodgkin lymphoma, spinal cord compression, 174

norepinephrine
    arterial pressure, 158
    septic shock, 355b
    vasopressor, 354–55

nosocomial meningitis, early sepsis, 357

nucleus, localization of the lesion, 319*t*

nursing care, persistent comatose states, 468

oculomotor palsy
  case of 40-year-old woman, 315*b*, 317, 320
  cause of, 321
  cranial nerves, 318
  diagnosis of, 317, 318*f*
  fixed and dilated pupil, 316–17
  funduscopy, 317
  neurologic examination of dilated pupil, 315*b*
  pain, 317
  posterior communicating artery aneurysms compressing nerve, 316*f*, 318–20
  rate of complete recovery, 319–20
  vascular abnormalities, 317
  visual loss and, 317
  See also pupil, fixed and dilated
ondansetron, 392
open craniotomy
  neurosurgical evacuation, 5
  traditional, 6–7
ophthalmoparesis, 250*f*
ophthalmoplegia, 317
opiates
  administration for headaches from brain tumors, 200
  confounding neurological examination, 358
  risk of delirium with, 324–26, 331
opioids, 243*t*
  failure to awaken postoperatively, 270
oral anticoagulation, traumatic brain injury (TBI), 26
orbit, localization of the lesion, 319*t*
organ donation
  case of 51-year-old man, 489*b*
  circulatory arrest and, 494, 497
  comfort medication, 493
  DCD donors, 496

DCD protocols, 496
donation after brain death (DBD), 490
donation after cardiac/circulatory death (DCD), 490–93
heart procurement from DCD donors, 494
key points to remember, 496–97
medical and social history, 492
mini apnea test, 495
multicenter study devising new score (DCD-N), 495*f*, 495–96
organ procurement coordinators, 493
organ procurement organization, 492
patient extubation, 493–94
point of no return, 490
protocol differences between DCD and DBD, 491*t*
TransMedics Organ Care System™ (OCS™), 494
waiting list in United States, 496
withdrawal of intensive care support, 490
ornithine transcarbamylase deficiency, 269
orolingual angioedema
  major complication of IV thrombolysis, 96*b*
  stroke patient, 92
osmotic demyelination, 243*t*
osmotic demyelination syndrome, 347–48
  differential diagnoses of posterior reversible encephalopathy syndrome (PRES), 236*b*
otitis media, 56–57
oxygenation, traumatic brain injury, 30*b*

pacemaker, Guillain-Barré syndrome (GBS), 398*b*
pain management, spinal cord compression, 175–78, 177*b*
parainfectious encephalitides, 245–46
paraneoplastic disease, 254

paraplegia
  flaccid, 182–83
  flaccid-type, 182–83
  postoperative, 184
parasitic infections, 243*t*
parenchymal intracranial hemorrhage,
    major complication of IV
    thrombolysis, 96*b*
parkinsonism, 283
paroxysmal sympathetic hyperactivity
    (PSH), 245, 380
  assessment measure for diagnosis
    of, 381*t*
  case of 22-year-old woman, 379*b*,
    384–86
  characteristics of spells, 380–83
  Clinical Feature Scale (CFS), 381*t*
  computed tomography (CT)
    scan, 379*b*
  Diagnosis Likelihood Tool
    (DLT), 381*t*
  differential diagnosis of, 383*t*
  episodes of, 380
  key points to remember, 386
  pharmacological options for treatment
    of, 385*t*
  treatment of, 384–86
patients. *See* triage communication
PCCs. *See* prothrombin complex
    concentrates (PCCs)
pembrolizumab
  immune-mediated myopathy, 250
  immune-related complications, 255
  lung cancer and, 250*f*
  metastatic melanoma treatment, 249*b*
  programmed death 1 (PD-1), 251–52
  treatment, 252
pembrolizumab/nivolumab, patients treated
    with, 250–51, 251*f*
pentobarbital
  aborting status epilepticus (SE), 193–94
  refractory status epilepticus (SE), 192*t*
pentose phosphate pathway, 350

percutaneous endoscopic gastrostomy
    (PEG)
  long-term support, 469
  precautionary measures, 466–67,
    467*b*
perfusion imaging, stroke patients, 116
perihematomal hypoperfusion, hematoma
    expansion, 5
perioperative atrial fibrillation, 267
perioperative stroke
  risk of, 266–67
  underlying mechanism, 267
peripheral nervous system, 252–53
peripheral neuropathy, 253
permissive hypertension, 364–65
persistent comatose states
  case of 43-year-old male, 463*b*
  categories of persistent disorders of
    consciousness, 465–66, 466*f*
  clinical signs of a vegetative state, 464,
    465*b*
  cognitive motor dissociation (CMD),
    465–66, 466*f*
  enteral feeding, 467
  functional magnetic resonance imaging
    (MRI), 464–66, 468–69
  higher-order cortex-motor dissociation
    (HMD), 465–66, 466*f*
  key points to remember, 468–69
  long-term care in facility, 468
  neurological examination, 464–66
  percutaneous endoscopic gastrostomy
    (PEG), 466–67, 467*b*, 469
  pneumoperitoneum, 467
  precautionary measures with gastrostomy
    and tracheostomy, 466–67, 467*b*
  predicting outcome of severe traumatic
    brain injury (TBI), 464
  tracheostomy, 466–68, 467*b*, 469
  See also coma
petechial hemorrhage in cerebral
    infarction, minor complication of IV
    thrombolysis, 96*b*

INDEX   549

phenobarbital
  aborting status epilepticus (SE), 191
  antiseizure drug, 284
  brain death determination and, 483–84
  management of status epilepticus (SE), 195*f*
  postresuscitation status myoclonus, 230–31
  treating patients with traumatic brain injury (TBI), 26
  treatment of delirium tremens, 342*t*
phenylephrine, 354–55
phenytoin, 237–38
  administration of, 283–84
  adverse effects and drug interactions, 281*t*
  postresuscitation status myoclonus, 230–31
pilocytic astrocytoma
  case of 40-year-old woman, 419*b*, 424
  causes of central diabetes insipidus (DI), 421*b*
  tumor resection, 419*b*, 420*f*
piperacillin-tazobactam
  cefepime and, 336–37
  septic shock treatment, 356*b*
pituitary adenoma, causes of central diabetes insipidus (DI), 421*b*
pituitary apoplexy
  acute care of, 209–10, 210*b*
  acute enlargement of tumor, 209
  care with endocrinologist, 211
  case of 73-year-old man, 116, 207*b*, 211
  computed tomography (CT) scan of heterogenous sellar and suprasellar mass, 207*b*, 208*f*
  concerns of cortisol and thyroid hormone deficiency, 210
  destruction of pituitary gland, 209
  key points to remember, 212
  magnetic resonance imaging (MRI), 212
  magnetic resonance imaging (MRI) studies, 208, 210–11

  outcomes of, 211
  pathophysiology of, 208–9
  symptoms of, 209
  transsphenoidal resection surgery, 210–11, 212
pituitary gland
  neurosurgical procedure in region of, 419*b*, 420
  preoperative imaging, 210–11
pituitary hormones, monitoring in pituitary apoplexy, 210*b*
pituitary ischemia, 208–9
plasma exchange (PLEX)
  immune checkpoint inhibitor-associated myopathy, 253
  immune therapy, 80
  immunosuppression, 77–78
  myasthenia gravis, 403*b*
  myasthenia gravis treatment, 406, 409
platelet transfusion(s), 16, 21
Platelet Transfusion Versus Standard Care After Acute Stroke due to Spontaneous Cerebral Hemorrhage Associated with Antiplatelet Therapy (PATCH) trial, 18–19
pneumococcal meningitis, 297*b*
polymerase chain reaction (PCR)
  herpes simplex virus (HSV), 73*b*
  screening multiple infectious agents on CSF, 62–64, 70
polyuria, neurological patient with, 420–21
Pompe disease, 87
positive end-expiratory pressures (PEEPs)
  pulmonary conditions after brain injury, 373, 375*t*
  sepsis patients, 355*b*, 358
positron emission tomography (PET)
  malignancy, 245
  myositis, 253
  rapidly progressive brain disease, 244–45
  tissue sampling, 68
postcardiac resuscitation syndrome
  clinical picture of, 452

neurological assessment, 452–53
See also prognostication after
cardiopulmonary resuscitation
postcraniectomy fluid collections, 49
postcraniectomy hydrocephalus, shunting,
49
posterior reversible encephalopathy
syndrome (PRES), 234–35
blood pressure fluctuations, 396–97
case of 48-year-old woman, 233*b*,
237–38
differential diagnoses of, 235–36, 236*b*
electroencephalogram (EEG), 237–38
ICU patients with, 327*t*
immune effector cell-associated
neurotoxicity syndrome (ICANS) and,
259
key points to remember, 238
magnetic resonance imaging (MRI),
234–35
mimicking other conditions, 235–36,
236*b*
onset of neurologic symptoms, 235
rapid recognition of, 236–37
recovery of patients, 237
recurrent seizures after, 237
risk factors for development of, 236*b*
white matter, 243*t*
postoperative hemorrhage
deterioration, 275
mechanical shift of brain
(sagging), 275
postoperative stupor, failure to waken after
surgery, 269, 270
postresuscitation encephalopathy, 230
post-traumatic hydrocephalus (PTH),
craniectomy, 47–48
prednisone
myasthenia gravis, 403*b*
myasthenia gravis treatment, 406
pregnancy. *See* eclampsia
PRES. *See* posterior reversible
encephalopathy syndrome (PRES)

primidone
posthypoxic myoclonus, 229–30
postresuscitation status myoclonus,
230–31
prognostication after acute ischemic stroke
and cerebral hemorrhage
case of 68-year-old woman, 443*b*, 444*f*,
448
clinical trials, 446–47
considerations for bedside
prognosticating, 447–48
importance of self-fulfilling prophecy,
447
importance of site of intracerebral
hematoma, 445
important observations, 448
intracerebral hemorrhage (ICH) score
(predicting 30-day mortality), 444–45,
445*t*
key points to remember, 449
main factors associated with worse
prognosis, 446, 446*t*
possibility of meaningful improvement,
448–49
premature withdrawal of life support,
447
speed of improvement, 448
treatment of disorders, 444
prognostication after cardiopulmonary
resuscitation
biomarker neuron-specific enolase
(NSE), 456
brainstem reflexes, 453–54
case of 60-year-old woman, 451*b*,
457–58
clinical picture of postcardiac
resuscitation syndrome, 452
diffusion-weighted imaging (DWI),
456–57
electroencephalography (EEG), 453,
454–55, 456*f*, 457–59
failure to awaken, 456–57
key points to remember, 459

INDEX   551

prognostication after cardiopulmonary
resuscitation (*cont.*)
laboratory tests, 454
magnetic resonance imaging (MRI),
456–57, 457*f*
motor response as prognosticator, 453
multimodality prognostication, 458–59
multisegmental myoclonus, 453
neuroimaging, 456
neurological assessment for comatose
patient, 452–53
poor outcome anticipated in
postresuscitation coma, 458*t*
somatosensory evoked potentials
(SSEPs), 454, 455*f*, 457–59
prognostication after traumatic brain injury
(TBI)
biomarkers as new tools, 440
case of 34-year-old woman, 435*b*–36,
440, 441
computed tomography (CT) scan
showing subarachnoid hemorrhage,
435*b*–36, 437*f*
Corticosteroid Randomization After
Significant Head Injury (CRASH)
model, 438
data points in, 439*t*
decision in neurocritical care, 438
ICP as indicator in trauma, 439–40
International Mission for Prognosis and
Analysis of Clinical Trials in Traumatic
Brain Injury (IMPACT), 437, 440
key points to remember, 441
magnetic resonance imaging (MRI),
438
neurosurgical intervention, 439
prediction models, 438–39
Transforming Research and Clinical
Knowledge in Traumatic Brain Injury
(TRACK-TBI), 439
progressive multifocal leukoencephalopathy
(JC virus), 243*t*
cause, diagnostic test and management, 65*t*

causes and neuroimaging, 63*t*
differential diagnoses of posterior
reversible encephalopathy syndrome
(PRES), 236*b*
treatment, 68–69
Propionibacterium acnes, postneurosurgical
meningitis, 49
propofol
alcohol withdrawal, 341–42
antiepileptic agent, 193
failure to awaken postoperatively, 270
ketamine and, 193
management of status epilepticus (SE),
195*f*
neuro-intensive care unit (ICU), 78
TBI treatment, 27–28
treatment of delirium tremens, 342*t*
propranolol
paroxysmal sympathetic hyperactivity
(PSH), 384, 385*t*, 386
prostate cancer, spinal cord
compression, 174
protamine, 16
low-molecular-weight heparin (LMWH)
and, 16, 20
prothrombin complex concentrates (PCCs)
administration of four-factor, 17–18
cost for treatment with four-factor,
17–18
four-factor, 16
four-factor, plus vitamin K, 26
protozoal infections, cause, diagnostic test
and management, 65*t*
Pseudomonas, 408
Pseudomonas aeruginosa, 334
psycho-polyneuritic syndrome, 349
ptosis, severe, 250*f*
pulmonary contusion, 372–73
pulmonary embolism
differential diagnosis of paroxysmal
sympathetic hyperactivity, 383*t*
paroxysmal sympathetic hyperactivity
(PSH), 386

pulmonary embolus
  acute pulmonary distress, 372–73
  after acute brain injury, 375*t*
pupil, fixed and dilated
  case of 40-year-old woman, 315*b*, 317, 320
  cerebral angiogram of posterior
    communicating artery aneurysm,
    315*b*, 316*f*
  complete right third-nerve palsy, 317,
    318*f*
  key points to remember, 321
  localization of the lesion, 318, 319*t*
  oculomotor palsy, 315*b*, 316–17,
    318–20, 321
  posterior communicating artery
    aneurysm, 315*b*, 318–20
  predicting aneurysmal rupture, 320
pupil reflexes, postresuscitation coma, 458*t*
pyridostigmine, myasthenia gravis
    treatment, 406, 409

quadriplegia, 182
quiet delirium, term, 324
quinolones, 392
  antibiotic-associated encephalopathy,
    334–35

rabies, cause, diagnostic test and
    management, 65*t*
radiation-induced encephalitis,
    noninfectious, 64
radiation therapy, malignant brain tumors,
    200
radiculitis, nivolumab/pembrolizumab,
    251*f*
randomized controlled trials, major stroke,
    110–11
Rapid Infusion of cold Normal Saline by
    paramedics during CPR (RINSE) trial,
    223–24
rapidly progressing hepatic encephalopathy,
    intracranial pressure (ICP) monitor,
    308–9

rapidly progressive brain disease
  brain biopsy, 244–45
  case of 36-year-old woman, 241*b*, 245
  cerebrospinal fluid (CSF), 241*b*, 242–44,
    246
  clinical history, 242–44
  computed tomography (CT) scans,
    244–45
  diagnosis of, 242, 245–46
  disease mechanisms, 244
  empiric therapy, 245
  infectious and inflammatory processes,
    244
  key points to remember, 246
  magnetic resonance imaging (MRI),
    241*b*, 242*f*, 242–44, 243*t*
  positron emission tomography (PET),
    244–45
rapid progressive dementia, common causes
    of, 242–44
ravulizumab, myasthenia gravis treatment,
    406
rebound edema, 309–10
recanalization, mechanical thrombectomy
    for, 100–1
recanalization therapy, endovascular, for
    acute stroke, 100–1, 101*b*
red blood cell transfusion, septic shock, 357
refractory status epilepticus, 75
relative hypotension, brain ischemia and,
    237–38
renal cancer, spinal cord compression, 174
renal failure
  azotemia from, 336
  drug neurotoxicity, 334–35
  opiates, 358
  posterior reversible encephalopathy
    syndrome (PRES), 237–38
reperfusion
  mechanical thrombectomy for, 100–1
  stroke, 107
reperfusion therapy, ischemic stroke not
    candidate for, 364–65

RESCUEicp trial, intracranial pressure (ICP), 28–29
RESPECT-CVT trial (Comparing Efficacy and Safety of Dabigatran Etexilate with Warfarin in Patients with Cerebral Venous and Dural Sinus Thrombosis), 142
respiratory failure
  acute neuromuscular disease, 84, 85–86, 88
  amyotrophic lateral sclerosis (ALS), 87
Restart or Stop Antithrombotics Randomized Trial (RESTART), 19–20
Restlessness, acute neuromuscular disorder, 83*b*, 84
retroperitoneal hemorrhage, major complication of IV thrombolysis, 96*b*
rhabdomyolysis, nivolumab/pembrolizumab, 251*f*
Richmond Acute Subdural Hematoma (RASH) score, 39–40, 39*t*
  grading scale, 39*t*
Richmond Agitation Sedation Scale (RASS), 324–26, 326*b*, 358
rickettsioses and ehrlichiosis, cause, diagnostic test and management, 65*t*
rituximab
  agitation and dysautonomia, 78–79
  immunosuppression, 77–78
  monoclonal antibody therapy, 253–54
  myasthenia gravis treatment, 406
rivaroxaban, 17, 26
  anti-factor Xa levels, 17–18
  reversal of DOACs, 17, 17*t*
Rocky Mountain spotted fever, 245–46
rozanolixizumab, myasthenia gravis treatment, 406

Safe Implementation of Thrombolysis in Stroke-Monitoring Study (SITS-MOST), 93
Sarcoidosis, diabetes insipidus (DI) in neurosciences ICU, 421*b*

schistosomiasis, 245–46
schizophrenia, autoimmune encephalitis and, 74
SE. *See* status epilepticus (SE)
sedation
  assessment of, 325*f*
  holidays, 358
  ICU stay, 324
  protocol, 358
  Richmond Agitation Sedation Scale (RASS), 324–26, 326*b*
sedative drugs
  brain death declaration and, 483–84
  clearance of, 483–84
seizures
  acute encephalitis, 62–64
  alcohol withdrawal, 341
  autoimmune encephalitis, 78–79, 80
  control for traumatic brain injury, 30*b*
  deterioration after brain surgery, 274–75
  differential diagnosis of paroxysmal sympathetic hyperactivity, 383*t*
  hemicraniectomy and, 133
  paroxysmal sympathetic hyperactivity (PSH), 386
  patients with cefepime neurotoxicity, 336
  posterior reversible encephalopathy syndrome (PRES), 237–38
  See also antiseizure medication; brain tumors
self-fulfilling prophecy, 447
  withdrawal of life support as, 476–77
sensory neuronopathy, 253
sepsis
  azotemia from renal failure, 336
  broad-spectrum antibiotics, 357, 358
  causes of toxic encephalopathy in, 335*f*
  differential diagnosis of paroxysmal sympathetic hyperactivity, 383*t*
  drug toxicity in ICU, 334
  encephalopathy, 334

high positive end-expiratory pressure (PEEP), 358

mean arterial pressure (MAP), 354–55, 355*b*

paroxysmal sympathetic hyperactivity (PSH), 386

recommendations from Surviving Sepsis Campaign, 355*b*

septic encephalopathy, 334

treatment, 354

See also encephalopathy

septic shock

broad-spectrum antibiotics, 356*b*, 357, 358

corticosteroids, 357

initial treatment of, 356*b*

key points to remember, 359

management principles, 359

recommendations from Surviving Sepsis Campaign, 355*b*

transfusion of red blood cells, 357

Sequential Organ Failure Assessment (SOFA) Score, 358–59

serotonin syndrome

differential diagnosis of paroxysmal sympathetic hyperactivity, 383*t*

ICU patients with encephalopathy, 327*t*

serum ammonia, 427*b*, 428, 431

See also liver cirrhosis

serum anti-factor Xa, low-molecular-weight heparin (LMWH), 16

serum osmolality, hyponatremia, 414*f*

serum osmolarity, 133–34

serum sodium, decreasing

case of 46-year-old woman, 411*b*, 416

hyponatremia, 412

See also hyponatremia; subarachnoid hemorrhage (SAH)

serum sodium, increasing

calculating change in, 422–23

case of 40-year-old woman, 419*b*, 424

See also diabetes insipidus (DI); hypernatremia

severe stress-induced cardiomyopathy, 373

severe subcortical leukoaraiosis, differential diagnoses of posterior reversible encephalopathy syndrome (PRES), 236*b*

Sheehan syndrome (postpartum ischemic pituitary necrosis), diabetes insipidus (DI) in neurosciences ICU, 421*b*

SIADH. *See* syndrome of inappropriate secretion of antidiuretic hormone (SIADH)

Simvastatin in aneurysmal subarachnoid hemorrhage (STASH) trial, 156–57

sinking skin flap syndrome, 48–49, 50

sinus bradycardia, treatment for, 393*t*

sinus tachycardia, treatment for, 393*t*

skin ecchymosis, minor complication of IV thrombolysis, 96*b*

small-fiber autonomic neuropathy, 253

sodium correction, central pontine myelinolysis (CPM), 347–48

sodium nitroprusside, Guillain-Barré syndrome (GBS), 397–98

solvents, 243*t*

somatosensory evoked potentials (SSEPs)

evaluating comatose patients after CPR, 454, 455*f*

postresuscitation coma, 458*t*

spinal cord compression

cancer and, 174*f*, 174

case of 70-year-old man, 173*b*, 178

key points to remember, 179

magnetic resonance imaging (MRI), 173*b*, 175

metastatic lesions and, 174*f*, 174

MRI Bilsky grading scale, 175, 177*t*

outcome of, 178–79

pain treatment, 175–78, 177*b*

radiotherapy, 175, 178

surgical decompression, 174–75

Tokuhashi scoring system, 174–75, 176*t*, 178

INDEX 555

spinal cord infarction (SCI)
aortic repair, 183–85
case of 58-year-old man, 181*b*, 186
complications of immobilization, 185–86
disabling, 186
magnetic resonance imaging (MRI) of thoracic and lumbar spine, 182*f*, 182
mechanisms contributing to, in perioperative period, 183–84
most common setting for, 183
myelopathy, 182
neurological examination, 182–83
owl eyes, 182*f*, 182
patients outcome with, 185–86
risk factors for, 183
spinal cord ischemia, 186
aortic repair, 186
corticosteroids, 185
fenestrated-branched endovascular aortic repair (F-BEVAR), 183–84
key points to remember, 186
management options for postoperative, 185*b*
myelopathy, 182
stepwise approach in confronting, 185*b*, 185
thoracic endovascular aortic repair (TEVAR), 183–84
spinal cord perfusion, treatment of, 186
spinal cord reflexes, brain death, 483*b*
Spinal Instability Neoplastic Score (SINS), 175
Staphylococcus aureus, postneurosurgical meningitis, 49
Start or Stop Anticoagulants Randomised Trial (SoSTART), 19–20
status epilepticus (SE)
algorithm for management of, 195*f*
benzodiazepines, 190–91, 192*t*
case of 42-year-old woman, 189*b*, 194–96
continuous infusion of barbiturates, 193

convulsive, 285
electroencephalographic (EEG) recording, 190
emergency department, 195*f*
Established Status Epilepticus Treatment Trial (ESETT), 190–91
Hypothermia for Brain Enhancement Recovery by Neuroprotective and Anticonvulsant Action after Convulsive Status Epilepticus (HYBERNATUS) trial, 194
ICU patients with encephalopathy, 327*t*
intensive care unit (ICU), 195*f*
key points to remember, 196
nonconvulsive, 269, 274–75, 277
posterior reversible encephalopathy syndrome (PRES), 237
prehospital, 195*f*
presence of nonconvulsive, 269
refractory, 190–91, 194, 196
successful treatment of, 190
therapeutic options for refractory, 192*t*
treatment of refractory, 196
treatment protocol, 194–96
status myoclonus, definition, 453
stereotaxic surgery, deep-seated hematomas, 6–7
steroids, high-dose, malignant brain tumors, 200–1
STICH. *See* Surgical Trial in Intracerebral Hemorrhage (STICH)
Streptococcus pneumoniae, bacterial meningitis, 53*b*, 54–55
stroke(s)
algorithm for control of hypertension, 363*f*
case of 82-year-old woman, 91*b*
hemorrhagic, 362
hypertension, 362
ischemic, 362
IV thrombolysis changing outcome for, 95–96
orolingual angioedema, 92–93

seizure mimicking, 93

treatment options for hypertension, 367*t*

See also acute stroke; hypertension; intravenous thrombolysis; ischemic stroke; "wake-up" major stroke

stupor after brain surgery

case of 23-year-old man, 273*b*, 277

cerebral angiogram showing cerebral vasospasm, 273*b*, 274*f*

cerebral infarction, 275

cerebral vasospasm, 276–77

computed tomography (CT) scan showing hyperdensities after surgery, 273*b*, 274*f*

deterioration after craniotomy, 274, 275*b*

hypernatremia, 275*b*, 275–76

hyponatremia, 275*b*, 275–76

key points to remember, 277

magnetic resonance imaging (MRI) showing large ependymoma in fourth ventricle, 274*f*

mechanism of deterioration, 275

neurosurgical procedures and complications, 275–76

postoperative complications, 276

postoperative hemorrhage, 275

postoperative seizures, 274–75, 277

seizures, 274–75

subarachnoid hemorrhage (SAH)

algorithm for control of hypertension, 363*f*

algorithm for evaluation and management of hyponatremia, 414*f*

angiographic-negative SAH patterns, 169

anterior communicating artery aneurysm, 411*b*

case of 44-year-old female, 165*b*, 170

case of 46-year-old woman, 411*b*, 416

cerebral angiogram for, 169–70

cerebral salt-wasting syndrome (CSW), 412, 413*f*, 414*f*

computed tomography (CT) scan, 165*b*, 166*f*, 167

differential diagnosis of paroxysmal sympathetic hyperactivity, 383*t*

fludrocortisone, 415, 416

hypertension treatment for aneurysmal, 366, 367

hyponatremia in, 412, 414*f*

intracranial pressure (ICP) monitor, 307–8

key points to remember, 170, 416

location of ruptured aneurysm, 166, 169–70

magnetic resonance imaging (MRI), 165*b*, 167

need for intracranial pressure (ICP) monitor, 307*b*

pretruncal nonaneurysmal, 167, 168*f*, 168

red blood cell transfusions, 357

SAH Study Group from Erasmus University, 166–67

serum sodium, 411*b*, 412

syndrome of inappropriate secretion of antidiuretic hormone (SIADH) and, 412, 413*f*, 414*f*, 415–16

treating patients with, 412–16

subarachnoid space, localization of the lesion, 319*t*

subcutaneous enoxaparin, 16

subdural hematoma

craniectomy, 45*b*

See also acute subdural hematoma

subdural hemorrhage, functional prognosis and cardiac risk, 289

subdural hygroma

complication after craniectomy, 46*f*, 46

computed tomography (CT) scans, 45*b*, 46*f*

sudden respiratory distress, 375–76

sulfonamides, antibiotic-associated encephalopathy, 334–35

surgery

acute subdural hematoma, 38

factors favoring, for ICH, 3*b*–5*b*

surgery (*cont.*)

malignant brain tumors, 201–3

See also failure to awaken after surgery; stupor after brain surgery

Surgical Trial in Intracerebral Hemorrhage (STICH), 5

STICH studies, 6

Surviving Sepsis Campaign, 354

recommendations from, 355*b*

sympathetic storms, 380

See also paroxysmal sympathetic hyperactivity (PSH)

symptomatic intracranial hemorrhage (sICH)

decision for reversing thrombolytic effect, 94, 95*f*

definition, 93

image of, in opposite hemisphere from stroke, 94*f*, 94

mortality rate for patients with, 94

reperfusion injury, 94

risks of, 104

risk with tenecteplase vs. tissue plasminogen activator, 95–96

See also intravenous thrombolysis

syndrome of inappropriate secretion of antidiuretic hormone (SIADH)

cerebral salt wasting (CSW) and, 413*f*

confusing free water and fluid restriction, 415–16

evaluation and management of hyponatremia, 414*f*

subarachnoid hemorrhage (SAH) and, 412

syndrome of the trephined, complication after craniectomy, 46*f*, 46, 48–49, 50

syphilis and spirochetes, cause, diagnostic test and management, 65*t*

takotsubo cardiomyopathy, 373

targeted temperature management

case of 62-year-old man, 221*b*, 224

clinical trials, 222, 223–24

concept of, 224

cooling devices in ICU, 222

current recommendations for, 225*b*

hypothermia and, 222–24

key points to remember, 225

patient treatment, 224

return on spontaneous circulation (ROSC), 221*b*

Targeted Temperature Management (TTM) trial, 222, 223–24

Targeted Temperature Management 2 (TTM2) trial, 222, 223–24

TBI. *See* traumatic brain injury (TBI)

TELL ME mnemonic, communication about triage over the phone, 502, 503*f*

TELSTAR trial, 299

temporal lobes, MRI in rapid progressive brain disease, 243*t*

Tenecteplase in wake-up ischemic stroke (TWIST), 112–13

Tenecteplase Reperfusion Therapy in Acute Ischemic Cerebrovascular Events-III (TRACE III) trial, 112–13

thalamic dementia, 140–41

thalamic hematoma

computed tomography (CT) scan of, 13*b*, 14*f*

enlargement of, 13*b*

fresh frozen plasma (FFP), 13*b*, 15–16

intravenous (IV) vitamin K, 13*b*, 15–16

Therapeutic Hypothermia After Cardiac Arrest in Non Shockable Rhythm (HYPERION) trial, 223–24

thiamine deficiency, Wernicke-Korsakoff encephalopathy, 349, 350

thiopental, brain death determination and, 483–84

third-nerve palsies, pupil-sparing, 318

thoracic endovascular aortic repair (TEVAR), 183–84

thrombocytopenia, anticoagulation reversal in ICH, 15*b*, 16

thrombolysis
    algorithm for control of hypertension, 363*f*
    ischemic stroke candidate, 362–64
    See also intravenous thrombolysis
Thrombolysis in Imaging Eligible, Late Window Patients to Assess the Efficacy and Safety of Tenecteplase (TIMELESS) trial, 112–13
thrombosis. *See* cerebral venous sinus thrombosis (CVST)
thrombotic vasculopathy, 58
thyroid hormone, pituitary apoplexy, 210
ticagrelor, duration of action, 18–19
tirofiban, reversal of, 290–91
tirofiban therapy, cerebral hemorrhage, 290–91, 291*f*
tocilizumab, cytokine release syndrome (CRS), 262
tocilizumab, intravenous, CAR T-cell infusion, 257*b*
Tolosa-Hunt syndrome, nivolumab/pembrolizumab, 252
tongue swelling, angioedema, 92
torsades de pointes, treatment for, 393*t*
toxicology screen, traumatic brain injury (TBI), 26
toxoplasmosis, cause, diagnostic test and management, 65*t*
tracheostomy
    advantages of, 467–68
    long-term support, 469
    placement, 467*b*, 469
    precautionary measures with, 466–67, 467*b*
tranexamic acid (TICH-2) trial, 446–47
Transforming Research and Clinical Knowledge in Traumatic Brain Injury (TRACK-TBI), 439
TransMedics Organ Care System™ (OCS™), 494
transsphenoidal neurosurgery, diabetes insipidus (DI) in neurosciences ICU, 421*b*

transsphenoidal resection surgery, 210–11
traumatic brain injury (TBI)
    active bleeding issues, 26
    alcohol intoxication leading to, 346–47
    brain death determination, 482
    case of 27-year-old patient, 23*b*
    comatose patients after severe, 463*b*, 464
    computed tomography (CT) scan, 23*b*, 24*f*
    CT scan showing subdural hematoma, 305*b*, 306*f*
    data points in prognostication of, 439*t*
    decompressive craniectomy (DECRA), 28–29
    definition of severe TBI, 27
    diabetes insipidus (DI) in neurosciences ICU, 421*b*
    emergency assessment, 24
    epidural hematoma, 37
    gunshot management, 25–26
    initial priorities after, 30*b*
    intracranial pressure (ICP) control and monitoring, 26–27
    intracranial pressure (ICP) monitor, 306
    intracranial pressure monitor, 311
    key points to remember, 31
    multiple hemorrhagic lesions (contusions) on admission CT scan of brain, 24*f*
    need for intracranial pressure (ICP) monitor, 307*b*
    paroxysmal sympathetic hyperactivity (PSH), 386
    patient with acute alcohol intoxication and, 340–41
    physicians managing, 24
    pulmonary edema in patient with, 373
    toxicology screening, 26
    treating increased ICP, 27–29, 28*f*
    treatment of, 29–31, 30*b*
    urgency of neurosurgical intervention, 24–26
    See also prognostication after traumatic brain injury (TBI)

INDEX   559

triage communication
diagnosis determination, 503
essential information, 504
information sharing, 503
key points to remember, 505
neurosciences intensive care unit (neuro-ICU) and, 504–5
sample, 501*b*
sorting information, 502
TELL ME mnemonic, 502, 503*f*
Triple M syndrome, myocarditis, myositis, and myasthenia gravis, 252–53
tuberculosis, causes and neuroimaging, 63*t*
tumor resection
case of 40-year-old woman, 419*b*, 424
pituitary gland region, 419*b*, 420
preoperative and postoperative MRI for, 419*b*, 420*f*
serum sodium of patient, 419*b*
See also diabetes insipidus (DI)

ubiquitin C-terminal hydrolase L1 (UCH-L1)
biomarker for prognostication, 440
ultra-early hematoma evacuation, concept of, 6–7
Ultra-early tranexamic acid after subarachnoid hemorrhage (ULTRA) trial, 149–50
uniform determination of death act (UDDA), 487
uremic encephalopathy, ICU patients with encephalopathy, 327*t*

valproate, disabling myoclonus, 231
valproate sodium, postresuscitation status myoclonus, 230–31
valproic acid
administration of, 283
adverse effects and drug interactions, 281*t*
carbapenems and, 283
management of status epilepticus (SE), 195*f*
postresuscitation status myoclonus, 230–31

refractory status epilepticus (SE), 192*t*
seizure therapy, 190–91
treatment in emergency room, 194–96
vancomycin, 333*b*
bacterial meningitis, 55*b*
Listeria monocytogenes, 54
meningitis patient, 53*b*
septic shock, 356*b*
varicella herpes zoster, causes and neuroimaging, 63*t*
varicella zoster virus (VZV)
cause, diagnostic test and management, 65*t*
IV acyclovir treating, 68–69
vasculitis, 58
vegetative state
clinical signs of, 464, 465*b*
See also persistent comatose states
venous thromboembolism, rivaroxaban for, 17
ventilator auto-triggering, brain death, 483*b*
ventricular tachycardia, treatment for, 393*t*
ventriculostomy, 8–9
acute hydrocephalus, 55*b*
bacterial meningitis, 56*t*
cerebral hemorrhage, 4–5
intracranial pressure (ICP) and, 26–27
lumbar drainage, 149, 153
placement, 48
placement of, 4–5, 8, 17–19
verapamil
cerebral vasospasm treatment option, 159*t*
intra-arterial therapy, 159–62
vigabatrin, postresuscitation status myoclonus, 230–31
viral encephalitides, 243*t*
viral encephalitis, diagnosis of, 74
viral infections, cause, diagnostic test and management, 65*t*
VISION (Vascular Events in Noncardiac Surgery Patients Cohort Evaluation) study, 266–67
vitamin K, 288–89, 290
patient with hematoma, 290
reversing antagonistic effect of warfarin, 15*b*, 15–16

von Willebrand factor, fibrinogen and, 290–91

"wake-up" major stroke
brain MRI showing area of infarction, 114*f*
case of 75-year-old man, 109*b*, 113*f*, 113, 114*f*
catheter cerebral angiogram, 114*f*
CT perfusion, 113*f*, 113
Efficacy and Safety of MRI-based Thrombolysis in Wake-Up Stroke (WAKE-UP) trial, 112–13
intravenous thrombolysis, 112–13
key points to remember, 116
mechanical thrombectomy, 110
proposed algorithm for emergency evaluation and management, 115*f*
randomized controlled trials, 110–11
Tenecteplase in wake-up ischemic stroke (TWIST) trial, 112–13
Tenecteplase Reperfusion Therapy in Acute Ischemic Cerebrovascular Events-III (TRACE III) trial, 112–13
thrombectomy in patients with large ASPECTS score, 111–12
Thrombolysis in Imaging Eligible, Late Window Patients to Assess the Efficacy and Safety of Tenecteplase (TIMELESS) trial, 112–13
See also stroke(s)
warfarin, 290
anticoagulation reversal in ICH, 15*b*
chronic anticoagulation, 287*b*
four-factor PCC reversing, 16, 20
patients anticoagulated with, 14
restarting, 19–20
traumatic brain injury, 26

Wernicke encephalopathy
malnourished alcoholic patients, 350
risk of, 350
Wernicke-Korsakoff encephalopathy
key points to remember, 350
thiamine deficiency, 349, 350
thiamine supplementation, 350
Wernicke-Korsakoff syndrome, 243*t*, 345*b*
alcoholism with malnutrition, 347
MRI showing restricted diffusion, 345*b*, 346*f*
thiamine deficiency, 349
West Nile virus
cause, diagnostic test and management, 65*t*
causes and neuroimaging, 63*t*
encephalitis, 62–64
lacking antiviral for infection, 68–69
outbreaks of encephalitis, 64
white matter, MRI in rapid progressive brain disease, 243*t*
withdrawal of life-sustaining treatment
allowing natural death, 478–79
case of 78-year-old woman, 471*b*, 478–79
cognitive and physical incapacity versus death, 477–78
DNR order, 478
key points to remember, 479
measures for, 478
morphine and lorazepam, 478
point of no return, 477
pulling the plug, 478–79
self-fulfilling prophecy, 476–77
withholding care, 478–79
See also do-not-resuscitate (DNR) order; organ donation
World Federation of Neurological Surgeons (WFNS), 147*b*

X-linked myotubular myopathy, 87

zilocuplan, myasthenia gravis treatment, 406